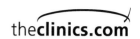

SURGICAL CLINICS
OF NORTH AMERICA

Current Practice in Pediatric Surgery

GUEST EDITOR
Mike K. Chen, MD

CONSULTING EDITOR
Ronald F. Martin, MD

April 2006 • Volume 86 • Number 2

SAUNDERS

An Imprint of Elsevier, Inc.

PHILADELPHIA   LONDON   TORONTO   MONTREAL   SYDNEY   TOKYO

W.B. SAUNDERS COMPANY
A Division of Elsevier Inc.

1600 John F. Kennedy Blvd., Suite 1800, Philadelphia, PA 19103-2899

http://www.theclinics.com

SURGICAL CLINICS OF NORTH AMERICA	Volume 86, Number 2
April 2006	ISSN 0039–6109
Editor: Catherine Bewick	ISBN 1-4160-3558-3

Reprints. For copies of 100 or more of articles in this publication, please contact the commercial Reprints Department Elsevier Inc., 360 Park Avenue South, New York, New York 10010-1710. Tel. (212) 633-3813, Fax: (212) 462-1935, email: reprints@elsevier.com

The ideas and opinions expressed in *The Surgical Clinics of North America* do not necessarily reflect those of the Publisher. The Publisher does not assume any responsibility for any injury and/or damage to persons or property arising out of or related to any use of the material contained in this periodical. The reader is advised to check the appropriate medical literature and the product information currently provided by the manufacturer of each drug to be administered to verify the dosage, the method and duration of administration, or contraindications. It is the responsibility of the treating physician or other health care professional, relying on independent experience and knowledge of the patient, to determine drug dosages and the best treatment for the patient. Mention of any product in this issue should not be construed as endorsement by the contributors, editors, or the Publisher of the product or manufacturers' claims.

Surgical Clinics of North America (ISSN 0039–6109) is published bimonthly by W.B. Saunders, 360 Park Avenue South, New York, NY 10010-1710. Months of publication are February, April, June, August, October, and December. Business and Editorial Offices: 1600 John F. Kennedy Blvd., Suite 1800, Philadelphia, PA 19103-2899. Accounting and Circulation Offices: 6277 Sea Harbor Drive, Orlando, FL 32887-4800. Periodicals postage paid at New York, NY and additional mailing offices. Subscription prices are $200.00 per year for US individuals, $315.00 per year for US institutions, $100.00 per year for US students and residents, $245.00 per year for Canadian individuals, $385.00 per year for Canadian institutions, $260.00 for international individuals, $385.00 for international institutions and $130.00 per year for Canadian and foreign students/residents. To receive student/resident rate, orders must be accompanied by name of affiliated institution, date of term, and the *signature* of program/residency coordinator on institution letterhead. Orders will be billed at individual rate until proof of status is received. Foreign air speed delivery is included in all *Clinics* subscription prices. All prices are subject to change without notice. POSTMASTER: Send address changes to *The Surgical Clinics of North America*, Elsevier Periodicals Customer Service, 6277 Sea Harbor Drive, Orlando, FL 32887-4800. **Customer Service: 1-800-654-2452 (US). From outside of the US, call 1-407-345-1000.**

The Surgical Clinics of North America is also published in Spanish by McGraw-Hill Interamericana Editores S.A., P.O. Box 5-237 06500 Mexico D.F. Mexico; and in Portuguese by Interlivros Edicoes Ltda., Rua Comandante Coelho 1085, CEP 21250, Rio de Janeiro, Brazil; and in Greek by Paschalidis Medical Publications, Athens Greece.

The Surgical Clinics of North America is covered in *Index Medicus, EMBASE/Excerpta Medica, Current Contents/Clinical Medicine, Current Contents/Life Sciences, Science Citation Index*, and *ISI/BIOMED*.

Printed in the United States of America.

CONSULTING EDITOR

RONALD F. MARTIN, MD, Staff Surgeon, Department of Surgery, Marshfield Clinic, Marshfield, Wisconsin; Clinical Associate Professor of Surgery, University of Vermont, Burlington, Vermont; Lieutenant Colonel, Medical Corps, United States Army Reserve

GUEST EDITOR

MIKE K. CHEN, MD, Associate Professor of Surgery and Pediatrics, Department of Surgery, College of Medicine, University of Florida, Gainesville, Florida

CONTRIBUTORS

KUMARI N. ADAMS, BS, University of Illinois College of Medicine at Chicago, Chicago, Illinois

KENNETH S. AZAROW, MD, FACS, Department of Surgery, Uniformed Services University of Health Sciences, Bethesda, Maryland

ELIZABETH A. BEIERLE, MD, Assistant Professor of Surgery, Division of Pediatric Surgery, Department of Surgery, University of Florida College of Medicine, Gainesville, Florida

DEBORAH F. BILLMIRE, MD, Associate Professor of Surgery, Indiana University School of Medicine, Indianapolis, Indiana

SCOTT C. BOULANGER, MD, PhD, Assistant Professor of Surgery, Division of Pediatric Surgery, University of Mississippi Medical Center, Jackson, Mississippi

MARY L. BRANDT, MD, Professor and Vice Chair, Michael E. DeBakey Department of Surgery, Baylor College of Medicine, Texas Children's Hospital Clinical Care Center, Houston, Texas

RANDALL S. BURD, MD, PhD, Assistant Professor of Surgery and Pediatrics, Departments of Surgery and Pediatrics, UMDNJ-Robert Wood Johnson Medical School, New Brunswick, New Jersey

MICHAEL C. CARR, MD, PhD, Associate Professor, Pediatric Urology, The Children's Hospital of Philadelphia; Associate Professor of Surgery in Urology, University of Pennsylvania School of Medicine, Philadelphia, Pennsylvania

MICHAEL G. CATY, MD, Chief of Pediatric Surgery, Surgeon-in-Chief, Pediatric Surgery, Women and Children's Hospital of Buffalo, Buffalo, New York.

EMILY R. CHRISTISON-LAGAY, MD, Research Fellow, Department of Surgery, Children's Hospital, Boston, Massachusetts

DAI H. CHUNG, MD, Associate Professor of Surgery and Pediatrics, Chief, Section of Pediatric Surgery, The University of Texas Medical Branch, Galveston, Texas

EDWARD DOOLIN, MD, Associate Professor of Surgery and Pediatrics, Children's Hospital of Pennsylvania, University of Pennsylvania, Philadelphia, Pennsylvania

STEVEN J. FISHMAN, MD, Co-Director, Vascular Anomalies Center, Senior Associate in Surgery, Children's Hospital; Associate Professor, Harvard Medical School, Boston, Massachusetts

JOHN R. GOSCHE, MD, PhD, Associate Professor of Surgery and Pediatrics, Chief, Division of Pediatric Surgery, University of Mississippi Medical Center, Jackson, Mississippi

EITAN GROSS, MD, Senior Lecturer in Pediatric Surgery, Department of Pediatric Surgery, The Hebrew University-Hadassah Medical School, Hadassah Medical Center, Jerusalem, Israel

JEFFREY H. HAYNES, MD, Associate Professor of Surgery and Pediatrics, Division of Pediatric Surgery, Medical College of Virginia, Virginia Commonwealth University Health System, Richmond, Virginia

MICHAEL A. HELMRATH, MD, Assistant Professor, Michael E. DeBakey Department of Surgery, Baylor College of Medicine, Texas Children's Hospital Clinical Care Center, Houston, Texas

AI-XUAN L. HOLTERMAN, MD, Associate Professor of Surgery, Department of Surgery, Division of Pediatric Surgery, University of Illinois at Chicago, Chicago, Illinois

THOMAS H. INGE, MD, PhD, FACS, FAAP, Assistant Professor of Surgery and Pediatrics Surgical Director, Comprehensive Weight Management Center, Division of Pediatric General and Thoracic Surgery, Cincinnati Children's Hospital Medical Center, Cincinnati, Ohio

SALEEM ISLAM, MD, Assistant Professor of Surgery, Division of Pediatric Surgery, University of Mississippi Medical Center, Jackson, Mississippi

DAVID W. KAYS, MD, Associate Professor of Surgery, Division of Pediatric Surgery, University of Florida College of Medicine, Gainesville, Florida

SUNGHOON KIM, MD, Attending Pediatric Surgeon, Children's Hospital and Research Center Oakland, Oakland, California

MAX R. LANGHAM, JR, MD, Professor of Surgery and Pediatrics and Chief, Division of Pediatric Surgery, University of Tennessee Health Science Center, Memphis; Director, Pediatric Surgery Residency Program, LeBonheur Children's Medical Center, Memphis; Consulting Surgeon, St. Jude Children's Research Hospital, Memphis, Tennessee

STANLEY T. LAU, MD, Research Fellow in Pediatric Surgery, Pediatric Surgery, Women and Children's Hospital of Buffalo, Buffalo, New York

DANIEL J. LEDBETTER, MD, Associate Professor of Surgery, Department of Surgery, Division of Pediatric Surgery, University of Washington, Seattle; Attending Surgeon, Children's Hospital and Regional Medical Center, Seattle, Washington

REBECCA M. McGUIGAN, MD, Department of Surgery, Madigan Army Medical Center, Tacoma, Washington

SCOTT J. MELLENDER, MD, Clinical Instructor in Surgery, Department of Surgery, UMDNJ-Robert Wood Johnson Medical School, New Brunswick, New Jersey

KRISTIN L. MEKEEL, MD, Fellow in Transplant Surgery, University of Florida College of Medicine, Gainesville, Florida.

BINDI NAIK-MATHURIA, MD, Resident, Michael E. DeBakey Department of Surgery, Baylor College of Medicine, Houston, Texas

OLUYINKA O. OLUTOYE, MBChB, PhD, Assistant Professor of Surgery and Pediatrics, Baylor College of Medicine, Texas Children's Hospital, Houston, Texas

RUTH A. SEELER, MD, Professor of Pediatrics, Department of Pediatrics, Division of Pediatric Hematology and Oncology, University of Illinois at Chicago, Chicago, Illinois

JEAN-YVES SICHEL, MD, Senior Lecturer in Otolaryngology, Department of Otolaryngology/Head and Neck Surgery, The Hebrew University-Hadassah Medical School, Hadassah Medical Center, Jerusalem, Israel

JOSEPH D. TOBIAS, MD, Professor of Anesthesiology and Child Health, Departments of Anesthesiology and Child Health, University of Missouri–Columbia, Columbia, Missouri

ROBERT D. WINFIELD, MD, Department of Surgery, University of Florida College of Medicine, Gainesville, Florida

LAURA VICK, MD, Resident in General Surgery, University of Mississippi Medical Center, Jackson, Mississippi

CONTENTS

evaluation of these topics is provided, with particular attention being paid to areas of controversy in the diagnosis and management of gastroesophageal reflux disease, fibrosing colonopathy, and hepatic disease.

information on three disorders commonly of interest to surgeons. These are biliary atresia, hepatoblastoma, and portal hypertension. Important new data have provided insight into the etiology of these disorders and resulted in changes in recommendations for their evaluation and surgical management.

Neuroblastoma and Wilms' tumor are two of the most common extracranial solid malignancies in infants and children. Despite intense basic science and clinical investigations, the overall survival for patients with advanced-stage neuroblastoma remains dismal. In Wilms' tumor, recent advances in the preoperative imaging have changed the operative approach to the routine contralateral kidney exploration. This article reviews the pathology, clinical presentation, diagnosis and treatment of neuroblastoma and Wilms' tumor.

This article describes the spectrum of germ cell tumors in children and adolescents. Differences in management principles for benign and malignant variants are discussed, and current survival rates for patients who have malignant tumors are addressed. The concept of organ sparing for certain gonadal germ cell tumors is explored. A discussion of the evolution and impact of prenatal diagnosis for fetal sacrococcygeal teratoma is included.

Children born with menigomyelocele have a compendium of neurologic disorders including a disrupted defecation process. Many of the multiple factors that contribute to an effective bowel movement are altered in meningomyelocele. Aggressive and proactive management using mechanical and pharmacologic therapies can result in functional and continent patients. This article reviews mechanical purgatives, diet and fiber, laxatives, and adjunctive therapy as methods to assist those who have meningomyelocele in maintaining a good clinical lifestyle.

Bladder function can simply be defined by two simple processes: storage and emptying. For children born with myelodysplasia, the developmental anomaly can affect both these processes, leading in some situations to upper tract deterioration if myelodysplasia is not recognized in a timely fashion. Clean intermittent catheterization can be employed to empty the bladder, thus improving the situation for children with poor bladder emptying. Pharmacologic measures have been used to improve bladder storage and the combination of pharmacotherapy and clean intermittent catheterization has become the mainstay technique for managing children with myelodysplasia. This article describes current trends in bladder management for children with myelodysplasia.

FORTHCOMING ISSUES

RECENT ISSUES

The Clinics are now available online!

www.theclinics.com

SURGICAL
CLINICS OF
NORTH AMERICA

Surg Clin N Am 86 (2006) xv–xvii

Foreword

Current Practice in Pediatric Surgery

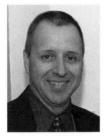

Ronald F. Martin, MD
Consulting Editor

The most singularly brilliant surgeon I have ever worked with, Dr. Albert W. Dibbins, was the first person to convince me that children are not small adults. And I, like many people, was in need of convincing. And he was, as always, right. It is largely for this reason—that children are not small adults—that I asked Dr. Chen to be Guest Editor for this issue on Pediatric Surgery and to tell the larger (no pun intended) surgical audience what we need to know about children.

Who cares or should care for children is a question that we need to discuss as a specialty. I, personally, would like to think that all children should be taken care of by the people who understand their problems best, but that may be an unreasonable tenet. As with many problems, reality and logistics get in the way. One inescapable observation is that children are generally healthier than adults, or at least less likely to require surgical care per capita. This leads to a much larger catchment area to support a fully committed pediatric surgeon. Adding to this dilemma, children are poor wage earners. So their care is paid for by their parents or their parents' insurers. Many of the uninsured persons in the United States are children. So from an economic standpoint, an even larger base of patients is required to support our pediatric surgical brethren financially. The need for a critical mass of pediatric surgical care coverage that is co-located to manage the realities of any surgical practice rounds out the strain on the system. This leads to centralization or regionalization, which

doi:10.1016/j.suc.2006.02.002

tends to translate into larger distances for patients to travel and subsequently places a burden on families who may be displaced from their homes, or on parents who are separated from one another while their child is being cared for. Although the Family and Medical Leave Act may help to mitigate some of the difficulties that present under these circumstances, many problems remain.

The issue of competent surgical training to care for children is also worth considering. Exposure to and participation in pediatric surgical training is a requirement of all of our approved postgraduate training programs. Whether this adequately qualifies a surgeon to operate upon children I shall leave for each reader to decide. In most situations, one can always transfer a stable patient to a system of greater capacity, but occasionally one encounters an unexpected problem, or a child may be too unstable for transfer. The problem is certainly not unique to children; we have heart centers, cancer centers, trauma centers, and others. But somehow, the problems seem magnified when it comes to children.

Institutional commitment to the care of children also has to be carefully considered in the care of the pediatric surgical patient. Dedicated nursing staffs, social service personnel, security personnel and procedures are all essential and, again, require a critical mass of patient volume to properly support.

There are many things that we as general surgeons can do to meet these infrastructural challenges. First, we can maintain familiarity with the maladies that commonly affect children and that may need our urgent intervention. Second, we should make every effort to ensure that our pediatric surgical colleagues are supported in their endeavors. That support could be economic support within larger practices or making sure that those who provide the "difficult" pediatric care also receive the referrals for the more straightforward care—the work that pays the bills but doesn't constrict one's coronaries. Or that support could be to work with government, hospitals, and third-party payers to ensure that every child has some form of health care insurance. We are willing to pay for basic public education for everyone through high school; why not health care? From a societal cost-benefit analysis, I cannot really see a difference.

There are many excellent reasons to have some understanding of the issues that face the pediatric population. The best may be that any of us who are likely to read this series may be called upon to deal with some of the more common ones at some point. Other reasons are that most children who fare well with their pediatric conditions will become adults and subsequently might need the services of the adult general surgeon, or that the American Board of Surgery requires us to have this knowledge for certification or re-certification, or that we ourselves may have or someday have children who will need surgical care. Whatever your reason for interest in this topic, it is hoped that this issue will be of help to you.

Ronald F. Martin, MD
Department of Surgery
Marshfield Clinic
1000 North Oak Avenue
Marshfield, WI 54449, USA

E-mail address: martin.ronald@marshfieldclinic.org

SURGICAL
CLINICS OF
NORTH AMERICA

Surg Clin N Am 86 (2006) xix–xx

Preface

Current Practice in Pediatric Surgery

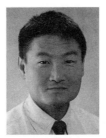

Mike K. Chen, MD
Guest Editor

The practice of pediatric surgery began nearly a century ago with William E. Ladd's service as a volunteer surgeon following the explosion in Halifax Harbor on December 6, 1917. That seminal event is thought to have spurred Dr. Ladd to develop an interest in the special needs of infants and children with surgical problems. Since then, the practice of pediatric surgery has changed a great deal, but to many of us who are devoted to this discipline, the principles and ideals have remained constant. For a variety of reasons, the care of infants and children and, more specifically, surgical procedures performed on them are more challenging and just mean more than the care of an adult. I certainly do not wish to imply that caring for an adult is not vital, but I would guess that the readers (particularly those who have or have had children) agree with me. Infants and children are vulnerable, and they are completely dependent on us for their welfare. For a group of professionals who are devoted to the care of other human beings, to focus on this particular fragile population is both gratifying and challenging.

Pediatric surgeons are devoted to the care of infants and children, but they also cherish the field for its variety. As evidenced by the number of topics presented in this issue of the *Surgical Clinics of North America*, the scope of pediatric surgery remains quite broad. It has been said that pediatric surgeons do everything except for "brain, bones, and heart." Nevertheless, this discipline continues to evolve, and teachers of my teachers may be a bit disappointed to see that this generation of pediatric surgeons is no longer caring for many of the diseases they were accustomed to seeing. On the

0039-6109/06/$ - see front matter © 2006 Elsevier Inc. All rights reserved.
doi:10.1016/j.suc.2006.02.001
surgical.theclinics.com

other hand, they might agree that progress has been made and could only have been derived from the solid foundation that they provided.

This issue is focused on the actual current practice of pediatric surgery, and I have asked the authors to present their own perspective. I challenged them to not recite the same information available in surgical texts, but to provide us with the latest thoughts and innovations. To that end, I am proud to have been associated with this issue. The topics covered are broad and contain most of the items seen by subspecialty-trained pediatric surgeons, but I am hopeful that the information is useful as well for the general surgeon who cares for infants and children.

Significant progress has been made in a variety of areas, although much controversy remains. Subjects covered in this issue range from perioperative considerations to congenital anomalies to common pediatric surgical problems. New embryologic information, pathophysiology, and other current thoughts on the etiology of many disorders are discussed. The latest therapies and innovations, which have significantly changed the practice of pediatric surgery, are presented. Some topics remain controversial and should stimulate further debate. Many of the infants and children formerly cared for by pediatric subspecialists are now adults who require the care of general surgeons and other adult caretakers. Problems in these patients include, for example, chest wall defects and meconium diseases (cystic fibrosis). Routine problems that can be confusing and that are more commonly encountered by general practitioners are nicely addressed in such articles as inguinal and scrotal disorders, vascular anomalies, and neck lesions. Adolescent bariatric surgery is covered as well. It is a timely topic, unfortunately a reflection of our lifestyle. The last articles on the care of bowel and bladder dysfunction in children with myelodysplasia present useful algorithms for the management of complex problems. They represent cogent examples of the outstanding outcomes that may be achieved when children with multiple medical problems are cared for by knowledgeable and dedicated caretakers.

Mike K. Chen, MD
Department of Surgery
College of Medicine
University of Florida
PO Box 100286
Gainesville, FL 32610, USA

E-mail address: chenmk@surgery.ufl.edu

ELSEVIER
SAUNDERS

SURGICAL
CLINICS OF
NORTH AMERICA

Surg Clin N Am 86 (2006) 227–247

Neonatal and Childhood Perioperative Considerations

Randall S. Burd, MD, PhD[a],*, Scott J. Mellender, MD[a],
Joseph D. Tobias, MD[b]

[a]Department of Surgery, Division of Pediatric Surgery,
Robert Wood Johnson Medical School, One Robert Wood Johnson Place, P.O. Box 19,
New Brunswick, NJ 08903, USA
[b]Departments of Anesthesiology and Pediatrics, University of Missouri–Columbia,
3W-27G Health Sciences Center, One Hospital Drive, Columbia, Missouri 65212, USA

The perioperative care of infants and children requires a team approach. Surgeons must recognize potential risk factors for adverse perioperative events and work with the anesthesiologist and other consultants to reduce or eliminate these factors to optimize the child's perioperative care. In the past decade, there has been considerable progress in perioperative management that now makes surgery safer and less distressing for children and their families. In this review, the authors cover recent advances in preoperative evaluation and intraoperative and postoperative management, focusing mainly on the immediate perioperative period for elective surgical procedures. Consistent with the authors' view that the optimal outcome is achieved by close collaboration of members of the surgical team, this review was written jointly by surgeons and an anesthesiologist.

Preoperative evaluation

Overview

Because many pediatric surgical procedures are elective and performed as same-day surgery, the preoperative evaluation and interventions aimed at reducing perioperative risks are commonly performed in an outpatient setting. Children who do not have acute illness or major chronic medical illnesses can be evaluated by the surgeon in the office and assessed by the anesthesiologist on the day of elective surgery. Although some institutions mandate a separate

---

* Corresponding author.
  E-mail address: burdrs@umdnj.edu (R.S. Burd).

surgical.theclinics.com

outpatient evaluation by an anesthesiologist, most have streamlined preoperative care by eliminating this additional visit. Some institutions even use telephone surveys to identify high-risk patients who may benefit from preoperative screening before the day of surgery. Although this practice increases the convenience for families, elimination of a preoperative anesthesia evaluation increases the importance of the surgeon's initial evaluation and can lead to delays or cancellations on the day of surgery when the evaluation is incomplete. The anesthesiologist working in the same-day surgery suite depends on accurate and timely information from the surgeon's outpatient evaluation to make an appropriate plan for perioperative management.

"One-stop" surgery

The interest in further streamlining the preoperative evaluation among children undergoing elective surgery can be seen in the development of "one-stop" surgery programs [1,2]. The focus of these programs is to increase convenience to families by eliminating the preoperative and postoperative visits. Children who are to undergo simple procedures such as umbilical or inguinal hernia repair, circumcision, or central line removal are prescreened by their primary care provider for major risk factors for adverse perioperative events. The children at low risk are evaluated by the surgeon and the anesthesiologist on the day of the scheduled procedure. Although one-stop surgery is associated with high parental satisfaction, it has several limitations. Despite adequate preparation, about 20% of one-stop procedures are cancelled or delayed because of failure to show up, parental decisions to forego surgery after surgical consultation, the surgeon's judgment about the need for surgery, or failure to follow preoperative feeding instructions [1,2]. This high cancellation rate requires modification of the processes used in the same-day surgery suite to avoid the costs associated with inefficient use of operating room resources.

Although major adverse events are less likely due to prescreening and the types of procedures selected for this approach, an expedited approach may not best serve the psychologic needs of many children and parents. A separate preoperative visit provides an opportunity for parents to meet with the surgeon in a less pressured environment, allows them more time to consider information about the appropriateness and potential outcomes of surgery, and may reduce parental anxiety [1,2]. In light of evidence that parental anxiety has a negative impact on the psychologic reaction of children to surgery [3], omission of the preoperative visit may not be the best choice for some families. Additional study of the impact of one-stop surgery is warranted before this option is more widely adopted.

Preoperative testing

Preoperative surgical evaluation should focus on identification of potential factors associated with frequently occurring perioperative complications and on those associated with high potential morbidity or mortality. In most cases, children at risk can be identified by a detailed history and physical examination without the need for additional laboratory studies or other investigations. In a cohort of 8772 healthy children undergoing minor surgical procedures, anesthesiologists requested laboratory studies in 2%, most often to evaluate for suspected anemia [4]. Although almost half of these studies were abnormal, surgery was not delayed or the anesthetic management modified based on these results. Furthermore, the incidence of minor and major perioperative complications was similar to a previous period during which routine laboratory studies were obtained on all children, suggesting that a policy of selective laboratory screening is safe. In a survey of members of the Society for Pediatric Anesthesia, it was found that the most common preoperative laboratory study requested was a hemoglobin or hematocrit, being performed in up to half of children depending on their age [5]. The utility of routine screening for anemia is low because only 0.5% of pediatric same-day surgery patients are anemic and the anesthetic plan is rarely modified because of anemia [5]. A more targeted approach is to obtain hemoglobin values on children at increased risk for anemia, including infants younger than 1 year (especially the former preterm infant in whom anemia is a risk factor for postoperative apnea), adolescent menstruating girls, or those who have chronic medical illnesses. A baseline study may also be useful among children who are undergoing procedures that have an anticipated high blood loss. A hemoglobin value can be obtained at the time of placement of the intravenous cannula in the operative room, avoiding the need for venipuncture in an awake patient. The usefulness of these recommendations has not been established.

In addition to screening for anemia, it has been shown that preoperative pregnancy testing and coagulation testing before tonsillectomy are also commonly performed at many institutions [5]. The value of these preoperative tests is controversial. In a study performed at a large children's hospital, Wheeler and Cote [6] found that routine pregnancy screening of 235 menarcheal adolescents detected pregnancy in 1%. Similar findings have been observed by others [7]. Routine pregnancy testing was favored by these investigators because of unreliable patient history, possible fetal or maternal complications related to the administration of anesthesia or the surgical procedure, and other potential liability that may occur as a result of unrecognized pregnancy. Nevertheless, there are other issues to consider, including the lack of demonstrated cost-effectiveness of routine testing, the uncertain effects of single anesthetic exposure on the fetus or mother, and the ethical and legal issues of pregnancy testing in minors [6]. Because of the controversy surrounding routine pregnancy screening in adolescents, each institution should develop recommendations that reflect the surgical team's views and that conform to state regulations [6]. If routine pregnancy testing is instituted, a specific policy should be in place that deals with the difficult task of informing the patient and her family about a positive test and providing counseling before the patient is discharged home.

Similar to pregnancy screening, routine coagulation screening before tonsillectomy is controversial. Tonsillectomy, commonly performed on otherwise healthy children, has a relatively high rate of postoperative bleeding (2%–4%) [8]. For many pediatric patients, this procedure is their first hemostatic "challenge." Because results from routine coagulation testing before tonsillectomy have been obtained in several large series, previous data allow a critical evaluation of the correlation between bleeding history and the results of coagulation testing. Most current evidence suggests that routine coagulation testing is not needed before tonsillectomy unless indicated by a bleeding history [8,9]. Extensive coagulation testing in this population has also revealed that most children who have a positive bleeding history do not have an identifiable bleeding disorder and that some children who have a coagulation disorder do not have a positive bleeding history [10,11]. Even patients who have normal routine coagulation studies and an insignificant history of bleeding may have identifiable coagulation disorders if tested more extensively [10]. The high false-positive rate of routine coagulation testing and the rarity of unrecognized coagulation disorders does not support routine coagulation testing for tonsillectomy.

Studies regarding coagulation testing before tonsillectomy provide a useful paradigm for the value of screening for bleeding disorders before other routine surgical procedures. Because of the absence of studies evaluating coagulation testing for other pediatric surgical procedures, it appears appropriate to follow the recommendation of obtaining coagulation testing only when indicated by history or physical examination for most procedures with similar or lower risk of hemorrhage compared with tonsillectomy. Data obtained from a large adult series showed that the most reliable factors for detecting bleeding disorders were a history of bleeding from minor wounds, frequent bruising, and the use of nonsteroidal anti-inflammatory drugs (NSAIDs) or platelet function antagonists [12]. In addition to children who have a positive bleeding history, coagulation studies should be considered in those undergoing procedures at high risk for bleeding; in those who have underlying medical conditions that increase the risk of coaguloapathy, such as liver disease or malabsorption; or in those receiving anticoagulants or other medications that increase the risk of a bleeding disorder.

Informed consent—surgical and anesthetic considerations

A critical aspect of preoperative preparation before pediatric surgical procedures is the informed consent process. Despite its importance, relatively little has been written about informed consent before pediatric surgical procedures. At the time of the preoperative surgical visit, families are presented with the nature of the condition, a description of the procedure, the risks associated with the procedure, and possible outcomes that may occur after surgery. Although it is the intention of every surgeon to provide patients and family with the information needed to make informed choices, the counseling provided by the surgeon may not be adequate or in a form that is preferred by some families. One survey in a pediatric surgical clinic revealed that most parents still had questions after the office visit was complete and many believed that they had a poor or average understanding of the potential outcomes of the planned operation [13]. Most parents use sources other than their surgeon to obtain medical information pertaining to their child. These sources include the primary care physician, books, magazines, newspapers, and the Internet [13]. In a study of parents of outpatients in a pediatric surgery clinic from 2003, 63% of parents obtained information pertaining to their child's condition using the Internet [14]. Because of the continued increase in Internet usage, this percentage is likely to be even higher today. Parents used the Internet to research several different topics including information about their surgeon (60%), treatment options (58%), the planned surgical procedure (37%), and the risks of treatment (34%) [14]. The importance of the Internet as an adjunct source of health care information for parents emphasizes the importance of accurate and updated Web site content, preferably developed with the contribution of pediatric surgeons. Although several studies have addressed the interactions between surgeons and their adult patients in an outpatient setting [15–17], this area has not been studied for pediatric surgery outpatient encounters in which parents most often serve as decision makers for their children.

Aspects of the anesthetic are similarly presented by the anesthesiologist on the day of the procedure or at a separate preoperative visit. Using interviews with a small cohort of parents of same-day surgery patients, Sobo [18] identified major themes of parental worries and fears. These worries included concerns about the child's fear or their possible noncooperativeness, their powerlessness as parents to control the child's safety, the risks of anesthesia, the risks related to performing procedures in younger patients, potential surgical or postoperative complications, and the potential need to alter the treatment plan intraoperatively or postoperatively. With regard to information about anesthesia, Wisselo and colleagues [19] identified specific areas of information needed by parents, the most frequent being information about induction, side-effects, emergence from anesthesia, and pain relief. Most parents like to know (or believe that they have a right to know) about all possible anesthetic complications, even those that are potentially life threatening. When parents were given highly detailed information about the conduct and potential complications of the planned anesthetic, no significant increase in parental anxiety was observed compared with those given less detailed information [20]. Most parents preferred a pamphlet or a preoperative visit with the anesthesiologist as a method for receiving information about anesthesia. Almost half of parents preferred receiving this information during the week before the procedure as opposed to the day before or the day of the operation [19].

Unique considerations arise when anesthesia is planned for the child who has a do-not-resuscitate (DNR) status. Although a DNR order may be in place, a child may require surgery to improve quality of life or to correct a self-limited medical condition. Examples of these procedures include placement of a gastrostomy for supplemental feeding, an appendectomy for appendicitis or the establishment of vascular access. In a recent report from the American Academy of Pediatrics, a panel that included pediatric surgeons and pediatric anesthesiologists developed recommendations for handling this problem [21]. An approach of "required reconsideration" of the DNR order is recommended when surgery is planned for any child who has DNR status. This approach includes a discussion with the child's parents or caregivers about the likelihood of requiring intraoperative resuscitation, the type of resuscitation methods that might be used, and the anticipated outcome should resuscitation be required. The potential benefits of perioperative suspension of DNR status should also be reviewed. Members of the perioperative team should be fully aware whether DNR status will be upheld or continued and should participate only if willing to uphold the wishes of the family. The child's perioperative DNR status and decisions to use other aspects of medical care such as ICU monitoring should be considered independently. When DNR status is held in the perioperative period, a plan should be in place should an arrest occur perioperatively and when continued support is likely to result only in prolonging the process of dying [21].

Perioperative adverse events

Overview

The goal of preoperative evaluation and perioperative management is to minimize morbidity and mortality. The focus should be to reduce uncommon but potentially life-threatening complications such as major respiratory events and to reduce common complications such as vomiting (Table 1). It is important to understand the frequency of these adverse events and the location at which they occur in the immediate perioperative period. In a review of 24,165 anesthetics administered over a 30-month period, Murat and colleagues [22] identified 1829 adverse events occurring in the operating room or recovery room. In the operating room, 724 adverse events were noted (31:1000 anesthetics). Most (53%) of these events were respiratory events. Adverse intraoperative events occurred more frequently in infants younger than 1 year than in older children. Respiratory and cardiac events were more frequent among infants and among those who had an American Society of Anesthesiologists (ASA) physical class higher than 2. In the recovery room, 1105 adverse events occurred (48:1000 anesthetics). Vomiting was the most common (77%) adverse event, and the incidence of vomiting increased with age. Respiratory events in the recovery room were more frequent in

Table 1
Perioperative adverse events among children

Perioperative complication	Types	Potential risk factors	Potential perioperative interventions
Respiratory events	Laryngospasm Bronchospasm Laryngeal edema Oxygen desaturation Aspiration/vomiting	Age Anesthetic not given by pediatric anesthesiologist Use of mask/LMA ENT procedure Acute respiratory infection	Preoperative optimization of major respiratory disease Postpone elective procedures 4–6 wk for acute URI Modify intraoperative airway management
Cardiac arrest	—	Age (particularly < 1 y) Emergency procedure ASA physical status > 2	Preoperatively identify cardiac anomalies Avoid halothane, particularly in infants Strategies to avoid adverse respiratory events
Perioperative anxiety	Preoperative anxiety Emergence delirium Postoperative behavioral changes	Parental anxiety Socially maladjusted child Shy/inhibited child	Preoperative preparation of child and parents Provide appropriate information for parents Selective parental presence on induction Premedication before induction
Postoperative nausea/ vomiting	—	Age Duration of anesthesia Duration of surgery History of postoperative vomiting Strabismus surgery History of postoperative vomiting in immediate family	Avoidance of emetogenic anesthetic agents Pre-emptive administration of antiemetics in high-risk children

Abbreviations: ASA, American Society of Anesthesiologists; ENT, ears, nose, and throat; LMA, laryngeal mask airway; URI, upper respiratory tract illness.

infants than in older children. Compared with children undergoing other types of procedures, intraoperative respiratory events and vomiting in the recovery room were more common among children undergoing ears, nose, and throat (ENT) procedures [22].

Respiratory complications

Two recent studies have identified potential independent risk factors for respiratory complications in children undergoing elective surgical procedures [23,24]. Mamie and colleagues [23] found that respiratory complications (laryngospasm, airway obstruction, bronchospasm, or oxygen desaturation) were less frequent in older children when anesthesia was administered by a pediatric anesthesiologist, when endotracheal intubation using a relaxant rather than a mask was used, or when a non-ENT procedure was being performed. The risk of respiratory complications decreased by 8% with each year of age. In a similar study, Bordet and colleagues [24] identified age less than 6 years, the presence of a respiratory tract infection, and the use of a laryngeal mask airway as independent factors associated with airway complications. Although each study described multivariate models constructed with different inputs, both showed the importance of age and the method of airway management as important factors contributing to respiratory complications.

The management of the child who has an acute upper respiratory tract illness (URI) and is scheduled for an elective procedure is a frequent problem because healthy children may have up to several URIs per year [25]. Children who have a recent (within 1 month) or active URI are more likely to have respiratory complications including breath holding, oxygen desaturation, and severe coughing [26,27]. Among those undergoing anesthesia during an active URI, significant independent risk factors for adverse respiratory events included copious secretions, the use of endotracheal intubation in children younger than 5 years, history of prematurity, nasal congestion, parental smoking, history of reactive airway disease, and surgery involving the airway [27].

Because URIs contribute to respiratory complications, the surgical team needs to decide when the morbidity of these events justifies postponement of surgery. When respiratory events related to a URI occur, most are easily managed and few lead to unplanned hospitalization (<0.5%) or other long-term sequelae [27,28]. There is considerable variation in the approach to this problem that reflects the diversity of patients, procedures, and practitioners involved. A survey of anesthesiologists showed that many factors are considered, including the presence of asthma, whether intubation is required, and the anesthesiologist's fear of potential litigation or past experience anesthetizing children who had a URI [29]. When surgery is postponed, the recommended time until rescheduled surgery ranges from 1 to more than 6 weeks, with most recommending a delay of 4 weeks or less. When a decision is made to proceed with surgery, modifications in the anesthetic technique include added hydration, use of an antisialogue, avoidance of endotracheal intubation, humidification of the anesthetic circuit, and the use of regional techniques [29]. Tait and Malviya [26] proposed an algorithm for managing the child who has a URI (Fig. 1). Factors considered include the urgency of the procedure, the likelihood that symptoms are due to an infectious etiology, the severity of symptoms, the planned mode of anesthesia administration, potential risk factors for respiratory complications, and related nonmedical factors.

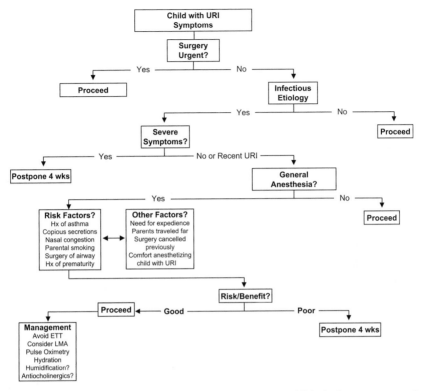

Fig. 1. Proposed algorithm for the preoperative management the child who has an upper respiratory tract infection. (*From* Tait AR, Malviya S. Anesthesia for the child with an upper respiratory tract infection: still a dilemma? Anesth Analg 2005;100(1):62; with permission.)

Cardiac complications

Although perioperative cardiac events are less common than adverse respiratory events, they are associated with significantly higher morbidity and mortality. The Pediatric Perioperative Cardiac Arrest (POCA) Registry was established in 1994 to identify risk factors for perioperative cardiac events and to develop strategies to reduce them [30]. In 2000, 289 cardiac arrests were reported to the POCA Registry [31]. Nearly half of these events (48%) were unrelated to anesthesia, occurring most commonly among children who failed to wean off bypass or who had early post-bypass heart failure or uncontrollable surgical bleeding. The incidence of anesthesia-related cardiac arrests was 1.4 events per 10,000 instances. Events related to medications or to cardiovascular events were most common [32]. Medication-related events were most often associated with the use of halothane and were more common among children who had an ASA physical class 1 to 2 than those with higher ASA classes. Although most (55%) anesthesia-related cardiac arrests occurred in infants younger than 1 year, sufficient data were not available to control for factors such as prematurity and congenital defects that may have had a confounding effect. Death occurred in 26% of children who had an anesthesia-related cardiac arrest. Independent factors associated with mortality included undergoing an emergency procedure and having an ASA physical class greater than 2, but did not include age [31].

Based on observations made from POCA Registry data, several strategies may help prevent cardiac arrest in children (see Table 1). Because medications are the leading cause of perioperative cardiac arrest, the medications used should carefully considered, particularly in infants [32]. Halothane was commonly used in anesthetic practice in the past because of its nonpungent effects that limited the potential for airway irritation. For this reason, it was the agent of choice for the inhalation induction of anesthesia in infants and children for many years. It has potent negative inotropic and chronotropic effects, which can lead to profound hypotension and bradycardia. These effects can be more problematic in dehydrated infants who had been nil per os for prolonged periods. Recently, sevoflurane has been introduced as an acceptable alternative that has fewer cardiovascular effects than halothane and is especially useful in the neonatal and infant populations who are at the greatest risk for halothane-induced cardiovascular depression.

Because of the importance of cardiovascular mechanisms as a cause of arrest, children who have cardiac disease must be identified preoperatively to appropriately modify the anesthetic plan. Although cardiac anomalies may already be known, occult defects may be found only at the time of the preoperative evaluation. One way that these defects are found is by the detection of a cardiac murmur. When a murmur is found, the main consideration is to identify occult cardiac lesions that (1) may have hemodynamic consequences during surgery (eg, pulmonary artery hypertension or left-to-right shunts) or (2) have no hemodynamic consequences but require administration of antibiotic prophylaxis (eg, a small ventricular septal defect). All infants younger than 1 year who have a murmur should undergo formal evaluation by a cardiologist before surgery because a significant cardiac lesion may have not yet become clinically apparent [33]. Most older children who have an "innocent" murmur without symptoms or signs of cardiovascular disease can safely undergo surgery. A preoperative cardiology evaluation is recommended for those discovered to have other types of murmurs or who have symptoms or signs of cardiovascular disease. Antibiotic prophylaxis should be considered before an emergency procedure not classified as clean when the etiology of the murmur is unclear [33].

Perioperative anxiety

Although uncommonly associated with major morbidity, perioperative anxiety and emergence delirium are disturbing for patients and their families. Significant anxiety is observed in as many as 65% of children before surgery and during induction [34]. In addition to leading to potential delays in induction, high levels of preoperative anxiety appear related to the development of emergence delirium and the postoperative development of new maladaptive behaviors and negative behavior changes, including general anxiety, separation anxiety, sleep anxiety, eating disturbances, aggression, and apathy/withdrawal [35]. Risk factors associated with perioperative anxiety include younger age, parental anxiety, lower social adaptive capabilities, and a temperament with low sociability [3].

Preoperative interventions to reduce anxiety are appropriate, particularly for children at risk (see Table 1). Preoperative preparation programs are now available in most hospitals but vary in content and approach [36]. These programs include child life preparation (coping skills instruction), modeling using a videotaped program, play therapy, tours of the operating room, and written materials [37]. Among these interventions, coping skills instruction is the most effective for reducing preoperative anxiety but also the most expensive to employ. Although child life preparation effectively reduces anxiety in the preoperative holding area and on separation from parents, this intervention has little impact on anxiety during induction, in the recovery room, or after hospital discharge [38]. Some methods of preoperative preparation such as modeling and operating room tours may increase perioperative anxiety, particularly among younger children and previously hospitalized children. For this reason, preoperative preparation must be modified to meet the needs of each child [37].

A common method that is used to decrease perioperative anxiety is allowing a parent to be present with the child during induction of anesthesia. This practice has significantly increased in the United States during the past decade [39]. The potential benefits include avoiding the need for premedication, avoiding the child's resistance to separation from parents, and decreasing perioperative anxiety and postoperative behavioral problems related to perioperative anxiety [37]. Although initial studies suggested that parental presence effectively reduced anxiety, more recent evidence suggests that this practice should be selectively applied and requires proper parental preparation to be effective. Children who most benefited from parental presence were those older than 4 years who had either a calm baseline personality or a mother who had a calm baseline personality [40]. To be effective, parents need to learn effective support techniques such as the use of distraction [41]. Although it has limitations, presence during induction is viewed favorably by parents; most believe that they have contributed to reducing their child's stress [42]. Compared with premedication with oral midazolam, however, parental presence during induction was found to be less effective at reducing anxiety [43]. The addition of parental presence did not significantly reduce anxiety more than using premedication alone [44]. Despite the appeal of parental participation for many parents, it is likely that parental presence will be applied more selectively and effectively in the future [37].

Postoperative management

Overview

Although outpatient surgery is appropriate for many pediatric surgical procedures, the surgical team needs to be alert to postoperative complications that require further management. Perioperative events may be identified in the hospital, leading to a prolonged recovery room stay or direct hospital admission. Other problems are identified only after discharge from the same-day surgery unit and require return to the hospital for admission. In a study of 3331 children undergoing day surgery, 130 (4%) had a prolonged recovery room stay and 61 (2%) were admitted to the hospital [45]. The main reasons for prolonged recovery room stays were nausea and vomiting or respiratory complications. Most children who had these complications recovered and were sent home, but 14% required admission to the hospital for further management. The most common reasons for unplanned hospital admission for the same-day surgery unit were respiratory complications or surgical reasons (including the surgeon's desire for a longer period of observation or a more extensive surgical procedure than planned). Although the ASA physical status of children did not differ between those who had a prolonged recovery room stay and those who did not, children admitted to the hospital after day surgery had a higher ASA physical status than those who were discharged. Although most children have an uneventful recovery after day surgery, the possibility of admission after day surgery should be communicated to families, particularly for children who have higher ASA physical status [45].

Postoperative nausea and vomiting

Although postoperative nausea and vomiting (PONV) is rarely associated with significant morbidity, it is the most frequent complication in the recovery room and is distressing to the child and parents [22]. Independent predictors of PONV include older age, duration of surgery more than 30 minutes, history of motion sickness, history of postoperative vomiting in the child or the child's immediate family, and strabismus surgery [46]. Management strategies used to reduce PONV include an alteration in the anesthetic technique to eliminate emetogenic factors and pre-emptive treatment strategies (see Table 1). Effective control of PONV begins with the elimination of factors or medications that may increase its incidence. Although not extensively studied in the pediatric population, experience in the adult population has demonstrated that specific anesthetic induction agents (etomidate, ketamine) and maintenance agents (nitrous oxide) increase the incidence of PONV. With the advent of shorter-acting, less soluble anesthetic agents such as sevoflurane or desflurane, the addition of nitrous oxide to the maintenance anesthetic adds little to ensure a rapid awakening. In addition, propofol (for anesthetic induction, maintenance, or just before emergence) can be added to the anesthetic technique to reduce PONV. Other risk factors for PONV include the reversal of neuromuscular blocking agents and the use of perioperative opioids. For many of the outpatient pediatric surgical procedures, postoperative pain can be effectively managed with a regional anesthetic technique (caudal or peripheral block) and acetaminophen or NSAIDs, thereby decreasing the need for opioids. In many centers, routine pre-emptive antiemetics (5-HT3 antagonists such as ondansetron) are used. In adults, small doses of dexamethasone have been shown to lessen the incidence of PONV when used alone and have a synergistic effect when administered with agents such as ondansetron. Alternatively, agents such as ondansetron or phenothiazines can be used to treat PONV when it occurs. Although phenothiazines are effective, adverse effects such as dystonic reactions, hypotension, sedation, and respiratory depression have limited their perioperative use of in some centers.

Postoperative pain management

The past 20 years have seen many changes in the understanding and treatment of acute pain in infants and children. The first step was to disprove the previously held misconceptions that neonates, infants, and children did not feel or react to pain like adults. This belief was based on the misconception that the immaturity of the central nervous system of infants made them less likely to perceive pain. This theory, compounded by fears of addiction and adverse effects from opioids, resulted in the inadequate treatment of pain. Recent studies have shown that infants and children experience a severity of postoperative pain similar to adults and that even premature infants demonstrate alterations in heart rate, blood pressure, and oxygen saturation in response to painful stimuli [47].

Considerations in the treatment of acute pain include the severity of the pain and the setting in which it is treated (inpatient versus outpatient). One approach is to use a three-step ladder (Box 1), initially described by the World Health Organization for the treatment of cancer-related pain [48]. Mild pain such as that following a soft tissue surgical procedure is initially treated with a nonopioid analgesic agent such as a prostaglandin synthesis inhibitor (acetaminophen, acetylsalicylic acid, or ibuprofen). Moderate pain such as that following a bony orthopedic procedure can usually be controlled with a combination of a prostaglandin synthesis inhibitor and a weak opioid (eg, a preparation of acetaminophen with codeine) for the outpatient or intravenous opioids or a regional anesthetic technique for the inpatient. More severe pain (thoracotomy or an exploratory laparotomy) generally requires a regional anesthetic technique or parenteral opioids. NSAIDs, acetaminophen, and salicylates act through the inhibition of the enzyme cyclooxygenase, thereby blocking the synthesis of prostaglandins that stimulate the free nerve endings of the peripheral nervous system. In distinction to opioids, these agents demonstrate a ceiling effect so that after a specific

---

Box 1. The World Health Organization ladder for pain treatment

Mild pain
1. NSAIDs
2. Acetaminophen
Moderate pain
1. NSAIDs or acetaminophen with a weak opioid (oxycodone, hydrocodone, codeine)
2. Intravenous opioids (with addition of fixed-interval NSAID or acetaminophen)
    A. Intravenous opioid by patient-controlled analgesia (PCA)
    B. Continuous infusion of opioid with as needed rescue doses of opioid
    C. Fixed-interval dosing of opioid
3. Regional anesthetic techniques
Severe pain (continue use of NSAID or acetaminophen)
1. Intravenous opioid by PCA
2. Regional anesthetic techniques

---

plasma concentration is achieved, no further analgesia is provided by increasing the dose. A more comprehensive review of the prostaglandin synthesis inhibitors can be found in other sources [49]. Those that are used most commonly in children and their various preparations are listed in Table 2.

Prostaglandin synthesis inhibitors can be used as the sole agent for minor pain, may be combined with weak opioids for oral administration to control moderate pain, and may be added to parenteral opioids and regional anesthetic techniques for severe pain. Its addition to opioids provides adjunctive analgesia and lowers the total amount of opioid required [50,51]. Because most opioid-related adverse effects are dose related, modalities that decrease total opioid consumption play a significant role in decreasing or preventing opioid-associated adverse effects. A technique used frequently by Tobias and colleagues [52] in the perioperative setting is the combination of the oral premedication (midazolam) with acetaminophen (15 mg/kg) or ibuprofen elixir (10 mg/kg). If preoperative administration is not chosen, then an acetaminophen suppository (40 mg/kg) can be placed following anesthetic induction. Because absorption is decreased with rectal administration, a larger dose of acetaminophen is required to achieve effective plasma levels [53]. A third option is the postoperative administration of ibuprofen or acetaminophen when the child complains of pain in the recovery room. This latter option is less desirable because the onset of activity of any of these agents following oral or rectal administration is 20 to 30 minutes. The

Table 2
Salicylate and nonsteroidal anti-inflammatory drug preparations

Medication	Preparation	Dosage forms
Ibuprofen	Oral suspension	100 mg/5 mL
	Infant drops	50 mg/1.25 mL
	Chewable tablets	50, 100 mg
	Children's caplets	100 mg
	Tablets	200, 400, 600, 800 mg
Choline magnesium	Liquid	500 mg/5 mL
trisalicilate	Tablets	500, 750, 1000 mg
Naproxen	Suspension	125 mg/5 mL
	Delayed-release tablets	275, 500 mg
	Tablets	250, 275, 375, 500, 550 mg
Tolmetin	Tablets	200, 600 mg
	Capsules	400 mg
Acetylsalicylic acid	Several different preparations available	

administration of a small dose of an intravenous opioid (fentanyl, 0.5 µg/kg; morphine, 0.02 mg/kg; or nalbuphine, 0.02–0.04 mg/kg) can be used to provide immediate analgesia while waiting for the onset of the oral/rectal acetaminophen or ibuprofen. When the patient is ready for discharge home, ongoing analgesia can be provided with acetaminophen or ibuprofen. Although it is most common to administer these agents on an "as-needed" basis, fixed-interval dosing may provide more effective analgesia. This process entails administering the medication around the clock for the first 24 to 48 hours and not waiting for the child to complain of pain. For this purpose, acetaminophen (10–15 mg/kg) every 4 hours or ibuprofen (10 mg/kg) every 6 hours can be used. If the patient is receiving acetaminophen as a fixed-interval dose and complains of pain, an "as needed" or supplemental dose of ibuprofen can be administered and vice versa. These techniques can be used for all types of acute pain.

When moderate pain needs to be treated on an outpatient basis or when the first step of the ladder fails in what was thought to be mild pain, the NSAID, aspirin, or acetaminophen can be combined with a weak opioid (codeine, oxycodone, or hydrocodone), which are available in tablet and liquid formulations. Acetaminophen with codeine elixir contains 120 mg of acetaminophen and 12 mg of codeine per 5 mL. Dosing is based on the codeine component, ranging from 0.5 to 1.0 mg/kg every 4 to 6 hours. Tablet preparations contain 325 mg of acetaminophen with 15, 30, or 60 mg of codeine. Codeine is metabolized by hepatic microsomal enzymes to morphine for a significant part of its analgesic effect. In a cohort of 96 children, Williams and colleagues [54] reported that 47% had genotypes associated with a reduction of the activity of the enzymes necessary for the conversion of codeine to morphine and that no morphine or metabolites were detected in 36% of the patients given codeine. Alternatives to codeine for oral administration include oxycodone or hydrocodone preparations, which are also available in liquid and tablet forms with acetaminophen or acetylsalicylic acid. Hydrocodone (7.5 mg) combined with 200 mg of ibuprofen is also available as a tablet. The dose should be based on the oxycodone or hydrocodone component, starting at 0.1 to 0.15 mg/kg every 4 to 6 hours. Regardless of the preparation used, increasing the dose may result in exceeding the amount of recommended acetaminophen (15 mg/kg/dose or 60–90 mg/kg/d).

In patients who cannot tolerate or will not accept oral or rectal medications, intravenous administration is possible with ketorolac, a parenteral NSAID. When first released, the initial clinical trails suggested that ketorolac was as effective as opioids in treating acute pain; however, its current clinical use is similar that of other NSAIDs as an adjunct to opioid analgesia [55]. Because ketorolac is more expensive than nonparenteral NSAIDs, future studies are needed to determine its advantages over more inexpensive agents and routes of delivery (oral or rectal) in various acute pain situations. The authors' current practice includes fixed-interval administration of ketorolac for the initial postoperative period or immediately following the acute pain issue, with the switch to acetaminophen or ibuprofen after the patient is able to tolerate oral or rectal medications. In the adult population, a ceiling effect has been reported so that no further analgesia was noted with doses of ketorolac higher than 7.5 to 10 mg [56]. Although there are no comparable studies in pediatric-aged patients, the authors' current practice includes dosing at 0.5 mg/kg up to a maximum of 10 mg every 6 hours. After the patient is able to tolerate oral medications, the switch is made to an oral NSAID or acetaminophen. Ketorolac is contraindicated in patients who have bleeding dyscrasias or in settings in which acute hemorrhage is a concern (eg, in patients who have abnormal coagulation function, in the trauma patient, or following intracranial or ENT surgery).

Opioids may act as pure agonists (bind and activate both μ and κ receptors) or as agonists/antagonists (bind and activate κ receptors while binding to but not activating μ receptors). Agonists/antagonists including nalbuphine, butorphanol, and pentazocine should not be administered to patients who have been chronically receiving opioids because these can precipitate withdrawal symptoms or reverse analgesia. Although these agents have a decreased potential to cause respiratory depression, there is also a ceiling effect for their analgesia. With dose escalation for increasing or persistent pain, there is a limit to the amount of analgesia achieved. Their potency and efficacy for severe pain is less than that of pure agonists. They may be useful for mild to moderate pain when oral administration of other agents such as acetaminophen with codeine is not feasible or when a more rapid onset of action is desired. The authors' practice frequently includes the intravenous administration of a single dose of these agents to treat moderate pain in the postanesthesia area, followed by the switch to oral agents when the patient is discharged home. An additional benefit of a drug such as nalbuphine is that it causes more sedation than other opioids and may be beneficial for the agitated postoperative patient. The agonists/antagonists should also be considered when supplemental intravenous analgesia is required in patients who are receiving or have received epidural or intrathecal opioids within the last 24 hours (see Tobias [49] for a full discussion of neuraxial opioids). The respiratory depression that can occur with the combination of intravenous and neuraxial opioids may be less if an agonist/antagonist is used rather than a pure agonist such as morphine. In these situations, the authors' practice is to administer incremental doses of nalbuphine (0.02–0.03 mg/kg) every 5 to 10 minutes as needed until the desired level of analgesia is achieved.

When opioids are chosen for postoperative analgesia, three choices must be made: (1) which opioid to use, (2) the mode of administration, and (3) the route of administration. Respiratory depression is similar if equipotent doses are administered. The authors' practice is to use morphine or hydromorphone. Meperidine is generally avoided given its higher incidence of dysphoric reactions and the potential for seizures related to the accumulation of the metabolite normeperidine. Morphine is metabolized in the liver to morphine-6-glucuronide, which is significantly more potent than the parent compound. Morphine-6-glucoronide is water soluble, penetrates the central nervous system poorly, and is of little consequence in most circumstances. It is cleared by the kidneys and can accumulate in patients who have renal insufficiency, resulting in respiratory depression. In such patients, alternative opioids such as hydromorphone (see later discussion), which has no active metabolites, should be considered. Hydromorphone may also be advantageous when adverse effects related to histamine release, such as pruritus, occur with morphine, which may be more common in adolescents and young adults.

The second decision regarding opioid analgesia is the mode of administration. Options include on demand (as-needed dosing), fixed-interval administration, continuous infusion, or patient-controlled analgesia (PCA) pumps. For optimal analgesia, opioids should be administered in a manner that maintains a steady-state serum concentration. For moderate to severe pain, on-demand administration generally does not provide adequate analgesia because of the delay in obtaining the medication. The optimal mode for the delivery of opioids remains PCA. PCA allows the patient to administer a preset amount of opioid at specific intervals. These devices may be used in children as young as 5 to 6 years [57,58]. Before instituting PCA administration of narcotics, pain must be controlled. An opioid is titrated in small, intravenous bolus doses (morphine 0.02 mg/kg every 5 minutes) to the desired level of analgesia before the PCA device is started. Its use may be limited in certain patients due to age, underlying illness, or mental capabilities. Many centers still use PCA in these types of patients, but allow the device to be activated by the bedside nurse. In this setting, the PCA device eliminates the delay in opioid administration that occurs while the nurse signs out the medication and draws it up. Murphy and colleagues [59] showed equivalent levels of analgesia and equivalent opioid consumption for PCA compared with nurse-controlled analgesia.

Regional anesthetic technique is an alternative that continues to increase in popularity. Depending on the site of surgery and the severity of the postoperative pain, this may include a neuraxial approach (caudal, lumbar, or thoracic epidural) or a peripheral nerve block. For unilateral surgery, a peripheral nerve block may be chosen. For outpatients, a single shot approach using only local anesthetic agents is used, such as a caudal epidural block with bupivacaine following inguinal hernorrhaphy. For the inpatient, more prolonged analgesia can be provided by a single shot approach using a combination of local anesthetic with opioid (morphine) or clonidine or by the placement of a catheter for a continuous infusion. Whenever neuraxial opioids are administered, ongoing monitoring of respiratory status is suggested given the potential for respiratory depression.

Summary

The safety of surgery and anesthesia for infants and children has improved over the past several decades. Same-day surgery is now feasible for most pediatric surgical procedures and has been widely adopted. The focus of preoperative management should be to identify children at high-risk for complications that are common and complications that are less common but potentially life-threatening. Psychologic preparation of children and their families is essential to reduce preoperative anxiety and the likelihood of short- and long-term adverse psychologic responses to surgery. Although additional work is needed, we have a better understanding of factors associated with major and minor adverse events that occur intraoperatively and postoperatively.

References

[1] Overdyk FJ, Burt N, Tagge EP, et al. "One-stop" surgery: implications for anesthesiologists of an expedited pediatric surgical process. South Med J 1999;92(3):308–12.

[2] Tagge EP, Hebra A, Overdyk F, et al. One-stop surgery: evolving approach to pediatric outpatient surgery. J Pediatr Surg 1999;34(1):129–32.

[3] Kain ZN, Mayes LC, Weisman SJ, et al. Social adaptability, cognitive abilities, and other predictors for children's reactions to surgery. J Clin Anesth 2000;12(7):549–54.

[4] Meneghini L, Zadra N, Zanette G, et al. The usefulness of routine preoperative laboratory tests for one-day surgery in healthy children. Paediatr Anaesth 1998;8(1):11–5.

[5] Patel RI, DeWitt L, Hannallah RS. Preoperative laboratory testing in children undergoing elective surgery: analysis of current practice. J Clin Anesth 1997;9(7):569–75.

[6] Wheeler M, Cote CJ. Preoperative pregnancy testing in a tertiary care children's hospital: a medico-legal conundrum. J Clin Anesth 1999;11(1):56–63.

[7] Azzam FJ, Padda GS, DeBoard JW, et al. Preoperative pregnancy testing in adolescents. Anesth Analg 1996;82(1):4–7.

[8] Howells RC II, Wax MK, Ramadan HH. Value of preoperative prothrombin time/partial thromboplastin time as a predictor of postoperative hemorrhage in pediatric patients undergoing tonsillectomy. Otolaryngol Head Neck Surg 1997;117(6):628–32.

[9] Asaf T, Reuveni H, Yermiahu T, et al. The need for routine pre-operative coagulation screening tests (prothrombin time PT/partial thromboplastin time PTT) for healthy children undergoing elective tonsillectomy and/or adenoidectomy. Int J Pediatr Otorhinolaryngol 2001;61(3):217–22.

[10] Gabriel P, Mazoit X, Ecoffey C. Relationship between clinical history, coagulation tests, and perioperative bleeding during tonsillectomies in pediatrics. J Clin Anesth 2000;12(4): 288–91.

[11] Windfuhr JP, Chen YS, Remmert S. Unidentified coagulation disorders in post-tonsillectomy hemorrhage. Ear Nose Throat J 2004;83(1):28–32 passim.

[12] Koscielny J, Ziemer S, Radtke H, et al. A practical concept for preoperative identification of patients with impaired primary hemostasis. Clin Appl Thromb Hemost 2004;10(3): 195–204.

[13] Noll S, Spitz L, Pierro A. Additional medical information: prevalence, source, and benefit to parents. J Pediatr Surg 2001;36(5):791–4.

[14] Semere W, Karamanoukian HL, Levitt M, et al. A pediatric surgery study: parent usage of the Internet for medical information. J Pediatr Surg 2003;38(4):560–4.

[15] Levinson W, Chaumeton N. Communication between surgeons and patients in routine office visits. Surgery 1999;125(2):127–34.

[16] Levinson W, Gorawara-Bhat R, Lamb J. A study of patient clues and physician responses in primary care and surgical settings. JAMA 2000;284(8):1021–7.

[17] Ambady N, Laplante D, Nguyen T, et al. Surgeons' tone of voice: a clue to malpractice history. Surgery 2002;132(1):5–9.

[18] Sobo EJ. Parents' perceptions of pediatric day surgery risks: unforeseeable complications, or avoidable mistakes? Soc Sci Med 2005;60(10):2341–50.

[19] Wisselo TL, Stuart C, Muris P. Providing parents with information before anaesthesia: what do they really want to know? Paediatr Anaesth 2004;14(4):299–307.

[20] Kain ZN, Wang SM, Caramico LA, et al. Parental desire for perioperative information and informed consent: a two-phase study. Anesth Analg 1997;84(2):299–306.

[21] Fallat ME, Deshpande JK. Do-not-resuscitate orders for pediatric patients who require anesthesia and surgery: American Academy of Pediatrics Section on Surgery, Section on Anesthesia and Pain Medicine, and Committee on Bioethics. Pediatrics 2004;114(6):1686–92.

[22] Murat I, Constant I, Maud'huy H. Perioperative anaesthetic morbidity in children: a database of 24,165 anaesthetics over a 30-month period. Paediatr Anaesth 2004;14(2):158–66.

[23] Mamie C, Habre W, Delhumeau C, et al. Incidence and risk factors of perioperative respiratory adverse events in children undergoing elective surgery. Paediatr Anaesth 2004; 14(3):218–24.

[24] Bordet F, Allaouchiche B, Lansiaux S, et al. Risk factors for airway complications during general anaesthesia in paediatric patients. Paediatr Anaesth 2002;12(9):762–9.

[25] Rosenstein N, Phillips WR, Gerber MA, et al. The common cold—principles of judicious use of antimicrobial agents. Pediatrics 1998;101(1 Suppl Pt 2):181–4.

[26] Tait AR, Malviya S. Anesthesia for the child with an upper respiratory tract infection: still a dilemma? Anesth Analg 2005;100(1):59–65.

[27] Tait AR, Malviya S, Voepel-Lewis T, et al. Risk factors for perioperative adverse respiratory events in children with upper respiratory tract infections. Anesthesiology 2001;95(2): 299–306.

[28] Parnis SJ, Barker DS, Van Der Walt JH. Clinical predictors of anaesthetic complications in children with respiratory tract infections. Paediatr Anaesth 2001;11(1):29–40.

[29] Tait AR, Reynolds PI, Gutstein HB. Factors that influence an anesthesiologist's decision to cancel elective surgery for the child with an upper respiratory tract infection. J Clin Anesth 1995;7(6):491–9.

[30] Posner KL, Geiduschek J, Haberkern CM, et al. Unexpected cardiac arrest among children during surgery, a North American registry to elucidate the incidence and causes of anesthesia related cardiac arrest. Qual Saf Health Care 2002;11(3):252–7.

[31] Morray JP, Geiduschek JM, Ramamoorthy C, et al. Anesthesia-related cardiac arrest in children: initial findings of the Pediatric Perioperative Cardiac Arrest (POCA) Registry. Anesthesiology 2000;93(1):6–14.

[32] Mason LJ. An update on the etiology and prevention of anesthesia-related cardiac arrest in children. Paediatr Anaesth 2004;14(5):412–6.

[33] McEwan AI, Birch M, Bingham R. The preoperative management of the child with a heart murmur. Paediatr Anaesth 1995;5(3):151–6.

[34] Kain ZN, Mayes LC, O'Connor TZ, et al. Preoperative anxiety in children. Predictors and outcomes. Arch Pediatr Adolesc Med 1996;150(12):1238–45.

[35] Kain ZN, Caldwell-Andrews AA, Maranets I, et al. Preoperative anxiety and emergence delirium and postoperative maladaptive behaviors. Anesth Analg 2004;99(6):1648–54.

[36] O'Byrne KK, Peterson L, Saldana L. Survey of pediatric hospitals' preparation programs: evidence of the impact of health psychology research. Health Psychol 1997;16(2):147–54.

[37] Kain ZN, Caldwell-Andrews A, Wang SM. Psychological preparation of the parent and pediatric surgical patient. Anesthesiol Clin North America 2002;20(1):29–44.

[38] Kain ZN, Caramico LA, Mayes LC, et al. Preoperative preparation programs in children: a comparative examination. Anesth Analg 1998;87(6):1249–55.

[39] Kain ZN, Caldwell-Andrews AA, Krivutza DM, et al. Trends in the practice of parental presence during induction of anesthesia and the use of preoperative sedative premedication in the United States, 1995–2002: results of a follow-up national survey. Anesth Analg 2004; 98(5):1252–9.

[40] Kain ZN, Mayes LC, Caramico LA, et al. Parental presence during induction of anesthesia. A randomized controlled trial. Anesthesiology 1996;84(5):1060–7.

[41] Blount R, Bachanas P, Powers S. Training children to cope and parents to coach them during routine immunizations: effects on child, parent, and staff behaviors. Behav Ther 1992;23: 689–705.

[42] Ryder IG, Spargo PM. Parents in the anaesthetic room. A questionnaire survey of parents' reactions. Anaesthesia 1991;46(11):977–9.

[43] Kain ZN, Mayes LC, Wang SM, et al. Parental presence during induction of anesthesia versus sedative premedication: which intervention is more effective? Anesthesiology 1998;89(5): 1147–56.

[44] Kain ZN, Mayes LC, Wang SM, et al. Parental presence and a sedative premedicant for children undergoing surgery: a hierarchical study. Anesthesiology 2000;92(4):939–46.

[45] D'Errico C, Voepel-Lewis TD, Siewert M, et al. Prolonged recovery stay and unplanned admission of the pediatric surgical outpatient: an observational study. J Clin Anesth 1998; 10(6):482–7.

[46] Eberhart LH, Geldner G, Kranke P, et al. The development and validation of a risk score to predict the probability of postoperative vomiting in pediatric patients. Anesth Analg 2004; 99(6):1630–7.

[47] Mather L, Mackie J. The incidence of postoperative pain in children. Pain 1983;15:271–82.

[48] Schug SA, Zech D, Dorr U. Cancer pain management according to WHO analgesia guidelines. J Pain Symptom Manage 1990;5:27–32.

[49] Tobias JD. Weak analgesics and nonsteroidal anti-inflammatory agents in the management of children with acute pain. Pediatr Clin North Am 2000;47:527–43.

[50] Maunuksela EL, Ryhanen P, Janhunen L. Efficacy of rectal ibuprofen in controlling postoperative pain in children. Can J Anaesth 1992;39:226–30.

[51] Sims C, Johnson CM, Bergesio R, et al. Rectal indomethacin for analgesia after appendectomy in children. Anaesth Intens Care 1994;22:272–5.

[52] Tobias JD, Lowe S, Hersey S, et al. Analgesia after bilateral myringotomy and placement of pressure equalization tubes in children: acetaminophen versus acetaminophen with codeine. Anesth Analg 1995;81:496–500.

[53] Birmingham PK, Tobin MJ, Henthorn TK, et al. Twenty-four hour pharmacokinetics of rectal acetaminophen in children. Anesthesiology 1997;87:244–8.

[54] Williams DG, Patel A, Howard RF. Pharmacogenetics of codeine metabolism in an urban population of children and its implications for analgesic reliability. Br J Anaesth 2002;89: 839–45.

[55] Vetter TR, Heiner EJ. Intravenous ketorolac as an adjuvant to pediatric patient-controlled analgesia with morphine. J Clin Anesth 1994;6:110–3.

[56] Reuben SS, Connelly NR, Lucie S, et al. Dose-response of ketorolac as an adjunct to patient-controlled analgesia with morphine in patients after spinal fusion surgery. Anesth Analg 1998;87:98–101.

[57] Doyle E, Robinson D, Morton NS. Comparison of patient controlled analgesia with and without a background infusion after lower abdominal surgery in children. Br J Anaesth 1993;71:670–3.

[58] Doyle E, Harper I, Morton NS. Patient-controlled analgesia with low dose background infusions after lower abdominal surgery in children. Br J Anaesth 1993;71:818–22.

[59] Murphy DF, Graziotti P, Chaldiadis G, et al. Patient-controlled analgesia: a comparison with nurse-controlled intravenous opioid infusion. Anaesth Intens Care 1994;22:589–92.

ELSEVIER
SAUNDERS

SURGICAL
CLINICS OF
NORTH AMERICA

Surg Clin N Am 86 (2006) 249–260

Gastroschisis and Omphalocele

Daniel J. Ledbetter, MD[a,b,]*

[a]*Department of Surgery, Division of Pediatric Surgery, University of Washington*
[b]*Department of Surgery, Children's Hospital and Regional Medical Center,
4800 Sand Point Way NE, P.O. Box 5371/G0035, Seattle, WA 98105-0371, USA*

The newborn who has an abdominal wall defect is one of the most dramatic presentations in medicine and offers many challenging problems to the pediatric surgeon. This article presents the basics of the two most common abdominal wall defects—gastroschisis and omphalocele—including principles and options of prenatal, postnatal, and surgical management. Although textbooks group the two entities together, they are separate and distinct and have many important differences in pathology and associated conditions that explain the differences in treatment plans and outcomes. Understanding the similarities and differences between gastroschisis and omphalocele is essential for patient management; therefore, the following sections first acknowledge the similarities and then emphasize the differences.

Definitions

Gastroschisis is a full-thickness defect in the abdominal wall usually just to the right of a normal insertion of the umbilical cord into the body wall. Rarely it is located in a mirror-image position to the left of the umbilical cord. A variable amount of intestine and occasionally parts of other abdominal organs are herniated outside the abdominal wall with no covering membrane or sac.

An omphalocele (also known as exomphalos) is a midline abdominal wall defect of variable size, with the herniated viscera covered by a membrane consisting of peritoneum on the inner surface, amnion on the outer surface, and Wharton's jelly between the layers. The umbilical vessels insert into the membrane and not the body wall. The hernia contents include a variable

---

* Department of Surgery, Children's Hospital and Regional Medical Center, 4800 Sand Point Way NE, P.O. Box 5371/G0035, Seattle, WA 98105-0371.
E-mail address: dan.ledbetter@seattlechildrens.org

amount of intestine, often parts of the liver, and occasionally other organs. The defect may be centered in the upper, mid, or lower abdomen and its size and location have important implications for management.

Abdominal wall development and the pathology of omphalocele and gastroschisis

The abdominal wall is formed by infolding of the cranial, caudal, and two lateral embryonic folds. As the abdominal wall is forming, the rapid growth of the intestinal tract leads to its migration outside the abdominal cavity through the umbilical ring and into the umbilical cord during the sixth week of gestation. By the 10th to 12th week, the abdominal wall is well formed and the intestine returns to the abdominal cavity in a stereotypical pattern that results in normal intestinal rotation and later fixation [1].

Gastroschisis is thought to result from an ischemic insult to the developing body wall. The right paraumbilical area is an area at risk because it is supplied by the right umbilical vein and right omphalomesenteric artery until they involute. If this ordered development and involution is disturbed in degree or timing, then a body wall defect could result from the resulting body wall ischemia [2,3]. An alternative hypothesis that may account for some cases of gastroschisis is that the defect results from an early rupture of a hernia of the umbilical cord [4].

In omphalocele, the bowel does not return to the abdomen but remains out in the umbilical cord. The exact sequence of events are not known but are presumed to involve a failure of abdominal wall infolding [1]. A variable amount of midgut and other intra-abdominal organs are herniated out of the defect depending on its size and relative location on the abdominal wall. Cranial fold deficits predominately result in epigastric omphaloceles that may be associated with additional cranial fold abnormalities such as anterior diaphragmatic hernia, sternal clefts, pericardial defects, and cardiac defects. When these elements occur together, they are known as the pentalogy of Cantrell [5]. When the infolding deficit involves the caudal fold, the omphalocele may be associated with bladder or cloacal exstrophy.

Epidemiology

There are regional differences in the incidence of abdominal wall defects and the relative proportions of gastroschisis and omphalocele; however, a rough estimate is that worldwide, the incidence of gastroschisis ranges between 0.4 and 3 per 10,000 births and seems to be increasing, whereas the incidence of omphalocele ranges between 1.5 and 3 per 10,000 births and is stable [6–8]. The etiology of both abdominal wall defects is unknown and most are sporadic, but there are rare familial (and possibly genetically determined) cases of gastroschisis and omphalocele. There are distinctive maternal risk factors for the different abdominal wall defects. Gastroschisis has a very strong association with young maternal age, with most of these mothers being age 20 years or younger [6]. In addition, gastroschisis has been linked to maternal exposure to cigarette smoking, illicit drugs, vasoactive over-the-counter drugs (such as pseudoephedrine), and environmental toxins [6]. These associations are consistent with the vascular insufficiency of the abdominal wall theories of the etiology of gastroschisis. In contrast, omphalocele is associated with advancing maternal age, with most of these mothers being over 30 years old [7].

Associated anomalies

Like all babies who have birth defects, children who have abdominal wall defects are at an increased risk for additional anomalies, but the relative risk and pattern of associated anomalies is a major difference between gastroschisis and omphalocele. These differences are very important in clinical management and long-term prognosis. In gastroschisis, the incidence of associated anomalies is between 10% and 20%, and most of the significant anomalies are in the gastrointestinal tract [9]. About 10% of babies who have gastroschisis have intestinal stenosis or atresia that results from vascular insufficiency to the bowel at the time of gastroschisis development or, more commonly, from later volvulus or compression of the mesenteric vascular pedicle by a narrowing abdominal wall ring [10]. Other less common associated anomalies include undescended testes, Meckel's diverticulum, and intestinal duplications. Serious associated anomalies outside the abdomen or gastrointestinal tract, such as chromosomal abnormalities, are unusual.

In contrast to the relatively low risk of associated anomalies mainly localized to the gastrointestinal tract seen in patients who have gastroschisis, patients who have omphalocele have a very high (up to 50%–70%) incidence of associated anomalies. The incidence of associated anomalies is lower in liveborn patients because those who have multiple and serious anomalies are more likely to be stillborn [11]. Chromosome anomalies, notably trisomy 13, 14, 15, 18, and 21, are present in up to 30% of cases. Cardiac defects are also common, being present in 30% to 50% of cases. Multiple anomalies are frequent and may be clustered in syndromic patterns. One important pattern is the Beckwith-Wiedemann syndrome that may be present in up to 10% of cases [12]. Beckwith-Wiedemann syndrome is marked by macroglossia, organomegaly, early hypoglycemia (from pancreatic hyperplasia and excess insulin), and an increased risk of Wilms' tumor, hepatoblastoma, and neuroblastoma developing later in childhood. The size of the abdominal wall defect in omphalocele does not directly correlate with the presence of other anomalies, as demonstrated by the finding that small defects found on prenatal ultrasound have a higher risk of associated chromosomal abnormalities and cardiac defects [13].

Prenatal diagnosis

Abdominal wall defects are often diagnosed by prenatal ultrasound done for routine screening or for obstetric indications such as evaluating an elevated maternal serum alpha fetoprotein (AFP). AFP is the fetal analog of albumin, and maternal serum AFP reflects the level of AFP in amniotic fluid. The testing was developed to evaluate the fetus for chromosomal abnormalities and neural tube defects, but AFP is also usually elevated with abdominal wall defects. The magnitude and likelihood of AFP elevation varies between gastroschisis and omphalocele [14]. In gastroschisis, maternal serum AFP is usually markedly abnormal, with an average elevation of more than nine multiples of the mean (MoM). In contrast, in omphalocele, AFP is elevated by an average of only four MoM, with a much wider range. This different pattern results in a lower sensitivity of maternal serum AFP for omphalocele than for gastroschisis. Like many screening tests, the sensitivity depends on the cutoff value chosen. For example, if abnormal is defined as greater than 3 MoM, then 96% of gastroschisis would be detected but only 65% of omphaloceles [15].

Prenatal ultrasound is done in most pregnancies in the United States and, when done, could potentially identify the overwhelming majority of abdominal wall defects and accurately distinguish omphalocele from gastroschisis. This identification would permit an opportunity to counsel the family and to prepare for optimal postnatal care. It is unfortunate, however, that the accuracy of prenatal ultrasound for diagnosing abdominal wall defects is affected by the timing and goals of the study, fetal position, and the experience and expertise of the operator. The specificity is high (more than 95%), but the sensitivity is only 60% to 75% for identifying gastroschisis and omphalocele [8,16]. Diagnostic errors may result because of (1) confusion with other rare abdominal defects (often away from the umbilicus, not covered by a membrane, and fatal); (2) ruptured omphaloceles that mimic a gastroschisis because of the lack of a covering membrane; or (3) rare cases of gastroschisis that start out as a covered defect and later rupture but are likely and more commonly simply missed during studies done for reasons other than screening for structural defects.

Prenatal management

A fetus with an abdominal wall defect is a high-risk pregnancy on many levels. For gastroschisis and omphalocele, there is an increased risk of intrauterine growth retardation (IUGR), fetal death, and premature delivery, so careful obstetric follow-up with serial ultrasounds and other tests of fetal well-being are indicated. In both cases, there is some controversy regarding the timing and mode of delivery.

In gastroschisis, the diagnosis of IUGR can be problematic because of the difficulty measuring the torso, but it probably affects 30% to 70% of fetuses. The cause of fetal growth failure in gastroschisis is unknown but presumed to be due to increased losses of protein from the exposed viscera, although inadequate supply of fetal nutrients is an alternative hypothesis. The exposed bowel is vulnerable to injury. The injury can range in severity from volvulus and loss of the entire midgut, to a more localized intestinal atresia and stenosis, to widespread inflammatory "peel" or serositis that can make the bowel loops indistinguishable from one another. The inflammatory peel develops after 30 weeks' gestation and is presumed to be due to bowel wall exposure to amniotic fluid or to intestinal lymphatic obstruction. The degree of the inflammatory peel is difficult to quantify on prenatal ultrasound and after delivery, so it has been difficult to correlate with clinical outcome variables [17]. Because bowel injury is a major predictor of postnatal mortality and morbidity, improved understanding and predictive testing would point the way toward potential interventions. Oligohydramnios is also common in gastroschisis, being present in up to 25% of cases. The cause is unknown and it is usually of moderate severity and associated with IUGR, fetal distress, and birth asphyxia. Cases of gastroschisis associated with oligohydramnios prompted investigation of amniotic fluid replacement with saline. Observations from these trials and experimental models supported the hypothesis that amniotic fluid was responsible for the inflammatory peel, and this has been investigated by amniotic fluid exchange transfusion. Preliminary reports have been promising, but additional experience is needed to confirm these results because of the previously noted difficulties in measuring the degree of bowel injury pre- and postnatally [18]. The most devastating prenatal complication with gastroschisis is the uncommon but unpredictable fetal death. It may be caused by an in utero midgut volvulus or probably more commonly by an acute compromise of umbilical blood flow by the eviscerated bowel. It is unfortunate that there are no reliable predictors of this complication [19]. It has been presumed that early ultrasound signs of bowel obstruction, such as increased bowel diameter, indicate a high-risk fetus, but whether it is a higher risk for fetal death and intestinal loss or only a higher risk for intestinal stenosis and atresia or inflammatory peel is not known. The uncommon but tragic fetal death or the patient who has major intestinal loss has been a strong motivating force for the early delivery of the fetus with gastroschisis before such complications happen [20]. It is still unclear whether a fetus with a high risk of prenatal complications can be reliably identified and whether the benefits outweigh the risks of early delivery [21,22].

Omphalocele also has an increased incidence of IUGR (5%–35%), fetal death (usually attributed to related to severe associated anomalies), and premature labor (5%–60%) [23]. Further prenatal diagnostic studies such as high-resolution ultrasound looking for structural defects (especially cardiac defects) and chromosomal studies are often done to diagnose associated anomalies and to help predict prognosis. Unlike gastroschisis, there is usually no reason to consider early delivery, although cesarean section is often done with giant omphaloceles to prevent rupture or dystocia during labor [24].

Newborn management

The initial management of newborns who have abdominal wall defects starts with the ABCs of resuscitation, and after these have been assessed and stabilized, attention is turned to the abdominal wall defect. Heat loss is an important problem, so care must be taken to dry the baby and maintain a warm environment while protecting the exposed viscera. Premature birth is frequently associated with both conditions and must be considered during the evaluation and treatment. Checking and maintaining serum glucose levels is part of any neonatal resuscitation but especially important in babies who have abdominal wall defects because of the associated prematurity, IUGR, and in omphaloceles, the possibility of Beckwith-Wiedemann syndrome. Prematurity, associated pulmonary hypoplasia, or the significant heart defects seen in omphalocele may lead to early intubation and mechanical ventilation [25]. Gastric decompression is important to prevent distention of the gastrointestinal tract and possible aspiration. Vascular access is obtained for intravenous fluids and broad-spectrum prophylactic antibiotics. Babies who have gastroschisis in particular have high fluid losses from evaporation and third-space losses and may require twice the maintenance volumes of fluids to maintain an adequate intravascular volume. A bladder catheter is useful to closely monitor urine output and guide the resuscitation. The umbilical artery and vein may be cannulated if needed during resuscitation but in omphalocele, placement may be difficult because of the abnormal insertion and course of the vessels. Even if umbilical cannulas are successfully placed, they may need to be removed during the repair of the defect.

When the ABCs have been accomplished, the abdominal wall defect can be assessed and treated. This process involves different considerations in gastroschisis and omphalocele. In gastroschisis, the exposed viscera are inspected and care is taken to avoid twisting of the mesenteric vascular pedicle. If there is vascular compromise because the abdominal wall opening is too small, then the defect should immediately be surgically enlarged, with care taken to avoid the adjacent umbilical vessels and mesentery. The exposed bowel needs to be protected and fluid and heat losses minimized. The easiest method is to place the exposed viscera and entire lower half the baby into a transparent plastic bowel bag. This is fast, requires no special skills or experience, and allows for ongoing assessment of bowel perfusion. Alternatively, the bowel alone can be wrapped with clear plastic wrapping but this can be technically more difficult. Finally, moist dressings over the bowel covered with a clear plastic wrapping is another strategy but requires judgment on how tight to wrap and it hides the bowel from view. Moist dressings alone should be avoided because of the increased evaporative heat losses. After the exposed bowel is covered, the entire mass is stabilized by placing the baby with its right side down to prevent kinking of the mesenteric pedicle [26].

With omphalocele, the care of the defect and its contents is different. The defect is inspected to make sure that the covering membrane is intact, and nonadherent dressings are applied and stabilized to prevent trauma to the sac. If the omphalocele sac is ruptured, then exposed bowel should be treated as it is for gastroschisis.

Surgical management

In gastroschisis and omphalocele, the ultimate goals are straightforward: to reduce the herniated viscera into the abdomen and to close the fascia and skin to create a solid abdominal wall with a relatively normal umbilicus while minimizing risks to the baby. To achieve these goals, many different techniques have been described. Treatment often varies depending on the size and type of the defect, the size of the baby, and the associated problems. Because there is little hard scientific evidence to favor one method over another, there is considerable variation in the surgical approach. What follows is the author's personal approach to gastroschisis and omphalocele, with discussion of some but not all of the alternative methods.

In gastroschisis, the ongoing fluid and heat losses of exposed bowel and the subsequent metabolic derangements make rapid coverage a high priority. During the initial resuscitation at delivery or as soon as possible thereafter, a prefabricated, spring-loaded Silastic silo is placed in the defect to cover the exposed bowel. This practice minimizes evaporative losses, prevents additional trauma, and allows for an ongoing assessment of bowel perfusion. These devices can be placed in the delivery room or at the bedside without anesthesia [27]. If the abdominal wall defect is too small to accommodate the device, then the defect can be enlarged under local anesthesia and sedation. If this device cannot be placed at the bedside, then as soon as possible after the initial resuscitation and stabilization, the baby is taken to the operating room for primary closure or silo placement. Formal closure in the delivery room is an intriguing concept that minimizes time and preoperative trauma but is only possible with planned delivery of a known defect and requires a significant commitment of resources [28]. Immediate primary repair without anesthesia has been reported for selected cases and may be the most dramatic example of minimally invasive and minimally traumatic surgery [29]. It is not known how often this approach is feasible.

After the placement of the spring-loaded silo, the baby is evaluated further and cared for in the ICU. With spontaneous diuresis, gastrointestinal tract decompression from above and below, and resolution of bowel wall edema, the volume of the exposed bowel in the bag markedly decreases in a short period of time. When the baby is otherwise stable and the spontaneous reduction of bowel into the abdomen has reached a plateau, the baby is taken to the operating room for an attempt at delayed primary closure. Serial reduction of the device at the bedside has been advocated, but the risk of displacing the coverage device makes this plan less appealing.

In the operating room, if the bowel can be reduced into the abdomen and the defect closed primarily (or by delayed primary repair), then it should be done. The decision of whether a baby can tolerate reduction and repair can be difficult and can be aided by measuring the intragastric pressure during attempted closure. A pressure of less than 20 mm Hg predicts successful closure without complications of excessive intra-abdominal pressure [30]. Other methods reported to help in the decision to close or not to close are measuring changes in central venous pressure, in ventilatory pressures, and in end-tidal carbon dioxide. If the baby is stable when the fascia is closed, then an umbilicus should be constructed at the level of the posterior iliac crest during the skin closure. Several different methods have been described that achieve an acceptable long-term contour by avoiding the long-term tendency of surgically sutured skin folds to flatten [31]. Creation of an umbilicus can always be deferred to a later time. If primary repair is not possible, then a formal Silastic silo is sutured to the fascia and serial reduction is done postoperatively. Several different methods of serial reduction have been described, but the author's preference is to use a specially designed wringer clamp with a guard that allows the Silastic sheets to be approximated while pushing the bowel down and away from the roller mechanism [32]. The incremental reduction steps are quick, easy, and easily reversible and can be done multiple times during the day and permit a gradual reclamation of abdominal domain. The reduction is done as tolerated over several days, with the goal to finish it within a week to 10 days to avoid the serious complications of wound infection and necrosis that result in separation of the Silastic sheets away from the fascia, creating an open abdomen. After the viscera have been reduced to the level of the abdominal wall, the baby is returned to the operating room for removal of the silo and closure.

Babies who have gastroschisis and associated intestinal atresia pose a serious challenge. If the bowel is in good condition and the abdomen can be closed without difficulty, then combined primary repair of both defects is possible, but such ideal circumstances are unusual. Therefore, when an atresia is present or suspected, the first priority is to close the abdomen by primary, delayed primary, or staged silo repair. The baby is maintained with gastric decompression and parenteral nutrition for several weeks until repeat laparotomy and repair of the intestinal atresia [10]. This staging of the repairs allows the inflammatory peel to resolve and the herniated contents to gain domain of the abdomen before opening the bowel and creating a vulnerable anastomosis.

For omphalocele, the strategy is markedly different. First, if the covering sac is intact, then there is no urgency to perform operative closure. So long as the viscera are covered with the membrane, a complete evaluation for associated defects can be done and other problems treated. When the baby is otherwise stable and if the defect is relatively small, then a primary repair can be done by excising the omphalocele membrane, reducing the herniated viscera, and closing the fascia and skin. Membrane overlying the liver that might be injured during excision can be left in place. When primary closure is not likely to be possible, there are many options, but the author's preference is to treat the omphalocele sac with topical silver sulfadiazine and allow it to epithelialize over the ensuing weeks to months [33,34]. Enteral feedings are usually tolerated after the baby recovers from any systemic problems. After the associated problems have been addressed, the family can be taught the relatively easy wound care, and the baby is followed in the outpatient clinic. When the sac is epithelialized or otherwise sturdy enough to withstand external pressure, compression is done with elastic bandages and serially increased until the abdominal contents are reduced. When the abdominal contents are reduced, the membrane is epithelialized, and the baby is well, a ventral hernia repair is done. This can usually be accomplished within 6 to 12 months, but there is little risk in waiting even longer. The fascial defect remains roughly the same size while the baby grows around it. This permits a relatively easy late closure of initially giant omphaloceles. This strategy was initially adopted for only those patients who had giant omphaloceles or serious associated problems but has worked so well in those difficult cases that it is now the author's preferred method for any defect that cannot be closed. It avoids problems of pulmonary compromise, wound breakdown, infection, and delayed enteral feedings that are encountered with a major operation in a vulnerable newborn. It is also especially useful for obtaining fascial closure in the epigastric region of large omphaloceles. Many alternative strategies for omphalocele closure have been described, including skin coverage only, staged Silastic silo reduction and repair, reduction within the omphalocele membrane, amnion inversion, and fascial patches. Each technique may have utility in certain circumstances, but in the author's experience, topical treatment with silver sulfadiazine and delayed repair of the epithelialized ventral hernia has been safe and effective.

Outcomes

The outcome of patients who have gastroschisis depends largely on the condition of the vulnerable bowel, whereas the outcome of patients who have omphalocele depends largely on the associated anomalies and medical conditions. Overall, patients who have gastroschisis have an excellent prognosis. Survival is at least 90% to 95%, with most of the deaths in patients who have catastrophic bowel loss, sepsis, and the long-term complications of short bowel syndrome. Patients who have atresia and relative short bowel syndrome may eventually do well despite a long initial hospitalization and prolonged dependence on hyperalimentation. Even babies who have intact intestinal tracts may require a prolonged hospitalization of weeks to months because of slow tolerance of enteral feeding [9]. A form of necrotizing enterocolitis manifested by pneumatosis intestinalis on abdominal radiograph is a unique form of intestinal injury that occurs in the postoperative period after gastroschisis repair when feedings are being advanced. Feedings are often complicated by gastroesophageal reflux that may be severe [35]. Long-term gastrointestinal function is usually good, although there is a 5% to 10% long-term risk of adhesive obstruction. Occasional patients have inexplicable long-term intolerance of enteral feedings. The outcome of babies who have omphalocele is much harder to generalize, but most mortality and morbidity is related to associated anomalies rather than the abdominal wall defect.

Summary

Although gastroschisis and omphalocele are distinct abdominal wall defects with many important differences, an understanding of the normal development of the abdominal wall and principles of intra-abdominal pressure evaluation and management and abdominal wall reconstruction are important for both conditions. Gastroschisis is likely the result of a discrete abdominal wall ischemic event and most of the morbidity is a result of acquired in utero bowel injury. The correction of gastroschisis may be accomplished by primary, delayed primary, or staged repair; the exact method is largely determined by the baby's general medical condition and capacity of the abdominal cavity relative to the herniated viscera. The long-term prognosis is excellent. Omphalocele is likely the result of a more general defect of body wall development and is associated with a much higher incidence of serious anomalies. The surgical correction of small defects is straightforward; for larger defects, a strategy of topical treatment of the membrane with silver sulfadiazine and late repair after epithelialization and external reduction of the hernia contents has simplified management and optimized outcomes. Rather than being related to the abdominal wall defect, the long-term outcome in gastroschisis is mainly related to the degree of associated intestinal injury, and the long-term outcome in omphalocele is mainly related to the associated anomalies.

References

[1] Vermeij-Keers C, Hartwig NG, van der Werff JF. Embryonic development of the ventral body wall and its congenital malformations. Semin Pediatr Surg 1996;5(2):82–9.
[2] deVries PA. The pathogenesis of gastroschisis and omphalocele. J Pediatr Surg 1980;15(3): 245–51.
[3] Hoyme HE, Higginbottom MC, Jones KL. The vascular pathogenesis of gastroschisis: intrauterine interruption of the omphalomesenteric artery. J Pediatr 1981;98(2):228–31.
[4] Glick PL, Harrison MR, Adzick NS, et al. The missing link in the pathogenesis of gastroschisis. J Pediatr Surg 1985;20(4):406–9.

[5] Cantrell JR, Haller JA, Ravitch MM. A syndrome of congenital defects involving the abdominal wall, sternum, diaphragm, pericardium, and heart. Surg Gynecol Obstet 1958; 107(5):602–14.

[6] Curry JI, McKinney P, Thornton JG, et al. The aetiology of gastroschisis. Br J Obstet Gynaecol 2000;107(11):1339–46.

[7] Tan KH, Kilby MD, Whittle MJ, et al. Congenital anterior abdominal wall defects in England and Wales 1987–93: retrospective analysis of OPCS data. BMJ 1996;313(7062):903–6.

[8] Rankin J, Dillon E, Wright C. Congenital anterior abdominal wall defects in the north of England, 1986–1996: occurrence and outcome. Prenat Diagn 1999;19(7):662–8.

[9] Molik KA, Gingalewski CA, West KW, et al. Gastroschisis: a plea for risk categorization. J Pediatr Surg 2001;36(1):51–5.

[10] Snyder CL, Miller KA, Sharp RJ, et al. Management of intestinal atresia in patients with gastroschisis. J Pediatr Surg 2001;36(10):1542–5.

[11] Hwang PJ, Kousseff BG. Omphalocele and gastroschisis: an 18-year review study. Genet Med 2004;6(4):232–6.

[12] Nicolaides KH, Snijders RJ, Cheng HH, et al. Fetal gastro-intestinal and abdominal wall defects: associated malformations and chromosomal abnormalities. Fetal Diagn Ther 1992; 7(2):102–15.

[13] Nyberg DA, Fitzsimmons J, Mack LA, et al. Chromosomal abnormalities in fetuses with omphalocele. Significance of omphalocele contents. J Ultrasound Med 1989;8(6):299–308.

[14] Palomaki GE, Hill LE, Knight GJ, et al. Second-trimester maternal serum alpha-fetoprotein levels in pregnancies associated with gastroschisis and omphalocele. Obstet Gynecol 1988; 71(6 Pt 1):906–9.

[15] Saller DN Jr, Canick JA, Palomaki GE, et al. Second-trimester maternal serum alpha-fetoprotein, unconjugated estriol, and hCG levels in pregnancies with ventral wall defects. Obstet Gynecol 1994;84(5):852–5.

[16] Walkinshaw SA, Renwick M, Hebisch G, et al. How good is ultrasound in the detection and evaluation of anterior abdominal wall defects? Br J Radiol 1992;65(772):298–301.

[17] Japaraj RP, Hockey R, Chan FY. Gastroschisis: can prenatal sonography predict neonatal outcome? Ultrasound Obstet Gynecol 2003;21(4):329–33.

[18] Luton D, Guibourdenche J, Vuillard E, et al. Prenatal management of gastroschisis: the place of the amnioexchange procedure. Clin Perinatol 2003;30(3):551–72 [viii].

[19] Salomon LJ, Mahieu-Caputo D, Jouvet P, et al. Fetal home monitoring for the prenatal management of gastroschisis. Acta Obstet Gynecol Scand 2004;83(11):1061–4.

[20] Fitzsimmons J, Nyberg DA, Cyr DR, et al. Perinatal management of gastroschisis. Obstet Gynecol 1988;71(6 Pt 1):910–3.

[21] Moir CR, Ramsey PS, Ogburn PL, et al. A prospective trial of elective preterm delivery for fetal gastroschisis. Am J Perinatol 2004;21(5):289–94.

[22] Puligandla PS, Janvier A, Flageole H, et al. The significance of intrauterine growth restriction is different from prematurity for the outcome of infants with gastroschisis. J Pediatr Surg 2004;39(8):1200–4.

[23] Hsieh TT, Lai YM, Liou JD, et al. Management of the fetus with an abdominal wall defect: experience of 31 cases. Taiwan Yi Xue Hui Za Zhi 1989;88(5):469–73.

[24] How HY, Harris BJ, Pietrantoni M, et al. Is vaginal delivery preferable to elective cesarean delivery in fetuses with a known ventral wall defect? Am J Obstet Gynecol 2000;182(6): 1527–34.

[25] Hershenson MB, Brouillette RT, Klemka L, et al. Respiratory insufficiency in newborns with abdominal wall defects. J Pediatr Surg 1985;20(4):348–53.

[26] Langer JC. Gastroschisis and omphalocele. Semin Pediatr Surg 1996;5(2):124–8.

[27] Minkes RK, Langer JC, Mazziotti MV, et al. Routine insertion of a silastic spring-loaded silo for infants with gastroschisis. J Pediatr Surg 2000;35(6):843–6.

[28] Coughlin JP, Drucker DE, Jewell MR, et al. Delivery room repair of gastroschisis. Surgery 1993;114(4):822–6 [discussion: 6–7].

[29] Bianchi A, Dickson AP, Alizai NK. Elective delayed midgut reduction—no anesthesia for gastroschisis: selection and conversion criteria. J Pediatr Surg 2002;37(9):1334–6.

[30] Yaster M, Scherer TL, Stone MM, et al. Prediction of successful primary closure of congenital abdominal wall defects using intraoperative measurements. J Pediatr Surg 1989;24(12):1217–20.

[31] Itoh Y, Arai K. Umbilical reconstruction using a cone-shaped flap. Ann Plast Surg 1992;28(4):335–8.

[32] Sawin R, Glick P, Schaller R, et al. Gastroschisis wringer clamp: a safe, simplified method for delayed primary closure. J Pediatr Surg 1992;27(10):1346–8.

[33] Hatch EI Jr, Baxter R. Surgical options in the management of large omphaloceles. Am J Surg 1987;153(5):449–52.

[34] Nuchtern JG, Baxter R, Hatch EI Jr. Nonoperative initial management versus silon chimney for treatment of giant omphalocele. J Pediatr Surg 1995;30(6):771–6.

[35] Beaudoin S, Kieffer G, Sapin E, et al. Gastroesophageal reflux in neonates with congenital abdominal wall defect. Eur J Pediatr Surg 1995;5(6):323–6.

ELSEVIER
SAUNDERS

SURGICAL
CLINICS OF
NORTH AMERICA

Surg Clin N Am 86 (2006) 261–284

Foregut Abnormalities

Bindi Naik-Mathuria, MD,
Oluyinka O. Olutoye, MBChB, PhD*

*Division of Pediatric Surgery, Michael E. DeBakey Department of Surgery,
Baylor College of Medicine, Texas Children's Hospital, 6621 Fannin CC 650.00,
Houston, TX 77030-2399, USA*

Pyloric stenosis

Hypertrophic pyloric stenosis (HPS) is among the most common surgical disorders in infancy and presents in approximately 3:1000 live births in the United States. There is a 4:1 male dominance, and white infants are more commonly affected. Birth order seems to play a role, because firstborn boys are more likely to be affected by the disorder than their siblings.

The precise cause of the pyloric circular muscle hypertrophy remains poorly understood. Some proposed causes include postnatal work hypertrophy, congenital delay of the pyloric sphincter opening, and milk curds obstructing the small channel, leading to redundancy in the pyloric mucosa and compensatory hypertrophy. Other researchers hypothesize that an increased production of gastrin or vasoactive intestinal peptide, either by the infant or mother, stimulates muscle hypertrophy or increases the intensity of pyloric contraction. An association with blood groups O and B, maternal stress, and systemic erythromycin (but not erythromycin ophthalmic ointment) given in the first 2 weeks of life have been suggested [1]. Environmental factors [2] and abnormalities in nitric oxide synthetase [3], interstitial cells of Cajal (gut pacemaker cells), neural cell adhesion molecule, or gastrointestinal hormones are believed to play a role. Despite these theories, none can explain fully the pathogenesis of pyloric stenosis, which implies that the cause may be multifactorial.

Diagnosis

The classic clinical presentation is projectile, nonbilious emesis in a 3- to 6-week-old infant, although it can present as early as 1 week or as late as

* Corresponding author.
E-mail address: oolutoye@bcm.tmc.edu (O.O. Olutoye).

doi:10.1016/j.suc.2005.12.011
surgical.theclinics.com

4 months of age. Shortly after emesis, an infant usually craves additional feedings. Significant dehydration, metabolic alkalosis (hypochloremic, hypokalemic), malnutrition, and gastritis can occur with prolonged symptoms. Jaundice may occur in approximately 2% of infants but resolves spontaneously within a week of pyloromyotomy. The typical physical findings include visible peristaltic waves in the epigastrium and a palpable mass or "olive," which can be discerned in 70% to 90% of cases by an experienced examiner. Unfortunately, the increased use of ultrasound for diagnosis has resulted in a gradual erosion of this art in younger practitioners. The ultrasound criteria for pyloric stenosis is a pyloric channel length >17 mm, pyloric muscle diameter >14 mm, and pyloric muscle wall thickness >3 to 4 mm (Fig. 1). A helpful pneumonic to remember these criteria is π, or 3.14 (ie, 3 mm thick, 14 mm wide). Ultrasound has been shown to be almost 100% sensitive for the diagnosis of pyloric stenosis. The most common abnormality that mimics HPS is pylorospasm. The sonographic double-track sign, which was once thought to be specific for HPS, also has been shown in cases of pylorospasm and no longer should be considered pathognomonic for HPS [4]. If ultrasound results are inconclusive, an upper gastrointestinal series can be performed. The series reveals the string sign or shoulders of the hypertrophied pyloric muscles bulging into the gastric lumen. Pylorospasm also can mimic HPS in this imaging modality.

Most referred patients have already undergone imaging for pyloric stenosis. However, finding a palpable "olive" on physical examination is a specific test for the disorder that can obviate the need for imaging, thus saving health care costs. Some institutions have developed guidelines that mandate surgical consultation before imaging is ordered when pyloric stenosis is being entertained. In a recent study, the amount of imaging performed did not differ significantly before and after the guideline was

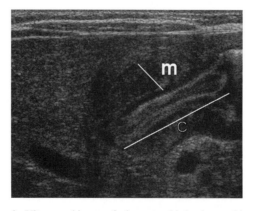

Fig. 1. Pyloric stenosis. Ultrasound image of a hypertrophied pylorus with a long pyloric channel (c) and thickened circular muscles (m). (Courtesy of Rajesh Krishnamurthy, MD, Department of Radiology, Texas Children's Hospital, Houston, Texas.)

set, but it proposed a cost-effective clinical pathway that can be adopted at individual centers [5].

Treatment

Initial management focuses on fluid and electrolyte replacement. Failure to correct preoperative alkalosis may result in postanesthetic apnea and respiratory arrest. The Fredet-Ramstedt extramucosal pyloromyotomy has been the classic surgical approach since early in the twentieth century. Since the original operation several alternative methods have been proposed. One is the pyloric traumamyoplasty, in which the pylorus is grasped with a Babcock clamp, which disrupts the hypertrophied circular muscles in two places. A randomized, prospective, controlled trial of traumamyoplasty and pyloromyotomy showed few complications, similar time to postoperative feeding, and similar rates of postoperative emesis in both groups. The traumamyoplasty group had significantly shorter operating room time than the traditional group, however [6]. The traditional small transverse upper abdominal incision for pyloromyotomy provides ease of access and avoids a moist umbilicus. This initially small scar tends to elongate with time, however. The more cosmetically appealing supraumbilical, semicircular incision introduced by Tan and Bianchi in 1986 [7] has gained wide acceptance. This approach is believed to be associated with a higher wound infection rate and incomplete pyloromyotomy because of the difficulty occasionally encountered delivering a large pylorus through the incision. Prophylactic antibiotics have been shown to decrease the wound infection rate [8]. A recent comparison of the right upper quadrant and umbilical incisions showed equal complication rates and much improved cosmesis in the latter group, however [9]. The umbilical incision can be modified to extend the skin or fascial incision in several ways, even by moving it to the right side of the umbilicus for better exposure for an exceptionally large pylorus [10]. Alternatively, using the supraumbilical approach, the pyloromyotomy can be performed intracorporeally. Traction sutures are placed on the anterior surface of the pylorus to bring it into view just beneath the incision. The pyloromyotomy is then performed under direct vision but without bringing the pylorus out of the abdomen. This method, when compared with the extracorporeal method, allowed quicker recovery of bowel function and shorter hospital stay while maintaining the cosmetic advantage of the supraumbilical incision [11]. One criticism of the supraumbilical incision is that the scar tends to rise on the abdominal wall as a child grows.

The ultimate scarless approach has been the laparoscopic approach. A small port through the existing umbilical defect and two small stab wounds leave virtually no scar. Several studies that compared laparoscopic and open pyloromyotomy were published, but most of these studies are single institution, retrospective reviews. A meta-analysis of several such studies showed that open pyloromyotomy has a higher efficacy and lower complication rate than laparoscopic pyloromyotomy, but the differences were not statistically significant [12]. Inadequate pyloromyotomy requiring reoperation, mucosal perforation and conversion to open are the complications frequently cited. There is a learning curve with the laparoscopic approach, with the incidence of complications decreasing with experience.

Surgery is the gold standard for treatment of HPS, and other nonoperative strategies are currently not recommended. Intravenous or oral atropine sulfate administration is reported to resolve the symptoms but requires prolonged hospitalization and intravenous nutrition [13,14]. Endoscopic treatment with balloon dilatation has been largely unsuccessful [15]. Endoscopic pyloromyotomy using an electroscopic needle knife or a sphincterotome also was described in ten patients with good results [16].

Postoperative care

Controversy remains regarding the ideal time to start feedings. Postoperative emesis is not uncommon after pyloromyotomy, presumably from pyloric edema and ileus. Most surgeons wait at least 2 to 6 hours after surgery to introduce either pedialyte and advance the amount given, or begin ad lib feedings with a formula of choice. No conclusive data show the benefit of any particular operative technique on postoperative feeding, although difficult supraumbilical cases tend to have a prolonged ileus. Most infants are discharged within 24 to 36 hours of surgery. Emesis or "wet burps" usually subside within the first week.

Outcomes

Surgery for HPS is usually successful and has minimal complications, with wound infections, small mucosal perforations, and inadequate pyloromyotomies being the main ones reported. Unidentified mucosal perforations can result in significant morbidity and mortality. If emesis persists beyond 2 weeks, concern should be raised for gastroesophageal reflux (GER) or inadequate pyloromyotomy. Radiographic studies are usually not useful because the appearance of HPS may persist postoperatively.

Duodenal obstruction

Duodenal atresia and stenosis are the most common causes of intestinal obstruction in newborns, with an estimated incidence of 1:10,000 live births. Causative theories of duodenal atresia include vascular disruption, abnormalities in neural cell migration, and failure of recanalization of the duodenal lumen from its solid cord stage. The latter theory is currently the most popular. Failure of recanalization, which occurs at 8 to 10 weeks' gestation, leads to either partial obstruction by an imperforate membrane or mucosal web or complete atresia. Fibroblast growth factor-10 is active in the duodenum at a late stage of development, and serves as a regulator in normal duodenal development. Fibroblast growth factor-10($-/-$) mutant mice demonstrate duodenal atresia with a variable phenotype similar to clinical findings in humans. The phenotype occurred in an autosomal-recessive pattern with incomplete penetrance (38%) [17], which suggested a genetic cause of duodenal obstruction, although few reports of a familial association exist (fewer than ten reports in the English language literature) [18].

Duodenal atresia and stenosis are frequently associated with other congenital abnormalities such as annular pancreas (most common), preduodenal portal vein, malrotation, biliary atresia, choledochal cyst, and anomalous bile duct communication between the proximal and distal ends of the duodenum [19]. Duodenal atresia is seen frequently in cases of Feingold syndrome, an autosomal-dominant inheritance of microcephaly and limb malformations [20]. Other rare associations include gastric antral web and esophageal atresia (EA) with unilateral lung agenesis [21,22]. The incidence of combined esophageal and duodenal atresia varies between 3% and 6% and is associated with significant morbidity and mortality. Duodenal atresia has a well-known association with Down syndrome (11%–33%) and cardiac anomalies (22%) [23]. Although Down syndrome does not directly increase the morbidity and mortality of duodenal obstruction, it carries a higher incidence of cardiac abnormalities, which in turn cause increased delayed mortality [23]. Vertebral, cardiac, renal, and gastrointestinal anomalies and deafness are seen in a minority of these patients, which is similar to the pattern of malformations seen in the VATER/VACTERL syndrome [20].

Duodenal atresias are classified into three types. Type I defect is the most common and represents a mucosal diaphragmatic membrane with an intact muscle wall. Occasionally, a membrane in the shape of a windsock may be noted, but the site of origin may be a few centimeters proximal to the perceived obstruction. The duodenal web almost always involves the opening of the bile duct at the ampulla of Vater. Type II defect has a short fibrous cord that connects the two ends of atretic duodenum. A type III defect, the rarest form, is one that involves a complete separation of the two ends of atretic duodenum with a mesenteric defect. Most of the unusual biliary duct anomalies coexist with this type of defect.

Diagnosis

Duodenal obstruction is increasingly diagnosed prenatally. Polyhydramnios and a dilated stomach and duodenum (sonographic double-bubble sign) may be seen by prenatal ultrasound by the seventh month of gestation or earlier. A detailed evaluation for other associated anomalies should be undertaken. Amniocentesis for chromosomal analysis is helpful for counseling. Bile-stained amniotic fluid further supports the diagnosis. If not diagnosed prenatally, the clinical presentation of duodenal obstruction is the onset of bilious emesis within a few hours of birth and intolerance of

attempted feedings. The abdomen is scaphoid because of the proximal obstruction. Plain radiographs demonstrate the classic double-bubble sign
(Fig. 2). In contrast to atresia, duodenal stenosis typically presents later in
life. Symptoms typically do not occur until a child eats more solid foods.
Failure to thrive may be the only presentation. It is not unusual to identify
a symptomatic duodenal stenosis in a child with trisomy 21 late in the teenage years. The diagnosis of duodenal stenosis is usually made by contrast
gastrointestinal studies.

Treatment

Once duodenal obstruction is diagnosed, nasogastric decompression and
fluid and electrolyte resuscitation should be started while the baby is more
thoroughly evaluated for associated anomalies. Kimble and colleagues
[24] proposed a comprehensive evaluation protocol that includes radiographs of the chest (two views) and abdomen to visualize the entire spine,
cardiac and renal ultrasonography, a micturating cystourethrogram in
babies who have an abnormal renal ultrasound or associated anorectal
anomaly, a sweat test (in babies who have jejunoileal atresia, specifically),
and a rectal biopsy in babies who have duodenal atresia and Down syndrome to rule out Hirschprung's disease. Most surgeons do not adhere to
such a strict evaluation, however. An echocardiogram may be the only study
needed. Surgical treatment for types II and III duodenal atresia is a duodenoduodenostomy, which can be performed in a side-to-side or proximal
transverse-to-distal longitudinal (diamond-shaped) anastamosis. If the
proximal duodenum is excessively floppy and distended, an antimesenteric

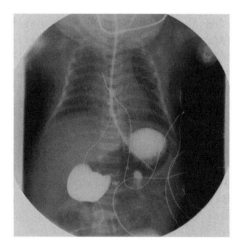

Fig. 2. Duodenal stenosis. Contrast study shows a dilated stomach and duodenal bulb, with
a trickle of contrast into the distal duodenum. (Courtesy of Rajesh Krishnamurthy, MD,
Department of Radiology, Texas Children's Hospital, Houston, Texas.)

tapering duodenoplasty can be performed. Type I defects can be corrected with a duodenoduodenostomy or merely by resecting the web. It is important to identify a windsock deformity when a type I defect is encountered, because the web may be proximal to the transitional segment of dilation. A longitudinal duodenotomy can be made to expose the web, and the web can be excised as long as the ampulla is preserved (which is found by applying pressure on the gallbladder to see where the bile exits). The duodenotomy is closed transversely. It is imperative to examine the distal bowel for other associated atresia or luminal obstructions. With advances in minimally invasive surgery, laparoscopic duodenoduodenostomies are being performed in neonates, but evaluation of distal internal webs is more difficult to accomplish laparoscopically [25].

Postoperative care

Nasogastric tube decompression is continued until bowel function returns. Some surgeons use a transanastomotic feeding tube to start feeding sooner, and others use short-term intravenous nutrition. There are conflicting reports on the benefits of transanastomotic feeding tube in enhancing the progression to full enteric (preanastomotic) feedings [26,27].

Outcomes

A comparison of surgical techniques reported no difference in postoperative feeding between duodenoduodenostomy and web excision with duodenoplasty. The duration of total parenteral nutrition, tolerance of early feeding, and onset of full feeding and hospital stay also did not vary between side-to-side and diamond-shaped anastomosis [27]. Early complications are rare (except for missed anomalies), but late complications are reported to occur in 12% to 15% of patients, with an associated 6% late mortality rate [28]. Complications include megaduodenum with abnormal motility, blind loop syndrome, duodenogastric reflux and esophagitis, pancreatitis, cholecystitis, and cholelithiasis. Megaduodenum can be avoided or corrected with a tapering duodenoplasty. A subtotal duodenectomy (which leaves only the basal portion that contains the ampulla of Vater) and a proximal jejunum onlay serosal patch have been described for the management of megaduodenum [29]. Blind loop syndrome occurs only in cases in which a duodenojejunostomy was performed, which is rarely performed anymore. A long-term follow-up study over 30 years reported that 20 of 169 patients required additional abdominal operations (eg, fundoplication, ulcer surgery, and adhesiolysis), 16 of 169 underwent revision of their original repair (redos or conversions), and ten late deaths were caused by complex cardiac malformations (5), central nervous system bleeding (1), pneumonia (1), leak (1), and multisystem organ failure (2) [28]. Overall, however, the success of surgery for duodenal obstruction is acceptable and continues to improve with advancements in neonatal intensive care, anesthesia, nutritional support, and an early evaluation to identify associated anomalies.

Duplication cysts

Most duplication cysts are really enteric cysts rather than true duplications of certain structures. They are found throughout the gastrointestinal tract, from mouth to anus. Duplication cysts vary widely in size and can be spherical or tubular in shape. They are composed of at least one layer of smooth muscle and a mucous membrane lining derived from some part of the gastrointestinal tract, not necessarily corresponding to the mucosa at the level of attachment. They are usually directly connected to the gastrointestinal tract and often share a common muscular wall. In the abdomen, they are usually found on the mesenteric border. Some thoracic duplication cysts may lie in a position distant to the esophagus, whereas others are connected to it. Completely isolated duplication cysts in the abdomen are rare, and only three to four cases have been reported thus far [30]. The thick wall of a duplication cyst usually makes it easy to differentiate from a thin-walled mesenteric cyst. Approximately 25% of duplication cysts contain ectopic mucosa, which is usually gastric mucosa. This condition can cause peptic ulceration and bleeding when the cysts are connected to the intestinal lumen. Duplications vary greatly in size and shape. Most are 2 to 4 cm in diameter and round, but can reach huge sizes that may fill the entire thorax. When tubular duplications involve the colon or rectum, associated anomalies, such as partial duplication of the external and internal genitalia, rectourethral or rectovaginal fistulas, and duplications of the urinary tract may be present. Approximately 75% of duplication cysts are located in the abdomen. Twenty percent occur within the thorax, 5% are thoracoabdominal, and the rest occur at unusual sites, such as the floor of the mouth.

Kong and colleagues [31] reported a case of a large floor-of-the-mouth cystic lesion that was prenatally diagnosed by ultrasonography and MRI. It displaced the tongue to the roof of the mouth and filled the entire oral cavity. The baby was delivered via an ex utero intrapartum treatment procedure to avoid airway obstruction at birth. Multiple theories exist regarding the origin of duplication cysts, but none can explain all the variations. Early theories hypothesized that duplications were caused by abnormal fetal luminal canalization or by the formation of abnormal diverticula and sequestration of portions of endoderm during development. Many authors have noted an association between vertebral anomalies, such as bifid or fused spines, and thoracoabdominal duplications. Foregut anomalies are also often associated with osseous abnormalities of the axial skeleton. These associations led to the widely accepted "split notochord theory," which proposed that the initial abnormality is duplication of the notochord, followed by herniation of the endoderm (the primitive gut) to adhere to the dorsal ectoderm between the duplicated notochords. This theory recently was confirmed by experimental reproduction of the anomaly in amphibian embryos [32]. Because duplications take so many different forms, it is possible that a multifactorial cause with a combination of these theories is responsible for the aberrations.

Diagnosis

Few reports of prenatal diagnosis exist [31,33]. The prenatal diagnosis allows prompt neonatal evaluation and surgical treatment [33]. One third of duplication cysts present in the newborn period and another third in the first few years of life. Clinical symptoms vary according to the size and location of the cysts. Abdominal cysts can cause intestinal obstruction, volvulus, intussusception, mesenteric ischemia, or pain. Cysts with gastric mucosa can cause severe bleeding. Colonic duplications are rare but can present with a picture similar to appendicitis. Thoracic cysts may cause serious respiratory problems from the trachea or lung compression or dysphagia if located in the wall of the esophagus. CT and MRI have been used with increasing frequency because they provide excellent anatomic details that aid in correct diagnosis and preoperative planning [34]. Despite advantages in imaging, however, CT scans still misclassify these lesions as soft tissue masses in up to 43% of patients and cannot determine the benign or malignant nature of the masses [35]. Endoscopic ultrasound-guided fine-needle aspiration that demonstrates detached ciliary tufts in cyst fluid and the absence of malignant cells confirms the benign nature of the cysts, which allows conservative and expectant management, if indicated [35].

Treatment

Treatment of duplication cysts is usually surgical excision. Except for rare cases in which urgent intervention is required, preoperative planning with precise diagnostic imaging is important [36]. Most lesions can be excised with minimal morbidity. Large gastric cysts sometimes require only partial cyst excision with mucosal stripping from the common wall or internal drainage of the cyst into the stomach. Duodenal cysts, when in a dangerous location for excision, can be managed by duodenotomy, partial excision and mucosal stripping, or drainage (internal or Roux-en-Y). Most small and large intestine cysts can be excised. In the case of a long tubular double colon cyst, internal drainage at the distal end may be sufficient. Thoracic duplication cysts also can be excised, but care must be taken not to injure the esophagus. Minimal access surgical techniques can be applied to the simpler duplication cysts, but thoracoabdominal and neurenteric cysts require careful preoperative delineation and more complex surgery.

Outcomes

When cysts are undiscovered or managed conservatively, they can cause problems. Peptic ulceration leading to serious gastrointestinal bleeding, hemoptysis from erosion into the bronchus, and mediastinitis from infection of a mediastinal cyst have been described [37]. Malignant transformation is also a potential hazard. A case of adenocarcinoma developing within a gastric duplication cyst that then invaded the stomach wall has been reported [38]. Malignant transformation also can occur after incomplete excision of a cyst, and total excision is recommended [37]. When complete resection is impossible, mucosal stripping should be done.

Esophageal atresia and tracheoesophageal fistula

Variants of esophageal atresia (EA) and tracheoesophageal fistula (TEF) are the most life-threatening congenital anomalies of the esophagus. The incidence of EA is approximately 1 in 4000 live births and is slightly more common in boys. The most common type accounts for 85% to 90% of cases and is composed of a proximal EA with distal TEF. Isolated (pure) EA is the next most common type and is seen in 5% to 7%. TEF without EA (the H-fistula) is seen in only 2% to 6% of cases. Other variations are much rarer. Congenital anomalies exist in approximately half the cases of EA, with cardiac anomalies being the most common, followed by musculo-skeletal, anal, and genitourinary anomalies. The presence of a cardiac malformation is a major determinant of mortality and often signals other associated anomalies. Tracheoesophageal anomalies are often part of the VACTERL complex (vertebral, anorectal, tracheoesophageal, cardiac, renal anomalies, and radial limb). Approximately 17.5% of babies who have EA have three components of this syndrome, and 1.5% have all of the components. EA is also associated with aneuploidies, specifically trisomies 13, 18, and 21. Other associated syndromes include CHARGE (coloboma, heart defect, choanal atresia, growth and mental retardation, genital hypoplasia, and ear anomalies), Potter's syndrome, and "schisis" syndrome (cleft lip and palate, omphalocele, and hypogenitalism).

EA and TEFs are believed to develop from an improper separation of the respiratory and digestive divisions of the primitive foregut. At approximately the twenty-second day of gestation, a ventral diverticulum of the foregut appears that elongates and separates into the trachea and esophagus by cephalad migration of the lateral foregut grooves. It is thought that EA is caused by abnormal growth of these grooves, whereas TEF is a result of the failure of the grooves to fuse in the midline [39]. This traditional theory has been challenged over the years. Different researchers have found lacking evidence for the fusion of the lateral ridges and have proposed alternate theories, such as disturbances in epithelial proliferation and apoptosis that are responsible for the separation of the esophagus and trachea [39]. The adriamycin rat model has been useful in studying EA/TEF in the early embryonic period [39,40]. Adriamycin has been shown to influence the sonic hedgehog protein (Shh) signaling pathway, which disrupts normal foregut development [40]. Other genes currently thought to play a role in the separation of the primitive foregut are retinoic acid receptors, which are associated with vitamin A, Gli family (zinc-finger transcription factors), forkhead family transcription factors, thyroid transcription factor-1, homeobox gene family, and T-box gene family [39].

Diagnosis

Prenatally, most cases of pure EA are associated with polyhydramnios, which may contribute to the high incidence of prematurity. A blind-ending proximal esophageal pouch and small or absent gastric bubble may be seen on ultrasound. In the presence of a distal TEF, the presence of polyhydramnios is variable. Pulmonary hypoplasia can develop if too much amniotic fluid leaks into the gastrointestinal tract through a distal fistula. The symptoms of EA/TEF present shortly after birth, when the infant is unable to swallow, drools saliva, spits up, and coughs or chokes. With EA, it is impossible to pass a nasogastric tube into the stomach. With TEF, the infant may become cyanotic and develop aspiration pneumonia. H-type fistula can be difficult to diagnose because the infant can swallow and a nasogastric tube is easily passed. These infants present with episodes of recurrent aspiration. Plain radiographs can make the diagnosis of EA by noting the end of the nasogastric tube in the chest. If a gas-filled stomach and intestinal loops are present, then a distal TEF is present. In a few cases, a distal fistula may exist but is occluded by mucus or other material.

An air-filled proximal esophageal pouch is sufficient to make the diagnosis of EA. A contrast study can be hazardous because of the risk of aspiration of contrast material. The preferred and most accurate approach for identifying a fistula is bronchoscopy. Rigid bronchoscopy is preferred because it provides a secure access to the airway and permits controlled ventilation as needed. The rigid bronchoscope can be positioned to occlude the fistula and permit adequate ventilation should respiratory deterioration occur during bronchoscopy. The diagnosis of an H-type fistula can be made with a prone "pull back" contrast study or by flexible or rigid bronchoscopy. The fistula is usually located in the upper thoracic or lower cervical region, and the tracheal orifice is usually more cephalad than the esophageal orifice. A Fogarty catheter can be used to probe irregularities to aid in discovery of the fistula and can be left in place in the esophagus so that it can be retrieved by esophagoscopy during the operation. Traction on the ends of the catheter can elevate the fistula into a cervical position, thus simplifying the repair. Alternatively, a flexible pediatric 2.2-mm bronchoscope through the endotracheal tube during surgery can be used to illuminate and localize the fistula tract [41].

Treatment

Preoperative treatment involves preventing pneumonitis and aspiration. The head of the bed should be elevated 30° to 45°, and a sump suction catheter should be placed in the proximal pouch. Other anomalies (especially in the setting of VACTERL syndrome) should be investigated. An echocardiogram is obtained to assess for cardiac anomalies and to determine the side of the aortic arch. Some surgeons opt to approach a TEF repair from the left chest if a right aortic arch is present. The distance between the proximal and distal ends of the esophagus should be determined carefully, because a long gap may preclude a simple repair. Accurate prediction of operative findings by routine preoperative chest CT scans has been shown to be a noninvasive method of determining the esophageal gap [42]. Further research must be done to establish the use and cost effectiveness of this modality. Historically, the Waterson classification, which is obsolete, stratified babies into three operative risk categories based on birth weight and associated anomalies. Although advances in neonatal surgical care have resulted in much improved outcomes, prematurity and respiratory distress syndrome still contribute significantly to morbidity and mortality in EA [43].

Esophageal atresia with distal tracheoesophageal fistula

The preference of the senior author is to perform a rigid bronchoscopy on all neonates who have EA to identify the location, size, and number of any associated fistulae and permit an initial evaluation of the degree of tracheomalacia. The preferred position of the endotracheal tube relative to the fistula and carina is determined. In the case of a pure (isolated) EA with a long (>3 vertebral bodies) gap, a gastrostomy is performed and the infant allowed to grow. For the commonest form, EA and distal TEF, a thoracotomy is performed.

A right-sided posterolateral extrapleural thoracotomy provides good exposure in most cases. Most surgeons prefer the extrapleural approach because it theoretically confines an anastomotic leak to an extrapleural location. A leak does not result in an empyema but rather in an esophagocutaneous fistula that generally closes spontaneously. In most cases of EA with distal TEF, the esophageal ends are close enough to permit a primary anastomosis. The fistula is divided flush with the trachea, which is closed with fine, permanent monofilament suture. The esophageal ends are anastomosed end to end, usually in a single layer. When there is a great deal of tension, the Haight two-layer, telescoping anastomosis can be performed. An alternative is the end-to-side anastomosis with ligation of the TEF. Recent modifications of this technique have resulted in a reduction of the high fistula recurrence that typically was associated with this approach [44]. A gastrostomy tube is not required for straightforward cases. Some surgeons place a transanastomotic soft feeding tube for early enteral nutrition. A drain/thoracostomy tube is left adjacent to the anastomosis.

In cases in which there is a long gap between the two esophageal ends, primary anastomosis may not be initially possible. A long gap is usually defined as a length that exceeds 2 cm or two vertebral body spaces or when the upper pouch level is above the thoracic inlet [45]. A gap of 3.5 cm or more is sometimes referred to as an "ultra-long" gap [46]. Although several strategies have been proposed to manage this condition, a delayed primary anastomosis is the favored approach. A delay of 2 to 3 months allows for esophageal growth. The upper pouch is suctioned and feeding occurs through a gastrostomy, which usually requires a long hospital stay. With adequate home nursing care, infants may be managed similarly at home and receive the benefits of parent-infant bonding and creation of a more compatible family environment [45]. Intermittent bougienage of the pouch is thought to promote growth, but no evidence exists for this. If the long gap is discovered at thoracotomy, both ends of the esophagus may be placed on tension with steel bars, stringed beads, magnets, or a high-tension anastomosis [47]. High-tension anastomoses result in fistulization of the two ends that can be serially dilated. Another method of esophageal lengthening involves continuous and progressive stretching of both esophageal ends using traction sutures. On average, primary esophagoesophagostomy can be done in 6 to 10 days [48]. The complications associated include fiber damage from overstretching the esophageal muscle, perforation or mediastinitis from suture detachment, and dysmotility of the repaired esophagus. It can be a useful adjunctive tool for the management of long gap atresia, however [49]. Proximal esophageal myotomy also has been used for esophageal lengthening but is associated with long-term esophageal dysfunction [47]. The Kimura procedure, first described in the 1980s, is currently performed in multiple centers [47,50]. This procedure is a multistaged, extrathoracic elongation of the proximal esophagus by translocation of the cervical esophagostomy along the anterior chest wall over weeks to months, followed by a definitive repair once an appropriate length is attained. The major benefit of this approach is the ability to provide oral sham feeds and prevent oral food aversion, a significant problem in this patient population. This procedure also can be used to bridge gaps as wide as seven vertebral bodies with the patient's native esophagus [47].

If esophageal reconstruction is not possible, esophageal replacement with a colon interposition graft, gastric tube [51], gastric pull-up [52], or small intestine interposition grafts [53] is an option. Because of small vessel size in infants, free revascularized grafts have not been used much. Esophageal replacement often exhibits early and late problems because of the loss of the transposed segment and the presence of the gastroesophageal junction in the chest or neck, which can cause metaplasia, Barrett's esophagus, and carcinoma [46]. Some authors believe that esophageal replacement should be used only after failure of a previous attempt of esophageal reconstruction (using the native esophagus) [46]. Spitz and colleagues [52] reported their large experience with gastric transposition at Great Ormond Street, noting a 12% leak rate, 30% swallowing dysfunction, and 8% incidence of delayed gastric emptying. Ninety percent of their patients had a good long-term outcome, with normal eating patterns and minimal symptoms. Patients who have an isoperistaltic gastric tube can develop Barrett's esophagus above the anastomosis and require lifelong endoscopic follow-up [52]. Thoracoscopic repair of EA/TEF is being performed via a transpleural [54] or extrapleural [55] approach in a few centers. The thoracoscopic approach also can be useful for ligation of a low H-type fistula not accessible through the neck [56]. Robotically assisted esophageal reconstruction in the neonate is shown to be feasible in pigs [57]; however, the current robotic models are too bulky and expensive to warrant routine use in neonates [54].

Postoperative care

Although some infants may be extubated in the operating room at the conclusion of the operation, recent trends favor a delayed extubation in the neonatal intensive care unit to avoid any emergent reintubation that may damage the tracheal repair. Some infants are maintained on neuromuscular blockade when there is significant concern for tension at the anastomosis, a strategy that is of unproven benefit. The head of the bed should be kept elevated. A contrast study is obtained approximately 4 to 5 days after surgery, after which time oral feeds can be instituted and the drain removed.

Outcomes

Anastomotic leak, strictures, and recurrent TEF are the principal complications. Leaks occur in approximately 5% to 10% of cases and are more common after a single-layer versus double-layer anastomosis. Stricture rate is higher with the double-layer anastomosis, however. Most leaks are minor and resolve spontaneously within 1 to 3 weeks with adequate drainage and intravenous nutrition. Complete disruption generally requires prompt repair. Historically, esophageal substitution procedure was performed at a later date, but more surgeons are attempting initial repair to save the native esophagus. Options for treatment include primary repair, placement of a pleural patch with or without an intercostal muscle flap buttress, and operative débridement with drainage alone. The outcome is generally good after a long healing period [58].

Strictures are common and result from ischemia at the anastomosis, leaks, and GER. Most patients respond to periodic dilations every 3 to 6 weeks over a 3- to 6-month period. When the response to dilations is poor, resection and reanastomosis or a stricturoplasty may be required. Almost all patients who have EA/TEF have some degree of GER and should be on antireflux medications. Untreated GER may worsen anastomotic strictures. The distal esophagus may be poorly innervated, and the typical symptoms of GE reflux may not be readily manifested. An analysis of 74 long-term survivors of EA repair who underwent routine endoscopies showed that approximately 40% of patients eventually had significant esophageal mucosal pathology or required a fundoplication before 3 years of age. Based on this finding, routine endoscopic follow-up of EA repair patients (regardless of symptoms) is recommended at least up to the age of 3 years in the setting of normal biopsies. In patients who have mild esophagitis, this follow-up should be continued to at least 6 years of age [59]. Koivusalo and colleagues [60] performed 18-hour esophageal pH monitoring 9 months after initial esophageal repair. Because 90% of patients with an abnormal test result developed significant GER, they proposed that postoperative pH monitoring may be a way to predict the occurrence of GER. Approximately one third of patients fail medical management and require a fundoplication. Because of the dyskinetic and shortened esophagus, the failure rate of the antireflux procedure is up to 30% in some studies [61].

Recurrent TEFs may present insidiously with a persistent cough or recurrent pneumonitis. They almost never close spontaneously and generally require reoperation. The lack of tissue to separate the trachea and esophageal suture makes the repair difficult and recurrence common. Treatment depends on closure of the fistula opening and placement of an intervening vascularized flap (intercostal muscle, pericardial patch).

Tracheomalacia occurs in up to 25% of patients who have EA and TEF. Respiratory symptoms, such as a "seal-bark" cough, noisy breathing, and apneic episodes related to eating, should prompt investigation for tracheomalacia by bronchoscopy [62]. The typical finding is fish-mouthing or tracheal collapse during spontaneous inspiration. Although in rare cases infants can develop chronic respiratory difficulty and arrest, most symptoms improve over time. Aortopexy should be considered if the trachea collapses to more than 80% of its maximal diameter during inspiration or if conservative therapy fails. If it fails, tracheal splinting or a tracheostomy may be required. When investigating tracheomalacia, it is important to define the contribution of gastroesophageal reflux disease (GERD) and exclude a vascular ring anomaly or a recurrent TEF. These conditions may present with similar symptoms [63].

With advances in neonatal surgical care, associated cardiac anomalies have become the most important risk factor for mortality. Mortality has decreased from 33% in the 1970s to 14% in the 1990s, and the incidence of stricture decreased significantly from 50% to 23% [64]. A health-related quality-of-life outcome study reported that most adult survivors of EA or TEF repair have a normal quality of life, with only 15% reporting impairment [65]. Finally, although only a few cases of esophageal carcinoma have developed in adults who have had EA/TEF, there are enough of these cases that one should remain vigilant of this potential [66].

Gastroesophageal reflux disease

The earliest description of GERD in children was in the 1940s, when it was known as chalasia, a benign condition that was managed with postural therapy and weaning slowly to solid foods. Although most symptoms disappear by 2 years of age, prolonged reflux can cause serious complications, such as recurrent regurgitation, growth retardation, intractable pain, esophageal stricture, Barrett's esophagus, and life-threatening respiratory symptoms. In infants, symptoms are reported to occur in approximately 70% of infants around the age of 4 to 5 months, declining to 20% by 6 to 7 months, and less than 5% by 12 months. This is referred to as physiologic reflux that will be outgrown [67]. In children aged 3 to 18 years, the prevalence of GERD symptoms ranges from 1.8% to 22%, and more than 25% of high school students reported GERD symptoms at least once a month [67]. In contrast to physiologic GER, GERD is a pathologic condition that causes complications. Severe or chronic GERD in children is thought to continue into adulthood and result in more serious complications if left untreated [67]. Factors thought to contribute to GERD include transient lower esophageal sphincter relaxation [68], low resting lower esophageal sphincter (LES) pressure, short intra-abdominal esophagus length, obtuse angle of His, and increased intragastric pressure.

Diagnosis

The diagnosis of GERD usually can be made clinically. In infants, persistent, nonbilious regurgitation of feeds with or without failure to thrive is the most common symptom. Many children who have GERD, however, are being identified because of respiratory symptoms, such as chronic cough, wheezing, stridor, choking, apnea, aspiration pneumonitis, chronic lung disease, and sudden infant death syndrome. Esophagitis associated with pain, dysphagia, hematemesis, irritability, and stricture is seen in approximately 10% to 20% of children who have GERD. Unusual neurologic symptoms or breath holding also may result from esophagitis. The association between GERD and asthma has been debated for some time. Vagally mediated laryngospasm and bronchospasm can result from acid stimulation within the esophagus, which mimics asthma. Studies report that the diseases can occur concurrently, however, and that GERD can exacerbate symptoms of asthma [69]. Asthma that occurs after the age of 3, reflux symptoms that precede pulmonary symptoms, family history negative for pulmonary disease but positive for GERD, and failure to exhibit pulmonary function improvement after medical therapy may indicate that GERD is the cause of asthma. In these patients, a 3-month trial of a proton pump inhibitor, administered in higher than standard doses and often twice daily, reportedly has been successful in reducing asthma symptoms [69]. GERD also has been associated with malrotation. In a series of 44 patients who had GERD, 54% were found to have associated malrotation, and they had significantly more delayed gastric emptying. Children who have GERD and delayed gastric emptying should undergo careful evaluation for malrotation [70].

Diagnostic studies include an upper gastrointestinal series, 24-hour pH monitoring, esophageal manometry, upper gastrointestinal endoscopy, and gastric emptying studies. Although the use of these studies varies, most centers consider the 24-hour pH probe as the gold standard for diagnosis. This test measures the frequency and duration of esophageal acid exposure and is especially useful in patients who present with uncharacteristic symptoms. A review of 72 children with chronic/recurrent otolaryngologic symptoms without an identified cause and refractory to medical treatment showed that most had underlying GER when they were evaluated using the pH probe [71]. Double probe pH monitoring is not usually used in children but may increase the sensitivity of the test, especially in children younger than age 2 [72].

A retrospective study that compared 24-hr pH probe and upper gastrointestinal series for the diagnosis of GERD cited that the 24-hr pH probe was almost twice as sensitive and specific than the upper gastrointestinal studies in all age groups and should be used as the first line of investigation [73]. Upper gastrointestinal studies are useful for detecting anatomic abnormalities or gastric outlet obstruction, however, and it remains useful to undergo this anatomic study before surgery.

Additional diagnostic modalities, such as endoscopy and gastric emptying studies, are used routinely in some centers or when warranted in special cases. Recently, other modalities have been used, such as intraluminal impedance catheters and a wireless pH recording system [68,74]. Impedance catheters evaluate the change in esophageal electrical resistance that occurs with the advancement of a bolus, regardless of the pH of the material. Combined multichannel intraluminal impedance and pH measurement has been shown to be highly specific for detecting the presence and pH of intraluminal materials. It also quantifies the proximal distribution and duration of nonacid reflux events, such as postprandially and after treatment. With further trials, this modality has the potential to become the new gold standard for diagnosis and an aid for guiding therapy in patients with ongoing symptoms after medical treatment [74–76]. The Bravo pH monitoring system consists of a small pH capsule that adheres to the esophageal mucosa and transmits intraluminal pH data to a receiver. Its sensitivity has been shown to be similar to the pH probe in adult studies. The advantage is that it lasts for several days and patients can continue their routine activities during monitoring, which provides a more representative pH recording. The size of the capsule currently limits its use in the pediatric population [68].

Treatment

Initial nonoperative treatment involves keeping the head of the bed elevated and providing thickened feedings. Prokinetic agents, antacids, or H-2 receptor blockers are the next line of therapy. Most infants respond to medical treatment and do not require a surgical procedure. Proton pump inhibitors have revolutionized medical therapy for GERD and ulcer disease in adults, and increasing evidence suggests their use in children. Among the five or more currently available proton pump inhibitors, only lansoprazole and omeprazole have been approved for use in children in the United States [69]. Children who have GERD have been shown to metabolize omeprazole faster than adults, and the dosage varies across studies [69,77]. Although proton pump inhibitors offer clear advantages over histamine-2 receptor antagonists in conditions such as severe esophagitis or eradication of *Helicobacter pylori*, their routine use in simple GERD is unsubstantiated and should be limited [78]. Large, multicenter controlled trials are necessary to determine the pharmacologic parameters at different ages, the efficacy profile, and the safety of chronic therapy in children [78,79].

After failure of medical treatment or in cases of serious complications from GERD, surgery is the best option. Although the Nissen fundoplication is the most popular operation in the United States, many others have been performed, such as the Nissen-Rossetti modification, the anterior (Thal) fundoplication, the Hill posterior gastropexy, the Boerema gastropexy, the Boix-Ochoa procedure, the Belsey Mark IV operation, and the posterior (Toupet) fundoplication. The goal of all operative techniques is to create an intra-abdominal high pressure zone. The Nissen fundoplication classically involves taking down the short gastric vessels and performing a full 360° wrap, whereas the Thal fundoplication is an anterior 270° partial wrap. The Nissen-Rossetti modification is popular in Europe and refers to the preservation of the short gastric vessels. The Mutaf procedure is a relatively simple alternative to the wrap technique and involves stapling the lesser curvature around a 26-30 Fr tube, which extends the esophagus approximately 60 mm into the stomach and creates a high-pressure zone [80]. Another alternative to fundoplication is total esophagogastric dissociation. When compared with fundoplication, the morbidity and mortality was similar, and failure rate was reported as less in the group that underwent total esophagogastric dissociation [81]. It may be a good option in neurologically impaired children or in cases of failed fundoplication.

The Nissen and Thal operations can be performed successfully laparoscopically. Nakajima and colleagues [82] described the left-sided Nissen fundoplication, in which crural dissection and repair are approached from the left side of the esophagus to provide better exposure than from the traditional right side. After mobilization of the fundus, the laparoscope is moved to the left mid-clavicular port, and crura approximation and intracorporeal knot-tying is performed in the relatively large subphrenic space. This approach is reported to work well in small infants but needs long-term follow-up [82]. Robotic-assisted fundoplication also has been attempted successfully; however, this technique is limited for small children because of the lack of adequate instrument size [83]. Computer-assisted telesurgery, which is the latest advancement in laparoscopic surgery that allows a surgeon to be submerged in the surgical field while seated at a distance from the patient, has been used in adults to perform fundoplications [84].

Endoluminal therapy as an alternative to surgery for GERD is being developed in adults and is increasing in popularity in the pediatric population. Endoscopic antireflux suturing (endocinch) is one of these methods. A small series of six children who underwent this procedure reported an improvement in symptoms, reduction in acid suppression therapy, and no complications at 6-month follow-up [85]. The Stretta procedure uses radio-frequency to induce collagen tissue contraction, which remodels and bolsters LES function. It also ablates nerves that relax the LES in the lower esophagus and cardia of the stomach [68,86,87]. For both of these new therapies, the durability, long-term results, and comparison to traditional surgical therapy have yet to be determined.

Outcomes

Although the immediate success rate after antireflux surgery is good, reports of recurrence range from 15% to as high as 45% in neurologically impaired children [86]. One study reported that reflux symptoms were still present in almost two thirds of children 2 months after fundoplication. Notably, 74% of these children had associated medical disorders, which may explain the poor success rate [88]. In the early postoperative period, symptoms similar to recurrent GERD can be the result of infection, poor swallowing, impaired esophageal emptying, slow or rapid gastric emptying, or overfeeding. A complete evaluation is warranted, including a contrast study, extended pH monitoring, and perhaps a gastric emptying study. If recurrent GERD is confirmed, it often requires a repeat antireflux operation. Reoperations are typically associated with a high incidence of complications, such as bleeding and vagal nerve injury, and can be technically challenging [86]. Successful revision surgery depends on the identification and correction of the reason for failure of the primary fundoplication. Wrap disruption, herniation of the gastroesophageal junction through the hiatus with or without the wrap, paraesophageal hernia, and esophageal dysmotility are some reasons for failure [89]. Although many surgeons attempt a redo fundoplication via an open approach, it can be accomplished successfully laparoscopically [89]. The Stretta procedure also has been used in patients who have recurrent GERD after failed initial surgery and may be a valuable tool for avoiding redo surgery. Larger trials and longer follow-up are required, however [86].

The Nissen fundoplication may be associated with the inability to vomit, dysphagia, dumping syndrome, diarrhea, and the development of gas bloat syndrome. These complications are less common after the Thal operation, but the recurrent reflux rate is higher. In one study, after open Nissen fundoplication, 85% of patients had no recurrent reflux, two patients with preoperative stricture developed wrap disruption, recurrent reflux, and re-stricture, and one patient developed esophagitis caused by wrap herniation. These results indicated that the open Nissen operation is effective for GERD [90]. Laparoscopic Nissen fundoplication was reported to have only a 4% wrap failure rate over a 10-year follow-up period and has significantly less morbidity and hospitalization stay than the open procedure [91]. Long-term outcomes of the laparoscopic Thal procedure are also favorable. Of 149 reviewed cases (half of which involved neurologically impaired children), only 5% required a redo operation [92]. These studies by experienced groups may not be reproduced easily by less experienced groups. Each surgeon and institution should determine their own success and complication rates periodically. This review should provide the basis for offering these procedures to patients, instead of merely relying on the excellent results reported in the literature.

Considerations in neurologically impaired children

Feeding difficulties and GERD are major problems in neurologically impaired children. Many of these patients are managed with a gastrostomy and often with a concomitant fundoplication to prevent new reflux or treat existing GER. The subject of a prophylactic fundoplication in a neurologically devastated child who may not tolerate silent aspiration or demonstrate such remains controversial. Some reports on these children have shown that laparoscopic fundoplication provided excellent outcomes in gastrointestinal symptoms and quality of life [93,94]. A retrospective review of 56 children treated with fundoplications reported that emesis and hematemesis were adequately controlled but that respiratory problems persisted. The recurrence rate of GER was high in these children, and many required many reoperations [94]. Many neurologically handicapped children have oropharyngeal discoordination in addition to GER. Treatment of GER with fundoplication cannot be expected to correct the respiratory symptoms because of poor oropharyngeal handling of saliva.

The long-term results of laparoscopic fundoplication in neurologically impaired children are not satisfactory, especially in terms of respiratory symptoms, and further refinements may be necessary to determine and prevent the real cause of these problems. A review that compared the outcomes of laparoscopically inserted gastrostomy tubes, with or without Nissen fundoplication, found that laparoscopic gastrostomy tube placement is associated with less morbidity, permits earlier enteric nutrition, and has a cosmetic advantage [95]. Another group reported success with a laparoscopically assisted jejunostomy tube. At 18-month follow-up, these patients had gained weight and had a high level of parental satisfaction. The authors believe that this method solves the feeding problem, even if reflux is not completely eliminated, and causes minimal surgical trauma and postoperative complications [96]. To determine the best way to manage this special group of children, a large controlled trial must compare the various methods of feeding tube placement and the necessity of fundoplication, including short- and long-term outcomes.

References

[1] Mahon BE, Rosenman MB, Kleiman MB. Maternal and infant use of erythromycin and other macrolide antibiotics as risk factors for infantile hypertrophic pyloric stenosis. J Pediatr 2001;139:380–4.

[2] To T, Wajja A, Wales PW, et al. Population demographic indicators associated with incidence of pyloric stenosis. Arch Pediatr Adolesc Med 2005;159:520–5.

[3] Subramanian R, Doig CM, Moore L. Nitric oxide synthase is absent in only a subset of cases of pyloric stenosis. J Pediatr Surg 2001;36:616–9.

[4] Cohen HL, Blumer SL, Zucconi WB. The sonographic double-track sign: not pathognomonic for hypertrophic pyloric stenosis, can be seen in pylorospasm. J Ultrasound Med 2004;23:641–6.

[5] Helton KJ, Strife JL, Warner BW, et al. The impact of a clinical guideline on imaging children with hypertrophic pyloric stenosis. Pediatr Radiol 2004;34:733–6.

[6] Ordorica-Flores R, Leon-Villanueva V, Bracho-Blanchet E, et al. Infantile hypertrophic pyloric stenosis: a comparative study of pyloric traumamyoplasty and Fredet-Ramstedt pyloromyotomy. J Pediatr Surg 2001;36:1000–3.

[7] Tan KC, Bianchi A. Circumumbilical incision for pyloromyotomy. Br J Surg 1986;73:399.

[8] Ladd AP, Nemeth SA, Kirincich AN, et al. Supraumbilical pyloromyotomy: a unique indication for antimicrobial prophylaxis. J Pediatr Surg 2005;40:974–7 [discussion: 977].

[9] Blumer RM, Hessel NS, van Baren R, et al. Comparison between umbilical and transverse right upper abdominal incision for pyloromyotomy. J Pediatr Surg 2004;39:1091–3.

[10] Alberti D, Cheli M, Locatelli G. A new technical variant for extramucosal pyloromyotomy: the Tan-Bianchi operation moves to the right. J Pediatr Surg 2004;39:53–6.

[11] Takamizawa S, Obatake M, Muraji T, et al. Supraumbilical pyloromyotomy: comparison between intracorporeal and extracorporeal approaches. Pediatr Surg Int 2004;20:101–4.

[12] Hall NJ, Van Der Zee J, Tan HL, et al. Meta-analysis of laparoscopic versus open pyloromyotomy. Ann Surg 2004;240:774–8.

[13] Huang YC, Su BH. Medical treatment with atropine sulfate for hypertrophic pyloric stenosis. Acta Paediatr Taiwan 2004;45:136–40.

[14] Sretenovic A, Smoljanic Z, Korac G, et al. [Conservative treatment of hypertrophic pyloric stenosis in children.] Srp Arh Celok Lek 2004;132(Suppl 1):93–6 [in Serbian].

[15] Hayashi AH, Giacomantonio JM, Lau HY, et al. Balloon catheter dilatation for hypertrophic pyloric stenosis. J Pediatr Surg 1990;25:1119–21.

[16] Ibarguen-Secchia E. Endoscopic pyloromyotomy for congenital pyloric stenosis. Gastrointest Endosc 2005;61:598–600.

[17] Kanard RC, Fairbanks TJ, De Langhe SP, et al. Fibroblast growth factor-10 serves a regulatory role in duodenal development. J Pediatr Surg 2005;40:313–6.

[18] Poki HO, Holland AJ, Pitkin J. Double bubble, double trouble. Pediatr Surg Int 2005;21: 428–31.

[19] Shih HS, Ko SF, Chaung JH. Is there an association between duodenal atresia and choledochal cyst? J Pediatr Gastroenterol Nutr 2005;40:378–81.

[20] Celli J, van Bokhoven H, Brunner HG. Feingold syndrome: clinical review and genetic mapping. Am J Med Genet 2003;122:294–300.

[21] Ferguson C, Morabito A, Bianchi A. Duodenal atresia and gastric antral web: a significant lesson to learn. Eur J Pediatr Surg 2004;14:120–2.

[22] Downard CD, Kim HB, Laningham F, et al. Esophageal atresia, duodenal atresia, and unilateral lung agenesis: a case report. J Pediatr Surg 2004;39:1283–5.

[23] Singh MV, Richards C, Bowen JC. Does Down syndrome affect the outcome of congenital duodenal obstruction? Pediatr Surg Int 2004;20:586–9.

[24] Kimble RM, Harding J, Kolbe A. Additional congenital anomalies in babies with gut atresia or stenosis: when to investigate, and which investigation. Pediatr Surg Int 1997;12:565–70.

[25] Rothenberg SS. Laparoscopic duodenoduodenostomy for duodenal obstruction in infants and children. J Pediatr Surg 2002;37:1088–9.

[26] Arnbjornsson E, Larsson M, Finkel Y, et al. Transanastomotic feeding tube after an operation for duodenal atresia. Eur J Pediatr Surg 2002;12:159–62.

[27] Ruangtrakool R, Mungnirandr A, Laohapensang M, et al. Surgical treatment for congenital duodenal obstruction. J Med Assoc Thai 2001;84:842–9.

[28] Escobar MA, Ladd AP, Grosfeld JL, et al. Duodenal atresia and stenosis: long-term follow-up over 30 years. J Pediatr Surg 2004;39:867–71 [discussion: 867–71].

[29] Endo M, Ukiyama E, Yokoyama J, et al. Subtotal duodenectomy with jejunal patch for megaduodenum secondary to congenital duodenal malformation. J Pediatr Surg 1998;33: 1636–40.

[30] Menon P, Rao KL, Vaiphei K. Isolated enteric duplication cysts. J Pediatr Surg 2004;39: e5–7.

[31] Kong K, Walker P, Cassey J, et al. Foregut duplication cyst arising in the floor of mouth. Int J Pediatr Otorhinolaryngol 2004;68:827–30.

[32] Emura T, Hashizume K, Asashima M. Experimental study of the embryogenesis of gastro-intestinal duplication and enteric cyst. Pediatr Surg Int 2003;19:147–51.

[33] Gul A, Tekoglu G, Aslan H, et al. Prenatal sonographic features of esophageal and ileal duplications at 18 weeks of gestation. Prenat Diagn 2004;24:969–71.

[34] Gupta AK, Guglani B. Imaging of congenital anomalies of the gastrointestinal tract. Indian J Pediatr 2005;72:403–14.

[35] Eloubeidi MA, Cohn M, Cerfolio RJ, et al. Endoscopic ultrasound-guided fine-needle aspi-ration in the diagnosis of foregut duplication cysts: the value of demonstrating detached ciliary tufts in cyst fluid. Cancer 2004;102:253–8.

[36] Azzie G, Beasley S. Diagnosis and treatment of foregut duplications. Semin Pediatr Surg 2003;12:46–54.

[37] Carachi R, Azmy A. Foregut duplications. Pediatr Surg Int 2002;18:371–4.

[38] Kuraoka K, Nakayama H, Kagawa T, et al. Adenocarcinoma arising from a gastric duplication cyst with invasion to the stomach: a case report with literature review. J Clin Pathol 2004;57:428–31.

[39] Felix JF, Keijzer R, van Dooren MF, et al. Genetics and developmental biology of oesopha-geal atresia and tracheo-oesophageal fistula: lessons from mice relevant for paediatric surgeons. Pediatr Surg Int 2004;20:731–6.

[40] Arsic D, Cameron V, Ellmers L, et al. Adriamycin disruption of the Shh-Gli pathway is associated with abnormalities of foregut development. J Pediatr Surg 2004;39:1747–53.

[41] Goyal A, Potter F, Losty PD. Transillumination of H-type tracheoesophageal fistula using flexible miniature bronchoscopy: an innovative technique for operative localization. J Pediatr Surg 2005;40:e33–4.

[42] Ratan SK, Varshney A, Mullick S, et al. Evaluation of neonates with esophageal atresia using chest CT scan. Pediatr Surg Int 2004;20:757–61.

[43] Deurloo JA, Smit BJ, Ekkelkamp S, et al. Oesophageal atresia in premature infants: an analysis of morbidity and mortality over a period of 20 years. Acta Paediatr 2004;93:394–9.

[44] Touloukian RJ, Seashore JH. Thirty-five-year institutional experience with end-to-side repair for esophageal atresia. Arch Surg 2004;139:371–4 [discussion: 374].

[45] Aziz D, Schiller D, Gerstle JT, et al. Can 'long-gap' esophageal atresia be safely managed at home while awaiting anastomosis? J Pediatr Surg 2003;38:705–8.

[46] Bagolan P, Iacobelli BB, De Angelis P, et al. Long gap esophageal atresia and esophageal replacement: moving toward a separation? J Pediatr Surg 2004;39:1084–90.

[47] Kimura K, Nishijima E, Tsugawa C, et al. Multistaged extrathoracic esophageal elongation procedure for long gap esophageal atresia: experience with 12 patients. J Pediatr Surg 2001; 36:1725–7.

[48] Foker JE, Linden BC, Boyle EM Jr, et al. Development of a true primary repair for the full spectrum of esophageal atresia. Ann Surg 1997;226:533–41 [discussion: 541–3].

[49] Lopes MF, Reis A, Coutinho S, et al. Very long gap esophageal atresia successfully treated by esophageal lengthening using external traction sutures. J Pediatr Surg 2004; 39:1286–7.

[50] Kimura K, Nishijima E, Tsugawa C, et al. A new approach for the salvage of unsuccessful esophageal atresia repair: a spiral myotomy and delayed definitive operation. J Pediatr Surg 1987;22:981–3.

[51] Borgnon J, Tounian P, Auber F, et al. Esophageal replacement in children by an isoperistaltic gastric tube: a 12-year experience. Pediatr Surg Int 2004;20:829–33.

[52] Spitz L, Kiely E, Pierro A. Gastric transposition in children: a 21-year experience. J Pediatr Surg 2004;39:276–81 [discussion: 276–81].

[53] Bax NM, Van Renterghem KM. Ileal pedicle grafting for esophageal replacement in children. Pediatr Surg Int 2005;21:369–72.

[54] Rothenberg SS. Thoracoscopic repair of tracheoesophageal fistula in newborns. J Pediatr Surg 2002;37:869–72.

[55] Tsao K, Lee H. Extrapleural thoracoscopic repair of esophageal atresia with tracheoesophageal fistula. Pediatr Surg Int 2005;21:308–10.

[56] Aziz GA, Schier F. Thoracoscopic ligation of a tracheoesophageal H-type fistula in a newborn. J Pediatr Surg 2005;40:e35–6.

[57] Lorincz A, Langenburg SE, Knight CG, et al. Robotically assisted esophago-esophagostomy in newborn pigs. J Pediatr Surg 2004;39:1386–9.

[58] Chavin K, Field G, Chandler J, et al. Save the child's esophagus: management of major disruption after repair of esophageal atresia. J Pediatr Surg 1996;31:48–51 [discussion: 52].

[59] Schalamon J, Lindahl H, Saarikoski H, et al. Endoscopic follow-up in esophageal atresia-for how long is it necessary? J Pediatr Surg 2003;38:702–4.

[60] Koivusalo A, Pakarinen M, Rintala RJ, et al. Does postoperative pH monitoring predict complicated gastroesophageal reflux in patients with esophageal atresia? Pediatr Surg Int 2004;20:670–4.

[61] de Lagausie P, Bonnard A, Schultz A, et al. Reflux in esophageal atresia, tracheoesophageal cleft, and esophagocoloplasty: Bianchi's procedure as an alternative approach. J Pediatr Surg 2005;40:666–9.

[62] Triglia JM, Guys JM, Louis-Borrione C. Tracheomalacia caused by arterial compression in esophageal atresia. Ann Otol Rhinol Laryngol 1994;103:516–21.

[63] Orford J, Cass DT, Glasson MJ. Advances in the treatment of oesophageal atresia over three decades: the 1970s and the 1990s. Pediatr Surg Int 2004;20:402–7.

[64] Tonz M, Kohli S, Kaiser G. Oesophageal atresia: what has changed in the last 3 decades? Pediatr Surg Int 2004;20:768–72.

[65] Koivusalo A, Pakarinen MP, Turunen P, et al. Health-related quality of life in adult patients with esophageal atresia: a questionnaire study. J Pediatr Surg 2005;40:307–12.

[66] Alfaro L, Bermas H, Fenoglio M, et al. Are patients who have had a tracheoesophageal fistula repair during infancy at risk for esophageal adenocarcinoma during adulthood? J Pediatr Surg 2005;40:719–20.

[67] Hassall E. Decisions in diagnosing and managing chronic gastroesophageal reflux disease in children. J Pediatr 2005;146:S3–12.

[68] Strople J, Kaul A. Pediatric gastroesophageal reflux disease: current perspectives. Curr Opin Otolaryngol Head Neck Surg 2003;11:447–51.

[69] Gold BD. Asthma and gastroesophageal reflux disease in children: exploring the relationship. J Pediatr 2005;146:S13–20.

[70] Demirbilek S, Karaman A, Gurunluoglu K, et al. Delayed gastric emptying in gastroesophageal reflux disease: the role of malrotation. Pediatr Surg Int 2005;21:423–7.

[71] van den Abbeele T, Couloigner V, Faure C, et al. The role of 24 h pH-recording in pediatric otolaryngologic gastro-oesophageal reflux disease. Int J Pediatr Otorhinolaryngol 2003; 67(Suppl 1):S95–100.

[72] Demir H, Ozen H, Kocak N, et al. Does simultaneous gastric and esophageal pH monitoring increase the diagnosis of gastroesophageal reflux disease? Turk J Pediatr 2005;47: 14–6.

[73] Al-Khawari HA, Sinan TS, Seymour H. Diagnosis of gastro-oesophageal reflux in children: comparison between oesophageal pH and barium examinations. Pediatr Radiol 2002;32: 765–70.

[74] Tutuian R, Castell DO. Use of multichannel intraluminal impedance to document proximal esophageal and pharyngeal nonacidic reflux episodes. Am J Med 2003;115(Suppl 3A): 119S–23S.

[75] Craig WR, Hanlon-Dearman A, Sinclair C, et al. Metoclopramide, thickened feedings, and positioning for gastro-oesophageal reflux in children under two years. Cochrane Database Syst Rev 2004;18(4):CD003502.

[76] Chicella MF, Batres LA, Heesters MS, et al. Prokinetic drug therapy in children: a review of current options. Ann Pharmacother 2005;39:706–11.

[77] Marier JF, Dubuc MC, Drouin E, et al. Pharmacokinetics of omeprazole in healthy adults and in children with gastroesophageal reflux disease. Ther Drug Monit 2004;26:3–8.

[78] Marchetti F, Gerarduzzi T, Ventura A. Proton pump inhibitors in children: a review. Dig Liver Dis 2003;35:738–46.

[79] Carcelen Andres J, Barroso Peez C, Fabrega Bosacoma C, et al. [Proton pump inhibitors in paediatrics.] Farm Hosp 2005;29:43–54 [in Spanish].

[80] Sanal M, Korkmaz M, Karadag E, et al. Results of the Mutaf procedure in patients with gastroesophageal reflux disease. Pediatr Surg Int 2004;20:326–8.

[81] Goyal A, Khalil B, Choo K, et al. Esophagogastric dissociation in the neurologically impaired: an alternative to fundoplication? J Pediatr Surg 2005;40:915–8 [discussion: 918–9].

[82] Nakajima K, Kawahara H, Wasa M, et al. Laparoscopic left-sided Nissen fundoplication in children. Surg Today 2004;34:562–4.

[83] Heller K, Gutt C, Schaeff B, et al. Use of the robot system Da Vinci for laparoscopic repair of gastro-oesophageal reflux in children. Eur J Pediatr Surg 2002;12:239–42.

[84] Aurora AR, Talamini MA. A comprehensive review of anti-reflux procedures completed by computer-assisted tele-surgery. Minerva Chir 2004;59:417–25.

[85] Cano Novillo I, Benavent Gordo MI, Garcia Vazquez A, et al. [Alternative treatment of gastroesophageal reflux: endoluminal gastric plication.] Cir Pediatr 2004;17:113–7 [in Spanish].

[86] Islam S, Geiger JD, Coran AG, et al. Use of radiofrequency ablation of the lower esophageal sphincter to treat recurrent gastroesophageal reflux disease. J Pediatr Surg 2004;39:282–6 [discussion: 282–6].

[87] Liu DC, Somme S, Mavrelis PG, et al. Stretta as the initial antireflux procedure in children. J Pediatr Surg 2005;40:148–51 [discussion: 151–2].

[88] Gilger MA, Yeh C, Chiang J, et al. Outcomes of surgical fundoplication in children. Clin Gastroenterol Hepatol 2004;2:978–84.

[89] Hatch KF, Daily MF, Christensen BJ, et al. Failed fundoplications. Am J Surg 2004;188: 786–91.

[90] Zeid MA, Kandel T, el-Shobary M, et al. Nissen fundoplication in infants and children: a long-term clinical study. Hepatogastroenterology 2004;51:697–700.

[91] Rothenberg SS. The first decade's experience with laparoscopic Nissen fundoplication in infants and children. J Pediatr Surg 2005;40:142–6 [discussion: 147].

[92] van der Zee DC, Bax KN, Ure BM, et al. Long-term results after laparoscopic Thal procedure in children. Semin Laparosc Surg 2002;9:168–71.

[93] Lima M, Bertozzi M, Ruggeri G, et al. Laparoscopic antireflux surgery in neurologically impaired children. Pediatr Surg Int 2004;20:114–7.

[94] Kawahara H, Okuyama H, Kubota A, et al. Can laparoscopic antireflux surgery improve the quality of life in children with neurologic and neuromuscular handicaps? J Pediatr Surg 2004; 39:1761–4.

[95] Wadie GM, Lobe TE. Gastroesophageal reflux disease in neurologically impaired children: the role of the gastrostomy tube. Semin Laparosc Surg 2002;9:180–9.

[96] Esposito C, Settimi A, Centonze A, et al. Laparoscopic-assisted jejunostomy: an effective procedure for the treatment of neurologically impaired children with feeding problems and gastroesophageal reflux. Surg Endosc 2005;19:501–4.

ELSEVIER
SAUNDERS

SURGICAL
CLINICS OF
NORTH AMERICA

Surg Clin N Am 86 (2006) 285–299

Midgut Abnormalities

John R. Gosche, MD, PhD*, Laura Vick, MD,
Scott C. Boulanger, MD, PhD, Saleem Islam, MD

*Department of Surgery, Division of Pediatric Surgery, University of Mississippi Medical
Center, 2500 North State Street, Jackson, MS 39216, USA*

The midgut is that portion of the intestinal tract that receives its principal blood supply from the superior mesenteric artery and extends from the level of the distal duodenum to approximately the mid-transverse colon. Altered midgut embryologic development accounts for abnormalities of rotation and fixation, intestinal atresias and stenoses, and persistence of vestigial structures. Congenital or acquired loss of absorptive capacity leads to inadequate absorptive capacity referred to as short bowel syndrome (SBS).

Intestinal atresia and stenosis

Jejunoileal atresia is a common cause of obstruction in newborns. Atresias and stenoses likely reflect the same etiology but with differing degrees of severity. Atresias outnumber stenoses by approximately 20 to 1. Reported incidence rates for intestinal atresias and stenoses have varied widely in the literature. In 1974, Ravitch and Barton [1] used an incidence rate of 1 in 2710 live births for intestinal atresia to predict manpower requirements for pediatric surgeons. A recent population-based study from Hawaii reported a similar incidence rate of 1 in 3448 live births [2].

Presentation

Patients who have intestinal atresia present with an intestinal obstruction in the first days of life. The most frequent symptom at presentation is bilious emesis. Other common symptoms include abdominal distension and failure to pass meconium. Less than one third of patients are diagnosed prenatally [3,4]. Intestinal atresias are usually detected during prenatal ultrasound evaluation for maternal polyhydramnios. Polyhydramnios is observed

---

* Corresponding author.
E-mail address: jgosche@surgery.umsmed.edu (J.R. Gosche).

more commonly in association with proximal atresias. Another common obstetric complication associated with intestinal atresia is premature birth. Patients who have proximal intestinal atresias also frequently are small for gestation age, presumably because of the inability to absorb swallowed amniotic fluid [5].

Depending on the degree of obstruction, patients who have stenoses of the midgut may present as newborns with intestinal obstruction or they may present weeks or months later with recurrent vomiting and failure to thrive.

Embryology

The embryologic origin of atresias and stenoses of the midgut is believed to be an ischemic insult to the developing bowel. This premise is based on the classic experiments by Louw and Barnard [6]. This mechanism explains the frequent association of atresias with mesenteric defects and with other conditions that may cause strangulating obstruction of the intestinal tract (eg, volvulus, intussusception, internal hernias, and gastroschisis). An ischemic etiology also may explain why intestinal atresia is associated with maternal smoking and vasoconstrictor drug exposure during pregnancy [7].

Some types of intestinal atresia, particularly the familial form of multiple atresias, may result from altered morphogenesis [8]. Recent evidence from an animal model suggests that disturbed separation of the gut and notochord during early midgut development may lead to multiple intestinal atresias [9].

Diagnosis

The diagnosis of an intestinal atresia is usually straightforward and can be made based on the presenting symptoms and plain abdominal radiographs. The number of dilated bowel loops usually indicates the level of obstruction. Contrast studies are not required to make the diagnosis in patients who have proximal atresias; however, a contrast enema may be useful to rule out the possibility of the rare associated colonic atresia. Patients with evidence of distal atresias frequently are evaluated by contrast enemas to rule out other nonoperative causes for a distal obstruction.

An upper gastrointestinal contrast study with small bowel follow through frequently is required to make the diagnosis in patients who present in a delayed fashion with a midgut stenosis. An upper gastrointestinal contrast study is also useful to rule out malrotation, with or without volvulus, as the cause of a partial obstruction.

Management

Treatment of an intestinal atresia requires operative intervention. Preoperatively, patients should be hydrated adequately, and electrolyte abnormalities must be corrected. A nasogastric tube should be passed to decrease the risk of vomiting with aspiration. Because of the low incidence of associated cardiac anomalies, patients who have intestinal atresias do not require a preoperative echocardiogram unless there are signs or symptoms that suggest a cardiac defect.

The surgical treatment of atresias and stenoses usually requires resection of the atretic segment with primary anastomosis. Occasionally a type I atresia or web and patients with stenoses can be treated by simple web excision or stricturoplasty. A common practice is to flush the distal intestinal lumen with saline to rule out the possibility of a second, more distal atresia. Infrequently, a patient who has atresia with vascular compromise of the intestine or meconium peritonitis requires resection and exteriorization. Patients who have multiple atresias (type IV) often require a staged approach.

After the atretic segment is resected, the surgeon is faced with the difficulty of creating an anastomosis between two intestinal segments with marked size discrepancies (Fig. 1). In patients who have an isolated atresia and a relatively short segment of dilated proximal intestine, resection of the dilated segment with primary end-to-oblique or end-to-side anastomosis is a good option. In patients who have a long segment of markedly dilated proximal intestine or multiple atresias, resection of the dilated segments may result in loss of too much absorptive capacity. A simple resection with reanastomosis in these patients is frequently associated with functional obstruction, however, because of poor peristalsis of the dilated proximal segment. One option for these patients is to perform an antimesenteric tapering enteroplasty to reduce the caliber of the proximal bowel to a more normal diameter. Alternatively, imbrication of the proximal intestine can be used to reduce the effective intraluminal diameter of the proximal segment. Most series, including a recent report from the United Kingdom [10], suggest that enteroplasty or plication is used in one third or less of patients. To date, no randomized studies have compared outcome in patients undergoing repair of intestinal atresias, with or without the addition of an enteroplasty or plication.

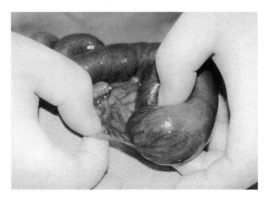

Fig. 1. Type II intestinal atresia. Note the size discrepancy between the proximal and distal bowel.

Totally laparoscopic and laparoscopic-assisted approaches for the surgical treatment of neonates with midgut atresia only recently have been reported [11].

Outcome

The reported survival rates for patients who have isolated, uncomplicated intestinal atresia approach 100%. Some patients who have multiple atresias and most patients with type IIIb atresias (apple-peel deformity) experience SBS.

Rotational anomalies

Rotational anomalies represent a spectrum of defects, from complete nonrotation, in which the entirety of the small intestine is on the right side of the abdomen and the colon is positioned on the left, to relatively minor abnormalities associated with incomplete fixation of the cecum and ascending colon. Anomalies of intestinal rotation are believed to arise during the second stage of midgut development (10–12 weeks' gestation), at which time the midgut returns to the abdominal cavity from the umbilical stalk. During this period, there is an orderly pattern of reduction in which the small bowel returns first and the cecum and proximal colon return last. Nonrotation is believed to result from laxity of the umbilical ring, which allows reduction en masse of the entire midgut during the tenth week of development. Recently, Kluth and colleagues [12] showed that localized growth of the duodenum seems to be the primary event in intestinal rotation, and they proposed that rotational anomalies result from localized growth failures of the duodenal loop.

The incidence of anomalies of intestinal rotation has been reported to be 1 in 6000 live births; however, the true incidence is unknown because many patients remain asymptomatic. In fact, complete nonrotation "is said to be found in 0.5% of autopsies" [13].

Presentation

Rotational anomalies may become symptomatic at any age, including late into adult life. However, eighty percent of patients who do become symptomatic do so in the first month of life. Symptoms associated with anomalies of rotation may be acute or chronic. The most feared complication associated with anomalies of intestinal rotation is midgut volvulus with intestinal ischemic necrosis (Fig. 2). Rotational anomalies, particularly nonrotation, predispose patients to midgut volvulus because of the narrowed mesenteric attachment of the small bowel. Most of these patients present with acute onset of severe abdominal pain associated with bilious emesis. Other presenting signs and symptoms may include abdominal distension, abdominal tenderness, and passage of blood or passage

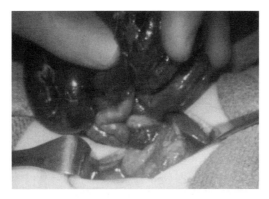

Fig. 2. Midgut volvulus. Note narrow mesenteric base. (Courtesy of R. Touloukian, MD, New Haven, Connecticut).

of sloughed mucosal tissue per rectum. Late signs include peritonitis and hypovolemic shock. Many patients who have acute midgut volvulus have no preceding symptomatology. Some patients have a history of intermittent crampy abdominal pain and vomiting, however, which suggests prior episodes of lesser degrees of volvulus.

Another cause of vomiting in patients who have anomalies of intestinal rotation may be compression of the duodenum by peritoneal bands (Ladd's bands) between the abnormally positioned cecum and the right retroperitoneum. These patients frequently present with a history of chronic vomiting (often bilious) associated with failure to gain weight.

The optimal management of patients who present with volvulus requires a high index of suspicion and an extreme sense of urgency. Patients who present with acute onset of bilious vomiting with peritonitis require no further diagnostic studies. Delaying operative intervention to obtain tests to confirm the diagnosis risks the opportunity to prevent irreversible intestinal damage. For patients who present with chronic or less acute symptoms, however, an upper gastrointestinal contrast series is the diagnostic study of choice to confirm or rule out a rotational anomaly. Other diagnostic tests, including plain abdominal radiographs, contrast enemas, and ultrasonography, are neither sensitive nor specific enough to make the diagnosis. An ultrasound finding of the superior mesenteric vein located to the left of the superior mesenteric artery highly suggests malrotation [14]. A normal relationship does not exclude the diagnosis, however [15].

Management

Patients who have peritonitis require emergent operative exploration after expeditious fluid resuscitation. Standard operative management involves several important steps: (1) evisceration of the entire midgut with inspection of the mesenteric root, (2) derotation of the midgut in a counterclockwise direction, (3) division of any peritoneal bands that are compressing the duodenum (Ladd's bands), (4) widening of the base of the mesentery, and (5) carefully returning the viscera to the abdominal cavity and placing the duodenum and proximal jejunum along the right gutter and the cecum in the left lower quadrant. Most surgeons also perform an appendectomy to prevent future diagnostic confusion related to an abnormally positioned appendix.

When intestinal ischemia or necrosis is encountered at the time of operative exploration, several options exist. Short segments of clearly necrotic bowel should be resected, with or without primary reanastomosis. Patients who have extensive ischemic involvement of the midgut should undergo initial detorsion and a period of intraoperative observation. If bowel perfusion improves but the viability remains questionable, a second-look procedure should be considered. The decision to perform an extensive resection is a difficult one and is based on several considerations, including the length of remaining bowel, the patient's condition, the ability of the environment to support a patient with SBS, and the surgeon's preference and beliefs. One option is to perform detorsion and Ladd's procedure and close the patient. A frank discussion with the family should follow. Consideration of re-exploration with resection can occur after 24 to 48 hours depending on the patient's condition and with input from the family and other health care providers.

Several small series of patients who underwent laparoscopic evaluation and treatment of malrotation without volvulus have been reported [16–18]. The laparoscopic Ladd's procedure incorporates the same steps that are performed during the open procedure. To date, no reports show that the long-term results with this approach, in terms of preventing future episodes of volvulus, are comparable to the open approach. Laparoscopic exploration is a valuable tool for assessing the location of the ligament of Treitz in patients with an equivocal upper gastrointestinal contrast study.

Any patient with symptoms attributable to malrotation should undergo operative treatment. An area of controversy involves whether a patient with asymptomatic malrotation should have a prophylactic Ladd's procedure performed. Most patients who have midgut volvulus present within the first 2 years of life; however, volvulus can occur at any age. A recent report showed that older children who present with malrotation frequently present emergently with potentially life-threatening complications, a significant proportion of whom had volvulus or required intestinal resection [19]. In a recent publication, however, the same authors used a Markov decision analysis model to show that performing prophylactic Ladd's procedures in patients age 18 or older did not increase quality adjusted life expectancy [20]. It seems appropriate to recommend a prophylactic Ladd's procedure for all patients 18 years of age. The decision to perform a prophylactic operation in asymptomatic adults should be individualized based on operative risk and patient preference.

Outcome

The mortality rate associated with operative treatment of malrotation depends on the presence and extent of intestinal necrosis, ranging from nearly 0% without necrosis to more than 50% for patients who have extensive necrosis. The most common postoperative complication after a Ladd's procedure is adhesive small bowel obstruction. Recurrent volvulus is unusual and is usually caused by inadequate widening of the mesenteric root. Most patients report improvement in their preoperative symptoms after a Ladd's operation. Some patients experience persistent vomiting, diarrhea, or abdominal pain, however, which may reflect pre-existing intestinal dysmotility.

Short bowel syndrome

SBS refers to a disorder in which the small intestine is incapable of supporting a patient's nutritional needs. SBS can be defined as the loss of small bowel below that necessary to support absorption of sufficient calories for adequate growth. This definition is a functional one and not anatomic, because the amount of small bowel needed to support adequate nutrition is different from individual to individual and depends not only on absolute length but also on other factors, such as type of bowel resected, presence of an ileocecal valve, and presence of the colon.

SBS can result from several etiologies, including disorders of motility or impairment of intestinal absorption. SBS most commonly results from massive resection of the small intestine, however. In infants, the most common cause of SBS is necrotizing enterocolitis [21]. In the past, the most common causes were intestinal atresias and midgut volvulus. Other causes include gastroschisis and volvulus associated with meconium ileus. Rare causes include vascular events associated with coagulopathies or invasive monitoring devices. In older children, SBS generally results from trauma, ischemia as a result of shock or inotropes, or Crohn's disease. Certain functional disorders also can lead to SBS (eg, long-segment aganglionosis and idiopathic intestinal pseudo-obstruction).

Medical management

The goal of medical management of SBS is to maximize intestinal adaptation while limiting complications. Aggressive enteral alimentation is the mainstay of therapy. Enteral nutrients have a potent trophic effect on the intestinal mucosa. Once the decision to start enteral feeds is made, an appropriate formula must be selected to meet the patient's needs. High carbohydrate loads can create an osmotic stress on the gut and lead to bacterial proliferation, inflammation, and osmotic diarrhea [22]. Fats stimulate secretion of antimotility hormones and may prolong intestinal transit time. Long-chain fats seem to be more trophic to the small intestine and are an important component of dietary manipulation to stimulate intestinal adaptation [23]. Enteral nutrition is begun slowly and advanced as tolerated. Continuous enteral infusion enhances absorption by permitting total saturation of gut transporters [24]. Parenteral alimentation is decreased isocalorically as enteral feedings are advanced. Tolerance can be determined by measuring reducing substances in the stool or by following stool output.

Pharmacologic interventions are frequently required. Antacids, type-2 histamine receptor blockers, or proton pump inhibitors are used to treat the gastric hypersecretion that occurs after massive small bowel loss. Medications that slow peristalsis (eg, loperamide, lomotil, codeine, paregoric, or tincture of opium) may help increase nutrient contact time with enterocytes and improve absorption [25]. Cholestyramine can be given to bind bile acids and reduce choleretic diarrhea in patients who have lost a large portion of the terminal ileum. Pharmacologic therapies may have negative effects. Suppression of gastric acid production can contribute to bacterial overgrowth. Similarly, antimotility agents can increase the risk of bacterial overgrowth. Although cholestyramine may help with choleretic diarrhea, malabsorption and steatorrhea may be exacerbated if bile acid loss exceeds the maximal hepatic synthesis, which causes a decrease in the bile acid pool and impairment of luminal fat digestion [26].

Supplemental enteral nutrients may improve absorption and stimulate intestinal adaptation. Although insoluble fiber contributes to stool bulk and decreases whole gut transit time, soluble fiber slows gastric emptying and gut transit. Bacterial fermentation of soluble fiber results in intraluminal release of short-chain fatty acids, which are trophic to the intestinal mucosa. Medium-chain triglycerides are frequently used in patients who have short bowel because of ease of absorption. Medium-chain triglyceride supplementation may improve enteral absorption but does not seem to stimulate intestinal adaptation. Long-chain fats seem to stimulate gut adaptation more than medium-chain triglycerides, probably in part by providing substrate for prostaglandin synthesis. Glutamine is an amino acid that is an energy source for enterocytes and colonocytes. Glutamine supplementation may induce mucosal hyperplasia and prevent deterioration in gut permeability and mucosal atrophy in patients who are receiving total parenteral nutrition.

Somatostatin and its synthetic analog, octreotide, have inhibitory effects on a wide array of gastrointestinal hormones and can decrease gastric acid secretion, gallbladder contraction, bowel motility, small intestine secretions, gastric emptying, and exocrine pancreas function [25]. These effects may help to improve fluid and electrolyte balance and increase substrate absorption in patients who have SBS. Somatostatin analogs reduce levels of several gastrointestinal hormones, however, including growth hormone, and can suppress enterocyte transport of glucose and several amino acids.

Finally, animal studies have identified several hormones and growth factors that may function as biologic modifiers of intestinal adaptation.

Few of these agents have been tested adequately in humans. The most extensively studied agents include epidermal growth factor, growth hormone, insulin-like growth factor, glucagon-like peptide 2, interleukin-11, and transforming growth factor- alpha.

Surgical management

Surgical intervention should be considered for patients who fail to wean from parenteral alimentation despite an adequate period of intestinal adaptation (Fig. 3). Although conservation of bowel length is a basic concept in SBS, motility takes precedence over bowel length [27]. The timing of operative intervention is key. Early operation may result in needless interventions on patients who would have adapted on their own, whereas late intervention may result in unnecessary complications and added total parenteral nutrition–related costs. Falcone and Warner [28] suggested a period of at least 1 year to allow for intestinal adaptation. Some patients, however, require earlier intervention. The major goal of any operative intervention is to increase intestinal absorptive capacity, which can be accomplished by increasing transit time, improving the function of the remaining bowel, or increasing the mucosal surface area of the bowel.

Operative approaches designed to slow intestinal transit include colonic interpositions, reversed small bowel segments, intestinal valves, intestinal pacing, and recirculating loops. Because of discouraging results and

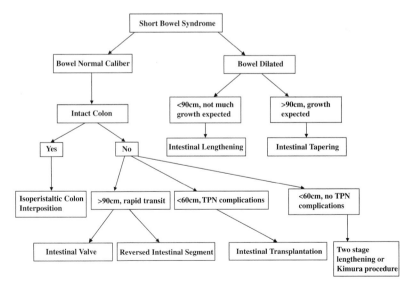

Fig. 3. Algorithm for the surgical management of patients with SBS. (*From* Falcone RA Jr, Warner BW. Short bowel syndrome. In: Ziegler MM, Azizkhan RG, Weber TR, editors. Operative pediatric surgery. New York: McGraw-Hill; 2003. p. 711; with permission.)

prohibitive morbidity, recirculating loops probably should not be performed. Colonic interpositions involve placing a segment of colon in continuity with the small intestine in either an isoperistaltic or antiperistaltic direction. Because the basic colonic rhythm is slower, intestinal transit time is increased [27]. The interposed colon also absorbs water, electrolytes, and nutrients. Colonic interposition is a good option in patients who have normal small bowel caliber and colon length.

Reversed small bowel segments also increase intestinal transit time. Proximally placed segments can result in a stagnant loop and accentuate malabsorption of fat-soluble vitamins and lipids [28]. The length of segment is critical. Although 10 cm has been used on average in adults, infants have had good results with as little as 3 cm being reversed.

Surgically created valves attempt to mimic the ileocecal valve. Valves create a partial obstruction and induce hypertrophy of all layers of the bowel wall, including the mucosa [29]. Intestinal valves are most commonly created as part of a staged intestinal lengthening procedure.

Reversed electrical intestinal pacing has been shown to improve net water absorption in experimental animals [30]. Only one human report of intestinal pacing is known, which showed no improvement [28].

Other procedures aim to normalize motility. Localized segments of dysmotile bowel should be resected. Mechanical causes of bowel dilation should be corrected. If the bowel is dilated but the inherent motility is retained, peristalsis may be improved by either tapering or plication [28].

Expanding the surface area allows more mucosal contact with lumenal nutrients. One way to expand surface area is to place bowel back in continuity. The downside to restoring continuity, however, may be prolonged diarrhea with perianal irritation. Bianchi [31] described a bowel lengthening procedure in 1980 that took advantage of the fact that the mesenteric blood supply bifurcates before entering the intestinal wall. In this procedure, dilated small bowel is divided along the long axis into two tubes. This procedure increases the overall length of the bowel and improves peristalsis. Chahine and Ricketts [32] described a modification of the Bianchi procedure that requires only one anastomosis. Overall, the results from these procedures are good, although some patients experience recurrent dilatation and patients who have motility disorders may experience complications related to stasis [27]. Kimura and Soper [33] described a two-stage procedure for bowel lengthening based on the blood supply being parasitized from the abdominal wall or liver. Clinical experience with this technique is limited.

Another approach to increasing mucosal surface area is neomucosa, which is mucosa grown from areas of normal bowel to adjacent surfaces. Initially the growth of neomucosa begins by lateral movement of columnar epithelial cells. Eventually complete coverage occurs, including villi and smooth muscle. This technique has been performed only in animal models.

The most recently described bowel lengthening procedure is the serial transverse enteroplasty. Described by Kim and colleagues [34], a gastrointestinal stapler is applied transversely onto the bowel in partially overlapping fashion from alternating and opposite directions to create a zigzag-like channel. Initial animal studies showed that animals gained weight and bowel length remained significantly longer than control bowel at harvest. Initial clinical experience with this procedure has been favorable [35].

In patients who have SBS who do not have sufficiently dilated bowel for the previously mentioned lengthening procedures, sequential lengthening procedures have been described [27]. At the initial operation, a nipple valve is created to induce bowel dilation. Once sufficient dilation ensues, a lengthening procedure can be performed.

Intestinal transplantation might be considered the ultimate surgical treatment for SBS. With advances in immunosuppressive therapy and operative technique over the past decade, intestinal transplantation has become clinically feasible [36]. Indications for intestinal transplantation in patients who have SBS include recurrent catheter sepsis, loss of venous access, and total parenteral nutrition–induced end-stage liver disease. Contraindications for transplant include active systemic infection and incurable malignancies [37]. Current patient and graft survival rates are 73% and 60% at 1 year, 58% and 50% at 3 years, and 45% and 37% at 5 years, respectively.

Meckel's diverticulum

The embryologic midgut is open to the yolk sac, which grows slower than the rest of the embryo. As a result of this growth differential, the connection becomes elongated and narrow and is termed the "omphalomesenteric duct" or the "vitelline duct." Usually this structure disappears by gestational week 9. When there is a persistence of this structure, several omphalomesenteric duct derived anomalies may occur, of which Meckel's diverticulum is the most common [38].

Anatomically, this structure is located within 75 cm of the ileocecal valve in 75% of cases. The vascular supply to a Meckel's diverticulum is a vestige of the vitelline artery and arises directly from the mesentery [38,39]. There is ectopic gastric and pancreatic mucosa found in a Meckel's diverticulum in 95% of resected specimens for gastrointestinal bleeding and in 30% to 65% of asymptomatic patients [39].

Presentation

Researchers estimate that approximately 2% of the population has a Meckel's diverticulum. Most individuals remain asymptomatic, with only 4% to 35% developing symptoms [40–42]. The symptoms that occur are primarily related to the presence of ectopic mucosa (bleeding, inflammation), fixation to the abdominal wall (bowel obstruction), or

patency of the duct. Most symptoms develop within the first 2 years of life
(Fig. 4).

Diagnosis

Attempts to diagnose a Meckel's diverticulum are usually in the setting
of symptoms. Most commonly, the clinical setting is bleeding or chronic
abdominal pain. Plain radiographs are of limited value. With improvements
in technology, ultrasonography and CT scans may demonstrate an acutely
inflamed diverticulum [43]. A commonly used test in a child with a lower
gastrointestinal bleed is a technetium 99m pertechnetate isotope scan, which
permits the visualization of ectopic gastric mucosa [44]. Ranitidine may
increase the sensitivity of the test [44,45]. Some authors recommend
laparoscopy as a more sensitive tool. In a child who continues to bleed in
the face of a negative result on a Meckel's scan, laparoscopic examination
may be indicated.

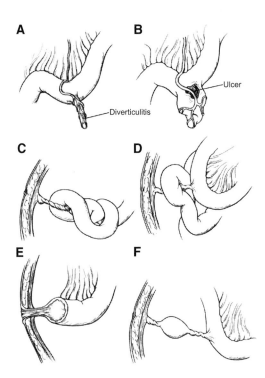

Fig. 4. Omphalomesenteric remnants. (*A*) Meckel's diverticulum with diverticulitis. (*B*) Meckel's diverticulum with ulceration and hemorrhage. (*C,D*) Bowel obstruction from volvulus
around attachments to the abdominal wall. (*E*) Patent omphalomesenteric duct. (*F*) Omphalomesenteric sinus and cyst. (*From* Sawin RS. Appendix and Meckel's diverticulum. In: Oldham
KT, Colombani PM, Foglia RP, et al, editors. Principles and practice of pediatric surgery. Philadelphia: Lippincott Williams and Wilkins; 2005. p. 1279; with permission.)

Treatment

In the symptomatic patient, there is no disagreement about treatment. Surgical resection is curative. An open operation may be chosen depending on the age of the patient and the indication. In infants with drainage from the umbilicus, a small umbilical exploration usually suffices. Laparoscopic approaches have become popular in the treatment of Meckel's diverticula. In most cases the diverticulum and attached ileum can be exteriorized via the umbilical port site for an extracorporeal resection. When possible, it is easier simply to remove the diverticulum. In cases of bleeding, it is mandatory to examine the adjoining segment of ileum, because the site of bleeding is usually in that location.

The management of an asymptomatic or incidental Meckel's diverticulum is more controversial [46]. A wide diverticulum with a thick palpable end is considered to have ectopic mucosa and should be removed [41,42]. Some authors have attempted to calculate an index based on the surface area of the patient as related to the dimensions of the Meckel's diverticulum [47]. The recommendations from a recent large cohort study were to perform incidental diverticulectomy in young patients (children), for large diverticula, and in the presence of abnormal (heterotopic) tissue [41]. One author recently reported the use of a Meckel's diverticulum as a Mitrofanoff in a patient with a previous appendectomy [48]. Thus, there may be value in preserving an asymptomatic Meckel's diverticulum.

References

[1] Ravitch MM, Barton BA. The need for pediatric surgeons as determined by the volume of work and mode of delivery of surgical care. Surgery 1974;76(5):754–63.

[2] Forrester MB, Merz RD. Population-based study of small intestinal atresia and stenosis, Hawaii, 1986–2000. Public Health 2004;118(6):434–8.

[3] Tam PK, Nicholls G. Implications of antenatal diagnosis of small-intestinal atresia in the 1990s. Pediatr Surg Int 1999;15(7):486–7.

[4] Basu R, Burge DM. The effect of antenatal diagnosis on the management of small bowel atresia. Pediatr Surg Int 2004;20(3):177–9.

[5] Surana R, Puri P. Small intestinal atresia: effect on fetal nutrition. J Pediatr Surg 1994;29(9): 1250–2.

[6] Louw JH, Barnard CN. Congenital intestinal atresia: observation on its origin. Lancet 1955; 269(6899):1065–7.

[7] Werler MM, Sheehan JE, Mitchell AA. Association of vasoconstrictive exposures with risks of gastroschisis and small intestinal atresia. Epidemiology 2003;14(3):349–54.

[8] Puri P, Fujimoto T. New observations on the pathogenesis of multiple intestinal atresias. J Pediatr Surg 1988;23(3):221–5.

[9] Gillick J, Giles S, Bannigan S, et al. Midgut atresias result from abnormal development of the notochord in an adriamycin rat model. J Pediatr Surg 2002;37(5):719–22.

[10] Kumaran N, Shankar KR, Lloyd DA, et al. Trends in the management and outcome of jejuno-ileal atresia. Eur J Pediatr Surg 2002;12(3):163–7.

[11] Garcia Vazquez A, Cano Novillo I, Benavent Gordo MI, et al. Jejunal diaphragm: laparoscopic treatment in newborns. Cir Pediatr 2004;17(2):101–3.

[12] Kluth D, Kaestner M, Tibboel D, et al. Rotation of the gut: fact or fantasy? J Pediatr Surg 1995;30(3):448–53.

[13] Skandalakis JE, Gray SW, Ricketts R, et al. The small intestines. In: Skandalakis JE, Gray SW, editors. Embryology for surgeons. 2nd edition. Baltimore: Williams & Wilkins; 1994. p. 184–241.

[14] Weinberger E, Winters WD, Liddell RM, et al. Sonographic diagnosis of intestinal malrotation in infants: importance of relative positions of the superior mesenteric vein and artery. AJR Am J Roentgenol 1992;159(4):825–8.

[15] Dufour D, Delaet MH, Dassonville M, et al. Midgut malrotation, the reliability of sonographic diagnosis. Pediatr Radiol 1992;22(1):21–3.

[16] Waldhausen JH, Sawin RS. Laparoscopic Ladd's procedure and assessment of malrotation. J Laparoendosc Surg 1996;6(Suppl 1):103–5.

[17] Gross E, Chen MK, Lobe TE. Laparoscopic evaluation and treatment of intestinal malrotation in infants. Surg Endosc 1996;10(9):936–7.

[18] Bass KD, Rothenberg SS, Chang JH. Laparoscopic Ladd's procedure in infants with malrotation. J Pediatr Surg 1998;33(2):279–81.

[19] Malek MM, Burd RS. Surgical treatment of malrotation after infancy: a population-based study. J Pediatr Surg 2005;40(1):285–9.

[20] Malek MM, Burd RS. The optimal management of malrotation diagnosed after infancy: a decision analysis. Am J Surg 2006;191:45–51.

[21] Falcone RA Jr, Warner BW. Short bowel syndrome. In: Oldham KT, Colombani PM, Foglia RP, et al, editors. Principles and practice of pediatric surgery. Philadelphia: Lippincott Williams and Wilkins; 2005. p. 1207–17.

[22] Vanderhoof JA, Young RJ. Enteral nutrition in short bowel syndrome. Semin Pediatr Surg 2001;10(2):65–71.

[23] Kollman KA, Lien EL, Vanderhoof JA. Dietary lipids influence intestinal adaptation following massive bowel resection. J Pediatr Gastroenterol Nutr 1999;28(1):41–5.

[24] Kelly DA. Liver complications of pediatric parenteral nutrition: epidemiology. Nutrition 1998;14(1):8–15.

[25] Schwartz MZ, Kuenzler KA. Pharmacotherapy and growth factors in the treatment of short bowel syndrome. Semin Pediatr Surg 2001;10(2):81–90.

[26] Jeppesen PB, Saun M, Tjellesen L, et al. Effect of intravenous ranitidine and omeprazole on intestinal absorption of water, sodium, and macronutrients in patients with intestinal resection. Gut 1998;43(6):763–9.

[27] Vernon AH, Georgeson KE. Surgical options for short bowel syndrome. Semin Pediatr Surg 2001;10(2):91–8.

[28] Falcone RA Jr, Warner BW. Short bowel syndrome. In: Ziegler MM, Azizkhan RG, Weber TR, editors. Operative pediatric surgery. New York: McGraw-Hill; 2003. p. 699–712.

[29] Collins J III, Vicente Y, Georgeson K, et al. Partial intestinal obstruction induces substantial mucosal proliferation in the pig. J Pediatr Surg 1996;31(3):415–9.

[30] Sawchuk A, Nogami W, Goto S, et al. Reverse electrical pacing improves intestinal absorption and transit time. Surgery 1986;100(2):454–60.

[31] Bianchi A. Intestinal loop lengthening: a technique for increasing small intestinal length. J Pediatr Surg 1980;12(2):145–51.

[32] Chahine AA, Ricketts RR. A modification of the Bianchi intestinal lengthening procedure with a single anastomosis. J Pediatr Surg 1998;33(8):1292–3.

[33] Kimura K, Soper RT. A new bowel elongation technique for the short-bowel syndrome using the isolated bowel segment Iowa models. J Pediatr Surg 1993;28(6):792–4.

[34] Kim HB, Fauza D, Garza J, et al. Serial transverse enteroplasty (STEP): a novel bowel lengthening procedure. J Pediatr Surg 2003;38(3):425–9.

[35] Javid PJ, Kim HB, Duggan CP, et al. Serial transverse enteroplasty is associated with successful short-term outcomes in infants with short bowel syndrome. J Pediatr Surg 2005;40(6):1019–24.

[36] Reyes J. Intestinal transplantation for children with short bowel syndrome. Semin Pediatr Surg 2001;10(2):99–104.

[37] Schwartz MZ, Prasad R. Intestine transplantation. In: Ziegler MM, Azizkhan RG, Weber TR, editors. Operative pediatric surgery. New York: McGraw-Hill; 2003. p. 1287–95.

[38] Sawin RS. Appendix and Meckel's diverticulum. In: Oldham KT, Colombani PM, Foglia RP, et al, editors. Principles and practice of pediatric surgery. Philadelphia: Lippincott Williams and Wilkins; 2005. p. 1269–82.

[39] Brown RL, Azizkhan RG. Gastrointestinal bleeding in infants and children: Meckel's diverticulum and intestinal duplication. Semin Pediatr Surg 1999;8(4):202–9.

[40] Vane DW, West KW, Grosfeld JL. Vitelline duct anomalies: experience with 217 childhood cases. Arch Surg 1987;122(5):542–7.

[41] Park JJ, Wolff BG, Tollefson MK, et al. Meckel's diverticulum: the Mayo Clinic experience with 1476 patients (1950–2002). Ann Surg 2005;241(3):529–33.

[42] Cullen JJ, Kelly KA, Moir CR, et al. Surgical management of Meckel's diverticulum: an epidemiologic, population based study. Ann Surg 1994;220(4):564–8.

[43] Baldisserotto M. Color Doppler sonographic findings of inflamed and perforated Meckel's diverticulum. J Ultrasound Med 2004;23(6):843–8.

[44] Poulsen KA, Qvist N. Sodium pertechnetate scintigraphy in detection of Meckel's diverticulum: is it usable? Eur J Pediatr Surg 2000;10(4):228–31.

[45] Rerksuppaphol S, Hutson JM, Oliver MR. Ranitidine enhanced 99m technetium pertechnetate imaging in children improves the sensitivity of identifying heterotopic gastric mucosa in Meckel's diverticulum. Pediatr Surg Int 2004;20(5):323–5.

[46] Soltero MJ, Bill AH. The natural history of Meckel's diverticulum and its relation to incidental removal: a study of 202 cases of diseased Meckel's diverticulum found in King County, Washington, over a fifteen year period. Am J Surg 1976;132(2):168–73.

[47] Karabulut R, Sonmez K, Turkyilmaz Z, et al. A new index for resection of Meckel's diverticula in children. Scand J Gastroenterol 2004;39(8):789–90.

[48] Boemers TM. Mitrofanoff procedure with Meckel's diverticulum. BJU Int 2001;88(7): 799–800.

ELSEVIER
SAUNDERS

Surg Clin N Am 86 (2006) 301–316

SURGICAL
CLINICS OF
NORTH AMERICA

Hindgut Abnormalities

Stanley T. Lau, MD, Michael G. Caty, MD*

Women and Children's Hospital of Buffalo, 219 Bryant Street, Buffalo, NY 14222, USA

Hindgut abnormalities encompass a broad range of congenital defects. This article focuses on defects in intestinal innervation and anorectal malformations. This article also touches on suppurative diseases as they pertain to pediatric surgery. During the last several decades, significant advances have been made in the understanding and treatment of Hirschsprung's disease and intestinal neuronal dysplasia as well as in the correction of anorectal malformations. The main aim of the surgical treatment for these patients is to create a reconstructed anatomy that functions as close to normal as possible, while treating the functional sequelae of these defects in an attempt to provide these children with a good quality of life.

Embryology

During the third week of gestation, the embryo undergoes cephalocaudal and lateral infolding, leading to the incorporation of the endoderm into the embryo and the formation of the primitive gut. The hindgut ultimately forms the distal third of the transverse colon, the descending colon, the sigmoid, the rectum, and the upper part of the anal canal. The endodermal lining of the hindgut also forms the internal lining of the bladder and urethra.

The end of the hindgut enters into the cloaca, an endoderm-lined cavity that is in direct contact with the surface ectoderm. The cloacal membrane forms the contact area between the endoderm and ectoderm. Classic teaching of human embryology describes the division of the cloaca by the descent of the urorectal septum separating the urogenital sinus and the hindgut at about 6 weeks of gestation. However, recent studies have demonstrated a separate primitive urogenital sinus and an anorectum as early as the fourth week of gestation [1,2]. Furthermore, the urorectal septum does not actively descend in humans. The cloaca remains intact as a single cavity until the

---

* Corresponding author.
E-mail address: caty@ascu.buffalo.edu (M.G. Caty).

0039-6109/06/$ - see front matter © 2006 Elsevier Inc. All rights reserved.
doi:10.1016/j.suc.2006.01.002

cloacal membrane ruptures through apoptotic cell death. The dorsal aspect of the cloaca becomes part of the amniotic cavity, and the tip of the urorectal septum becomes the perineal body. The anorectal canal later occludes due to adhesion and subsequent epithelial plugging and is then recanalized through apoptotic cell death.

The anal membrane is surrounded by an ectodermal depression, known as the anal dimple or the proctodeum. During the eighth week, the anal membrane ruptures and forms a patent anal canal. Thus, the upper portion of the anal canal is formed from endodermal origins and is supplied by the inferior mesenteric artery, which is the blood supply for the hindgut. The lower third of the anal canal comes from ectodermal origins and is supplied by the rectal arteries, which are branches of the internal pudendal artery. The pectinate line marks the junction between the endodermal and ectodermal parts [3].

The circular muscle of the hindgut forms at the caudal end by the ninth week of gestation, spreading over the entire colon by the tenth week. The ganglion cells of the myenteric plexus reach the colon during the seventh week and complete innervation occurs by the twelfth week. The longitudinal muscle fibers appear at the anal canal by the end of the tenth week, progressing cranially up to the cecum by the eleventh week [3,4].

Anatomy

The colon can be divided into the cecum and the ascending, transverse, descending, and sigmoid colon. The arterial supply arises from the superior and inferior mesenteric arteries. The marginal arteries connect the branches of these two arteries, extending from the ileocolic junction to the distal sigmoid colon.

The rectum is the terminal end of the colon, beginning anterior to the level of the third sacral vertebra and extending to the anal canal. The inferior mesenteric artery feeds the superior rectal artery, which supplies the superior portion of the rectum. The middle rectal arteries are branches of the internal iliac arteries, and supply the middle and inferior portions of the rectum. The inferior rectal arteries supply the inferior portion of the rectum and arise from the internal pudendal arteries.

The anal canal extends from the anorectal junction to the anal verge. The lining is comprised of different types of epithelium at various levels. As the rectum merges into the anal canal, the tissue forms longitudinal folds known as the columns of Morgagni. The anal glands are found at the distal end of these folds, emptying into the anal crypts located between the columns of Morgagni.

The mucosa of the upper anal canal is lined by columnar epithelium. However, over the area of the dentate line, the lining transitions from columnar to squamous epithelium. This transition area is known as the cloacogenic zone. Below the cloacogenic zone, the anoderm extends to the anal verge. This anoderm is analogous to skin, although it lacks accessory skin structures. The true skin begins at the anal verge [5].

The classic anatomic teaching of the pelvic floor musculature describes a funnel-shaped pelvic diaphragm comprised of individual muscles, including the two coccygeous muscles as well as the levator ani muscles, which are divided into three parts. These are the puborectalis, the pubococcygeous, and the iliococcygeous muscles. Recent advances in surgical techniques used in hindgut reconstruction have shown that these distinctions are in fact artificial (Fig. 1). Instead, these muscles are continuous and surround the rectum in a funnel-shaped structure and extends parallel to the rectum down to the perianal skin. The external sphincter is comprised of parasagittal muscle fibers that meet anterior and posterior to the anus. These fibers are joined by fibers running parallel to the rectum. These fibers are perpendicular to the parasagittal fibers and join the upper portion of the muscle structure, or the levator muscle. These perpendicular fibers define the anterior and posterior borders of the anus [6,7].

Innervation of the hindgut involves both the sympathetic and parasympathetic nervous systems. The first three lumbar segments supply the sympathetic innervation to the rectum, with fibers running through the sympathetic chain and along the preaortic plexus, extending to the upper rectum via the inferior mesenteric plexus. The parasympathetic innervation derives from the nervi erigentes, which come from the second, third, and fourth sacral nerves. Motor innervation of the internal sphincter also involves both the sympathetic and the parasympathetic systems. The anorectal muscle complex extending from the levator to the external sphincter is

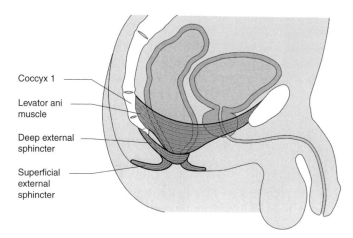

Fig. 1. Normal relationship of the levator ani to the deep and superficial external sphincters. (*Adapted from* deVries PA, Pena A. Posterior sagittal anorectoplasty. J Pediatr Surg 1982;17:642.)

supplied by the internal pudendal nerve and the fourth sacral nerve. The cutaneous sensation of the perianal area and anal canal distal to the dentate line runs along the inferior rectal nerves [5].

Physiology

The normal colonic motility produces a slow transit that facilitates fluid absorption and a mass movement that aids in defecation. Local segmental contractions slowly move the feces forward, peristaltic contractions produce both retrograde and slow forward movement, and mass contractions empty long segments of the colon in a forward fashion.

Intestinal contents typically reach the colon in about 3 to 6 hours, entering the cecum in a liquid state. Within the next 24 hours, the feces reach the rectum and become solid. The rectosigmoid colon acts as a reservoir, holding the fecal material for variable periods of time. As the rectal contents move distally, the sensory ability of the anal canal allows the individual to voluntarily relax or contract the voluntary sphincter, maintaining continence or allowing gas or stool to escape.

Fecal continence depends on muscle structures, sensation, and bowel motility. The primary muscles involved are the internal anal sphincter and the muscle complex extending from the levator to the external sphincter. Sensory afferents are located in the anal mucosa, providing pain, touch, temperature, and pressure sensations.

The internal anal sphincter is predominantly a slow-twitch, fatigue-resistant smooth muscle. At rest, this muscle contracts with a frequency of 15 to 35 cycles per minute, contributing 70% to 85% of the resting sphincter pressure. The percent contribution of the internal anal sphincter decreases during rectal distention as the muscle reflexively relaxes. This intrinsic neural reflex stems from an intrinsic innervation located in the intramural plexuses and the myenteric and submucosal ganglia [8]. Thus, the internal anal sphincter is primarily responsible for maintaining anal continence at rest [9].

The voluntary muscle complex extends from the levator to the external sphincter. As the involuntary peristaltic contraction of the rectosigmoid pushes the fecal mass into the anorectal area, the individual will voluntarily relax these muscles and allow the contents to migrate into the sensitive anal canal. Normal individuals have an exquisitely sensitive anal canal that can provide a wealth of information regarding stool consistency and amount, differentiating between gas, liquid, and solid. The voluntary muscles can push the rectal contents back into the rectosigmoid for storage until a socially acceptable time. When defecation is desired, the individual relaxes the voluntary muscles, allowing passage of the stool into the anorectum.

The emptying of the rectosigmoid is primarily driven by peristaltic contractions that can be augmented with a Valsalva maneuver. If this motility is impaired, as in most patients with anorectal malformations, a megarectum can develop. The resulting hypomotility leads to severe constipation and the development of overflow incontinence.

Hirschsprung's disease

In 1888 Harold Hirschsprung, a pediatrician from Copenhagen, described the autopsies of two infants who died of congenital megacolon. Although the condition had been described previously, Hirschsprung's name became attached to the disease that is characterized by an absence of ganglion cells in the affected portion of the hindgut [3]. This defect includes the myenteric Auerbach's plexus, the deep submucosal Henle's plexus, and the submucosal Meissner's plexus. The result is a physiologic obstruction at the level of the aganglionic segment. At birth, the infant is constipated, without evidence of physical obstruction. With time, secondary dilation and hypertrophy of the colon develops above the narrowed distal abnormal portion.

Approximately 1 in 5000 newborns are born with Hirschsprung's disease, with 80% of them male [10]. There is some hereditary factor, with an overall risk to a sibling of 4%. The extent of aganglionosis varies, with the internal anal sphincter involved in all cases and the entire rectum involved in most cases. However, the longer the aganglionic segment, the higher the risk to siblings and the lower the ratio of males to females affected. The risk to siblings is highest and the ratio closest to even with total aganglionosis of the colon (ie, Zuelzer-Wilson syndrome). Furthermore, a mother with colonic aganglionosis is more likely to transmit the disease than the father [11].

While description of the anatomy and physiology of Hirschsprung's disease has improved tremendously over recent years, the etiology remains elusive. The role of genetic defects has become more important in providing insight into this disease. To date, nine gene mutations have been associated with Hirschsprung's disease, including RET, GDNF, NRTN, EDNRB, EDN3, ECE-1, PHOX2b, SOX10, and ZFHX1B [12,13]. The RET gene is the major gene involved in the development of the disease, but all of these genes are required early in the development of the enteric nervous system. However, the abnormalities in these genes only account for about 50% of the cases of Hirschsprung's disease. The precise mechanism by which these genes cause this defect is not well understood. Perhaps many mutations lead to the same end point in Hirschsprung's disease, or perhaps all of the genes are necessary for differentiation of early precursors of enteric neurons. A loss in the function of any of these genes might lead to a pan-neuronal lesion resulting in aganglionosis [12].

Most children with Hirschsprung's disease present with intestinal obstruction or severe constipation during the neonatal period. The symptoms typically include failure to pass meconium within the first 24 hours of life, abdominal distention, and vomiting. This presentation is a spectrum that ranges from minimal symptoms developing within the first weeks or months of life to complete neonatal intestinal obstruction. Children diagnosed later in life often have a long history of constipation, enterocolitis, and frequently develop growth retardation [11].

In a patient suspected of having Hirschsprung's disease, a contrast enema should be administered. A digital rectal exam or a rectal irrigation should be withheld before the contrast enema, as these maneuvers might lead to a false-negative radiologic result. The classic contrast enema shows either a normal caliber or narrowed rectum with a dilated transition zone into a dilated proximal colon. Retention of the contrast medium in the colon for longer than 24 hours is also suggestive of the diagnosis.

Anorectal manometry offers another diagnostic modality, with accuracy reported as high as 85% [11,14]. In normal individuals, inflation of a rectal balloon distends the rectum and causes relaxation of the internal sphincter. In patients with Hirschsprung's disease, the pressure curve of the anal canal and distal rectum has characteristic changes that include a multisegmental rhythmic contraction with a lack of internal sphincter relaxation.

The official diagnosis of Hirschsprung's disease should be made histologically with a rectal biopsy. The characteristic appearance includes an absence of ganglion cells in the myenteric and submucosal plexuses as well as the presence of hypertrophied nerve trunks in the space normally occupied by the ganglion cells [15].

The first surgical treatment for Hirschsprung's disease was a diverting colostomy. While this was a life-saving maneuver, it was an undesirable long-term solution. Before our understanding of the disease improved, early unsuccessful attempts were made to remove the dilated abnormal-appearing colon. In 1946, Ehrenpreis suggested that the proximal colonic dilation was due to a distal obstruction [16]. The theory that the distal colon was the abnormal segment was confirmed in 1948 when Whitehouse and Kernohan described a lack of ganglion cells in the distal nondilated colon [17].

In 1948, Swenson and Bill described an operation known today as the Swenson procedure, involving removal of the aganglionic portion of the colon and rectum. They first performed this operation on a 6-year-old child who had previously undergone a diverting colostomy. Later, Duhamel described the use of a retrorectal anastamosis, and Soave developed the endorectal pull-through [18,19]. The Duhamel and Soave procedures theoretically offer less risk to the neurovascular plexus surrounding the rectum.

Traditionally, all three procedures have been performed in two or three stages. The first stage is a leveling colostomy or ileostomy, with intraoperative biopsies performed to determine the level of the transition zone from ganglionated to aganglionated colon. The second stage is performed between 3 to 12 months of age. At this operation, the ganglionated bowel is anastamosed to the anus. If a protecting proximal stoma is performed, then a third stage is planned to close the stoma.

Recently, many surgeons have moved toward performing a single-stage pull-through. So and colleagues first described the single-stage pull-through in 1980 [20,21], and since then the single-stage repair has been performed using the Swenson [22], Soave [23,24–26], and Duhamel [27–29] repairs as well as laparoscopically [30–33] and with a transanal [24,25,29] approach (Figs. 2 and 3).

Despite the growing volume of literature supporting the safety and efficacy of performing an open or laparoscopic single-stage definitive procedure, there is still a role for a multistaged approach. A single-stage procedure is contraindicated in patients with associated life-threatening anomalies, an overall deterioration of general health, severe enterocolitis, or a severe dilation of the proximal bowel [33]. In these patients, the surgeon should use a multistaged approach with a leveling colostomy followed by a definitive operation later. The presence of a pathologist capable of identifying ganglion cells on frozen section is also required to carry out the one-stage technique.

While recent advances in critical care and the early diagnosis of both Hirschsprung's disease and enterocolitis have lowered the impact of Hirschsprung's-associated enterocolitis, enterocolitis remains the major source of morbidity and mortality in Hirschsprung's disease [34,35]. The incidence of Hirschsprung's-associated enterocolitis is approximately 25%, occurring before surgical intervention as well as in the immediate postoperative period and several years after a definitive operation [35]. Swenson and colleagues reported a higher risk of developing enterocolitis within the first year after a definitive operation with 92% of these patients developing enterocolitis within 2 years [36]. Several risk factors for Hirschsprung's-associated enterocolitis have been described, including a delay in diagnosis of Hirschsprung's disease beyond 1 week of age, the presence of trisomy 21, and postoperative anastamotic complications, such as a stricture or a leak. Other studies have suggested an increased incidence of enterocolitis with a long

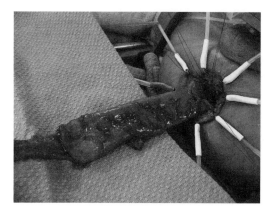

Fig. 2. Incisionless pull-through with transanal mobilization of full-thickness rectum.

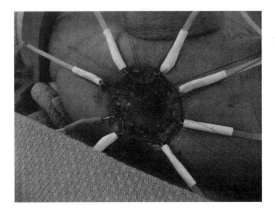

Fig. 3. Incisionless pull-through with a finished anastamosis.

segment of aganglionosis, a genetic predisposition, and with previous episodes of enterocolitis [35].

In patients with Hirschsprung's-associated enterocolitis, decompression of the bowel must be achieved in a timely fashion. This decompression is often possible with the use of a nasogastric tube as well as repeated rectal irrigations. The irrigations should be repeated two to three times per day until decompression has been achieved. This regimen can often provide a conservative management method until a definitive surgical procedure can be performed. If adequate intestinal decompression cannot be achieved using a nasogastric tube and rectal irrigations, the surgeon should perform a laparotomy with a leveling colostomy just proximal to the transition zone. A definitive operative procedure can be performed once the patient has recovered from the enterocolitis.

Intestinal neuronal dysplasia

Intestinal neuronal dysplasia (IND) is a clinical entity that resembles Hirschsprung's disease. First described in 1971, IND was further characterized in 1983 by Fadda and colleagues [37] into two separate subtypes. Type A occurs in less than 5% of cases and involves a congenital aplasia or hypoplasia of the sympathetic innervation. Type B occurs in over 95% of cases and is characterized by a defect in the parasympathetic submucosal and myenteric plexuses. Histologically, a biopsy specimen shows hyperganglionosis of the submucosal and myenteric plexuses with giant ganglia, ectopic ganglion cells in the lamina propria, and an increased acetylcholinesterase (AChE) activity in the mucosa, muscularis mucosa, and surrounding submucosal vessels. Clinically, both types of IND present in the neonatal period with intestinal obstruction and bloody diarrhea [15,38].

Since its first description, the histologic diagnosis of IND has been controversial. This confusion was due in part to the age-dependent changes in the histologic appearance of the enteric nervous system. Currently, the accepted histologic criteria include the presence of hyperganglionosis and giant ganglia as well as the presence of at least one of the following: ectopic ganglia in the lamina propria, increased AChE-positive nerve fibers around the submucosal blood vessels, and increased AChE-positive nerve fibers in the lamina propria. One must keep in mind, though, that hyperganglionosis can be a normal finding in a newborn [37,39,40].

The mainstay treatment for IND is conservative management with laxatives and enemas. In the majority of patients, the clinical manifestations resolve over time or at least are manageable. If conservative management fails after a period of time (ie, at least 6 months), then the surgeon should consider an internal sphincter myectomy. One rarely needs to resort to a resection and pull-through operation [37].

Recently, several different animal models have been developed that demonstrate submucosal plexus abnormalities similar to that seen in human IND. Two different Hox11L1 knockout mouse models were shown to have clinical, histological, and immunohistochemical characteristics similar to IND patients. However, analysis of this gene in human IND patients did not show any mutation [37]. Another mouse model involving a heterozygous mutation in the endothelin B receptor was recently shown to resemble IND patients [37,41]. While no clear genetic link has been defined yet, these studies suggest that the etiology of IND may lie in a genetic defect.

Anorectal malformations

The first description of imperforate anus was by Aristotle, who described the condition of an imperforate anus with a rectourethral fistula in a cow. In the seventh century, Paul of Aegina, a Byzantine physician, successfully incised the perineum of an infant born without an anus [3]. In 1835, Jean-Zulema Amussat described the dissection of the perineum with mobilization of the end of the rectum to the skin, emphasizing the necessity of mucosal continuity with the skin [3].

Imperforate anus occurs in 1 out of every 4000 to 5000 live births [42–44], most commonly with a rectourethral fistula in boys and a rectovestibular fistula in girls [45]. Previously, imperforate anus with a rectovaginal fistula was considered a relatively common defect. In retrospect, these malformations were likely either a misdiagnosed rectovestibular fistula or a persistent cloacal malformation, where the urinary tract, vagina, and rectum form a common channel. In fact, a true rectovaginal fistula is quite rare, occurring in less than 1% of all cases [46]. Imperforate anus occurring without a fistula occurs in only about 5% of patients [42]. The incidence of a subsequent sibling also having an anorectal malformation is approximately 1% [42,47,48].

Male defects

Imperforate anus with a rectourethral fistula is the most common defect in male patients. The fistula is located at the lower (ie, bulbar) or upper (ie, prostatic) urethra. The anorectal muscle complex is typically well developed in patients with rectobulbar fistulas. They also usually have a well-formed sacrum, a prominent midline groove, and a prominent anal dimple. In contrast, boys with a rectoprostatic fistula are more likely to have poorly developed musculature, an abnormal sacrum, and a flat perineum (ie, a poor midline groove with only a subtle anal dimple).

The fistulas associated with imperforate anus can also extend to the perineum (ie, cutaneous fistula) or to the bladder neck. The rectum of patients with a rectoperineal fistula is located within most of the sphincter mechanism, and only the most distal portion of the rectum is anteriorly misplaced. Imperforate anus with a rectovesical fistula to the bladder neck is the most common "high" defect, and occurs in about 10% of all male patients. These patients have a poorly developed anorectal muscle complex as well as an abnormal sacrum. Because the rectum of these patients is unreachable through a posterior sagittal incision, an abdominal approach must be added to the posterior sagittal incision. Imperforate anus without a fistula is more commonly associated with trisomy 21. These patients typically have a well-developed sacrum and good muscles with the rectum ending about 2 cm from the perineal skin [45,42].

Recently, Georgeson and colleagues [49] described a new technique of a laparoscopically assisted anorectal pull-through for the repair of a high imperforate anus. A laparoscopic dissection of the rectum is performed, dividing the fistula to the genitourinary tract. The bowel is then retracted out of the pelvis, allowing clear visualization of the pelvic musculature. The external perineum is inspected using transcutaneous electrostimulation and the limits of the proposed anal opening are determined. Through a small external perineal incision at this site, the intrasphincteric plane is bluntly dissected toward the light emanating from the laparoscopic light source. A Veress needle is passed under direct laparoscopic visualization into the middle of the pelvic musculature. This tract is then dilated, and the rectum is pulled through this path and an anorectal anastamosis is performed.

Rectal atresia is a rare defect occurring in 1% of all patients with an anorectal malformation. The anal canal is small but normally located, and the upper rectum is dilated. The separation of the rectum and anal canal can vary from a thin membrane to a dense fibrous tissue.

Female defects

The most common anorectal malformation in girls is imperforate anus with a rectovestibular fistula. Previously, many of these patients were misdiagnosed as having a rectovaginal fistula. Careful inspection reveals a normal urethral opening and vagina, with the fistula entering just below into the vestibule. A true rectovaginal fistula shows a fistula opening in the posterior wall of the vagina, within the hymenal ring. This malformation occurs in about 1% of all girls with anorectal malformations [46].

Girls with rectal atresia, those with imperforate anus and a rectoperineal fistula, and those with imperforate anus without a fistula are all similar to boys in both the surgical approach and the prognostic implications.

A persistent cloaca occurs once in 50,000 births [50], encompassing a spectrum of malformations with a confluence of the urinary, genital, and gastrointestinal tracts. Cloacal anomalies have a much broader range of anatomic anomalies than any other congenital malformation [51] and require a complex reconstruction.

Patients with a persistent cloaca have a common channel that empties the rectum, the vagina, and the urinary tract. At the mild end of the spectrum, the patient might have a persistent urogenital sinus, draining the vagina and bladder, with an anteriorly displaced anus adjacent to this sinus. With more severe malformations, the three tracts join in the pelvis, with varying lengths of the common channel. Low cloacal malformations with shorter channels (ie, <3 cm) are typically less complex while higher malformations with longer channels are often associated with a more complex defect requiring a more complicated surgical repair [42,45].

At birth, these children might appear to have imperforate anus and small genitalia. Careful inspection, however, reveals a single perineal orifice. If the colon is obstructed, the infant may become distended. Furthermore, as urine fills the common channel, it might flow retrograde into the vagina, distending the vagina and displacing the bladder forward. This occurs in more than 50% of the cases [52], and can lead to bladder outlet obstruction and hydronephrosis [50].

Cloacal exstrophy is a different anatomic problem than a persistent cloaca. Cloacal exstrophy was first described by Littre in 1709, but the first long-term survivor was first reported by Rickham in 1960 [53]. The incidence of this malformation is approximately 1 in every 300,000 live births [54]. The classic description of cloacal exstrophy includes an omphalocele, imperforate anus, exstrophy of two small hemibladders surrounding a lateral cecal fissure, and ambiguous genitalia. Often, the terminal ileum prolapses through the cecal fissure. The colon usually connects with the cecum and blindly ends in the pelvis.

Management

The initial management of a neonate with an anorectal malformation should include evaluations to exclude associated defects, including vertebral anomalies, cardiac malformations, esophageal atresia, and urinary defects. An echocardiogram should be obtained, as well as spine radiographs, a spinal ultrasound, and an abdominal ultrasound. As previously mentioned, a thorough perineal examination is crucial. Observation over the first 24 hours of life may be required to determine the presence or absence of a perineal fistula [52]. The intraluminal pressure of the bowel increases over this time, forcing the meconium through the fistula and allowing it to be seen on clinical examination. If one suspects a rectovesicular fistula in a male, with the presence of meconium in the urine, an abnormal sacrum, and a flat bottom, a descending colostomy should be considered. Similarly, if a persistent cloaca is identified, a colostomy is indicated. In both cases, a formal reconstruction can then be performed later.

Most pediatric surgeons now use a posterior sagittal approach to repair anorectal malformations. Recently, pediatric surgeons have increasingly favored a primary reconstruction of an anorectal malformation without a protective colostomy. An electrical stimulator is used to demonstrate muscle contraction and keep the incision in the midline. The fibers of the muscle complex are divided in the midline, and the rectum is separated from the urogenital structures. The limits of the anal canal are delineated anteriorly and posteriorly by using the electrical stimulator. The rectum and anus are then placed within the muscle complex. The perineal body is repaired and the muscle complex is reapproximated, incorporating the rectal wall at the anterior and posterior edges to avoid rectal prolapse.

A decompressive colostomy is usually required in patients with a persistent cloaca. Hendren recommends a right transverse colostomy, as a more distal colostomy could compromise a subsequent pull-through procedure or subsequent vaginal reconstruction [50,51]. Intermittent catheterization of the urogenital sinus might be needed to drain the vagina of urine and mucus in patients with hydrocolpos and resulting bladder outlet obstruction. Before attempting a definitive reconstruction, one can define the anatomy using contrast studies of the cloaca and distal limb of the colostomy. Endoscopic examination of the common channel can give valuable information about the length of the channel, as the level of the confluence can have a substantial implication for surgical repair. Magnetic resonance imaging of the spinal cord will reveal any evidence of a tethered cord, which is present in one third of persistent cloacal patients and in nearly all cloacal exstrophy patients [50].

Definitive repair of the persistent cloaca can be done between 6 and 24 months of age [50]. If the confluence of the urinary, genital, and gastrointestinal tracts occurs low (ie, common channel less than 3 cm), most surgical reconstructions can be done with a posterior sagittal approach. Higher malformations may require the addition of an abdominal approach and a vaginal reconstruction [42,45,50].

Previous efforts in the repair of a persistent cloaca involved complete separation and individual mobilization of the rectum, vagina, and urinary tract. Pena, however, described the technique of a total urogenital mobilization in patients with a low malformation and a short common channel. This maneuver involves separating the rectum from the vagina and mobilizing the vagina and urethra as a single unit, allowing a shorter operative time and avoiding some of the complications of a urethrovaginal fistula or a vaginal stricture [55]. According to Hendren, the surgeon should perform a pull-through procedure and address the genitourinary tract at the same operation because doing them separately is an onerous task [56].

As previously mentioned, a cloacal exstrophy is anatomically different from a persistent cloaca, and requires different surgical management. The gastrointestinal tract should be separated from the urinary tract, allowing the two hemibladders to be joined and closed. The omphalocele should be closed, and the divergent pubis approximated. The cecum should be separated from the bladder and closed, keeping the hindgut in continuity with the gastrointestinal tract. This rudimentary colon has the capacity to enlarge and lengthen, ultimately providing satisfactory colonic absorptive function. An end colostomy can be performed, especially in children with sacral agenesis and a lack of perineal muscle. Alternatively, a pull-through procedure could be performed either immediately or later. One should consider a protective ileostomy in either case [50]. The child will likely require further reconstruction later in life with bladder augmentation, continent diversion, and vaginal reconstruction.

Suppurative anorectal disorders

Perianal or perirectal abscesses typically occur in infants [57,65]. Usually, the infant develops a tender mass lateral to the anus. If the abscess is not fluctuant, one can manage the problem with sitz baths, but most (67%) will need surgical drainage. Approximately 20% to 40% of the perianal abscesses will develop into a fistula in ano [57–61].

A fistula in ano is a relatively common condition in infants. While not limited to the pediatric population, there are certain characteristics that distinguish it from the fistulae that occur in the adult population. A fistula in ano typically develops in male infants less than 1 year of age [57,59,60,62], developing from a progressing perianal abscess. These fistulae are rarely complex and have a low incidence of recurrence [59]. While a fistulectomy is the accepted treatment for adult patients, recent studies have shown that there may be some role for conservative treatment in infants [63,64]. Watanabe and colleagues [64] suggested that this might be a self-limiting disease that spontaneously resolves, allowing expectant management and avoidance of an operation. Most pediatric surgeons do not recommend routine fistulotomy or excision in an infant or child.

References

[1] Nievelstein RA, van der Werff JF, Verbeek FJ, et al. Normal and abnormal embryonic development of the anorectum in human embryos. Teratology 1998;57:70.

[2] Paidas CN, Morreale RF, Holoski KM, et al. Septation and differentiation of the embryonic human cloaca. J Pediatr Surg 1999;34:877.

[3] Skandalakis J, Gray S, Ricketts R. The colon and rectum. In: Skandalakis J, Gray S, editors. Embryology for surgeons. Baltimore (MD): Williams & Wilkins; 1994. p. 242.

[4] Sadler T. Langman's medical embryology. 6th edition. Baltimore (MD): Williams & Wilkins; 1990.

[5] Gordon PH. Anorectal anatomy and physiology. Gastroenterol Clin North Am 2001;30:1.

[6] deVries PA, Pena A. Posterior sagittal anorectoplasty. J Pediatr Surg 1982;17:638.

[7] Pena A, deVries PA. Posterior sagittal anorectoplasty: important technical considerations and new applications. J Pediatr Surg 1982;17:796.

[8] Weinberg G, Boley S. Anorectal continence and management of constipation. In: Ashcraft K, Holcomb G III, Murphy JP, editors. Pediatric surgery. 4th edition. Philadelphia: Elsevier Saunders; 2005. p. 518.

[9] Rao SS. Pathophysiology of adult fecal incontinence. Gastroenterology 2004;126:S14.

[10] Angrist M, Kauffman E, Slaugenhaupt SA, et al. A gene for Hirschsprung disease (megacolon) in the pericentromeric region of human chromosome 10. Nat Genet 1993;4:351.

[11] Holschneider A, Ure B. Hirschsprung's Disease. In: Ashcraft K, Holcomb G III, Murphy JP, editors. Pediatric surgery. 4th edition. Philadelphia: Elsevier Saunders; 2005. p. 447–95.

[12] Gershon MD, Ratcliffe EM. Developmental biology of the enteric nervous system: pathogenesis of Hirschsprung's disease and other congenital dysmotilities. Semin Pediatr Surg 2004;13:224.

[13] Tam PK, Garcia-Barcelo M. Molecular genetics of Hirschsprung's disease. Semin Pediatr Surg 2004;13:236.

[14] Ure BM, Holschneider AM, Meier-Ruge W. Neuronal intestinal malformations: a retro- and prospective study on 203 patients. Eur J Pediatr Surg 1994;4:279.

[15] Puri P. Hirschsprung Disease. In: Oldham K, Colombani P, Foglia R, editors. Surgery of infants and children: scientific principles and practice. Philadelphia: Lippincott-Ravin Publishers; 1997. p. 1277.

[16] Ehrenpreis T. Hirschsprung's disease. Am J Dig Dis 1971;16:1032.

[17] Whitehouse F, HKernohan J. Myenteric plexus in congenital megacolon. Arch Intern Med 1948;82:75.

[18] Duhamel B. A new operation for the treatment of Hirschsprung's disease. Arch Dis Child 1960;35:38.

[19] Soave F. A new surgical technique for treatment of Hirschsprung's disease. Surgery 1964;56: 1007.

[20] So HB, Becker JM, Schwartz DL, et al. Eighteen years' experience with neonatal Hirschsprung's disease treated by endorectal pull-through without colostomy. J Pediatr Surg 1998;33:673.

[21] So HB, Schwartz DL, Becker JM, et al. Endorectal "pull-through" without preliminary colostomy in neonates with Hirschsprung's disease. J Pediatr Surg 1980;15:470.

[22] Santos MC, Giacomantonio JM, Lau HY. Primary Swenson pull-through compared with multiple-stage pull-through in the neonate. J Pediatr Surg 1999;34:1079.

[23] De la Torre-Mondragon L, Ortega-Salgado JA. Transanal endorectal pull-through for Hirschsprung's disease. J Pediatr Surg 1998;33:1283.

[24] Langer JC, Durrant AC, de la Torre L, et al. One-stage transanal Soave pullthrough for Hirschsprung disease: a multicenter experience with 141 children. Ann Surg 2003;238: 569.

[25] Langer JC, Minkes RK, Mazziotti MV, et al. Transanal one-stage Soave procedure for infants with Hirschsprung's disease. J Pediatr Surg 1999;34:148.

[26] Langer JC, Seifert M, Minkes RK. One-stage Soave pull-through for Hirschsprung's disease: a comparison of the transanal and open approaches. J Pediatr Surg 2000;35:820.

[27] Jung PM. Hirschsprung's disease: one surgeon's experience in one institution. J Pediatr Surg 1995;30:646.

[28] Mir E, Karaca I, Gunsar C, et al. Primary Duhamel-Martin operations in neonates and infants. Pediatr Int 2001;43:405.

[29] Pierro A, Fasoli L, Kiely EM, et al. Staged pull-through for rectosigmoid Hirschsprung's disease is not safer than primary pull-through. J Pediatr Surg 1997;32:505.

[30] Georgeson KE. Laparoscopic-assisted pull-through for Hirschsprung's disease. Semin Pediatr Surg 2002;11:205.

[31] Georgeson KE, Cohen RD, Hebra A, et al. Primary laparoscopic-assisted endorectal colon pull-through for Hirschsprung's disease: a new gold standard. Ann Surg 1999;229:678.

[32] Georgeson KE, Fuenfer MM, Hardin WD. Primary laparoscopic pull-through for Hirschsprung's disease in infants and children. J Pediatr Surg 1995;30:1017.

[33] Georgeson KE, Robertson DJ. Laparoscopic-assisted approaches for the definitive surgery for Hirschsprung's disease. Semin Pediatr Surg 2004;13:256.

[34] Engum SA, Grosfeld JL. Long-term results of treatment of Hirschsprung's disease. Semin Pediatr Surg 2004;13:273.

[35] Vieten D, Spicer R. Enterocolitis complicating Hirschsprung's disease. Semin Pediatr Surg 2004;13:263.

[36] Swenson O, Sherman JO, Fisher JH, et al. The treatment and postoperative complications of congenital megacolon: a 25 year followup. Ann Surg 1975;182:266.

[37] Puri P. Intestinal neuronal dysplasia. Semin Pediatr Surg 2003;12:259.

[38] Puri P, Rolle U. Variant Hirschsprung's disease. Semin Pediatr Surg 2004;13:293.

[39] Meier-Ruge WA, Ammann K, Bruder E, et al. Updated results on intestinal neuronal dysplasia (IND B). Eur J Pediatr Surg 2004;14:384.

[40] Wester T, O'Briain DS, Puri P. Notable postnatal alterations in the myenteric plexus of normal human bowel. Gut 1999;44:666.

[41] von Boyen GB, Krammer HJ, Suss A, et al. Abnormalities of the enteric nervous system in heterozygous endothelin B receptor deficient (spotting lethal) rats resembling intestinal neuronal dysplasia. Gut 2002;51:414.

[42] Pena A, Levitt M. Imperforate anus and cloacal malformations. In: Ashcraft K, Holcomb G III, Murphy JP, editors. Pediatric surgery. 4th edition. Philadelphia: Elsevier Saunders; 2005. p. 496.

[43] Santulli TV. The treatment of imperforate anus and associated fistulas. Surg Gynecol Obstet 1952;95:601.

[44] Trusler GA, Wilkinson RH. Imperforate anus: a review of 147 cases. Can J Surg 1962;5:269.

[45] Levitt MA, Pena A. Outcomes from the correction of anorectal malformations. Curr Opin Pediatr 2005;17:394.

[46] Rosen NG, Hong AR, Soffer SZ, et al. Rectovaginal fistula: a common diagnostic error with significant consequences in girls with anorectal malformations. J Pediatr Surg 2002;37:961.

[47] Anderson RC, Reed SC. The likelihood of recurrence of congenital malformations. J Lancet 1954;74:175.

[48] Murken JD, Albert A. Genetic counselling in cases of anal and rectal atresia. Prog Pediatr Surg 1976;9:115.

[49] Georgeson KE, Inge TH, Albanese CT. Laparoscopically assisted anorectal pull-through for high imperforate anus—a new technique. J Pediatr Surg 2000;35:927.

[50] Hendren WH. Cloaca, the most severe degree of imperforate anus: experience with 195 cases. Ann Surg 1998;228:331.

[51] Hendren WH. Cloacal malformations: experience with 105 cases. J Pediatr Surg 1992;27:890.

[52] Pena A, Hong A. Advances in the management of anorectal malformations. Am J Surg 2000; 180:370.

[53] Rickham P. Vesico-intestinal fissure. Arch Dis Child 1960;35:97.

[54] Tank ES, Lindenauer SM. Principles of management of exstrophy of the cloaca. Am J Surg 1970;119:95.

[55] Pena A. Total urogenital mobilization—an easier way to repair cloacas. J Pediatr Surg 1997; 32:263.

[56] Hendren WH. Management of cloacal malformations. Semin Pediatr Surg 1997;6:217.

[57] Ashcraft K. Acquired anorectal disorders. In: Ashcraft K, Holcomb G III, Murphy JP, editors. Pediatric surgery. 4th edition. Philadelphia: Elsevier Saunders; 2005. p. 527.

[58] Macdonald A, Wilson-Storey D, Munro F. Treatment of perianal abscess and fistula-in-ano in children. Br J Surg 2003;90:220.

[59] Oh JT, Han A, Han SJ, et al. Fistula-in-ano in infants: is nonoperative management effective? J Pediatr Surg 2001;36:1367.

[60] Poenaru D, Yazbeck S. Anal fistula in infants: etiology, features, management. J Pediatr Surg 1993;28:1194.

[61] Serour F, Somekh E, Gorenstein A. Perianal abscess and fistula-in-ano in infants: a different entity? Dis Colon Rectum 2005;48:359.

[62] Shafer AD, McGlone TP, Flanagan RA. Abnormal crypts of Morgagni: the cause of perianal abscess and fistula-in-ano. J Pediatr Surg 1987;22:203.

[63] Rosen NG, Gibbs DL, Soffer SZ, et al. The nonoperative management of fistula-in-ano. J Pediatr Surg 2000;35:938.

[64] Watanabe Y, Todani T, Yamamoto S. Conservative management of fistula in ano in infants. Pediatr Surg Int 1998;13:274.

[65] al-Salem AH, Laing W, Talwalker V. Fistula-in-ano in infancy and childhood. J Pediatr Surg 1994;29:436.

ELSEVIER
SAUNDERS

Surg Clin N Am 86 (2006) 317–327

SURGICAL
CLINICS OF
NORTH AMERICA

Pediatric Surgical Issues in Meconium Disease and Cystic Fibrosis

Robert D. Winfield, MD[a], Elizabeth A. Beierle, MD[b],*

[a]Department of Surgery, University of Florida College of Medicine, P.O. Box 100286,
JHMHSC, Gainesville, FL 32610-0286, USA
[b]Division of Pediatric Surgery, Department of Surgery,
University of Florida College of Medicine, P.O. Box 100286, JHMHSC,
Gainesville, FL 32610-0286, USA

This article provides a summary of gastrointestinal surgical entities associated with meconium disease and cystic fibrosis (CF). Many of these conditions have standard treatments, which are discussed briefly. The primary focus is on the more current or controversial issues encountered. In addition, the authors review the recent findings associated with prenatal diagnosis of meconium disease. Finally, because many patients who have CF are enjoying a longer life span, new issues associated with gastroesophageal reflux (GER), hepatobiliary disease, and the controversial entity of fibrosing colonopathy (FC) are discussed.

Meconium plug syndrome

Meconium plug syndrome (MPS) was described originally by Clatworthy and colleagues [1] as referring to a temporary large bowel obstruction alleviated by the passage of meconium plugs. The usual presentation is that of a newborn who has abdominal distention, emesis, and failure to pass meconium for 24 to 48 hours. The diagnosis is made on the basis of suspicion and plain radiographs demonstrating distended loops of bowel with air-fluid levels. An enema with a soluble contrast agent such as diatrizoate meglumine, as initially described by Noblett [2], is often diagnostic and therapeutic, and most babies who have MPS pass a series of meconium pellets following the enema. The hyperosmolarity of the diatrizoate meglumine enema causes fluid to shift into the intestinal lumen and mandates careful monitoring of fluid status and renal function [3]. The fluid shifts may be

---

* Corresponding author.
E-mail address: beierea@surgery.ufl.edu (E.A. Beierle).

doi:10.1016/j.suc.2005.12.007
surgical.theclinics.com

dramatic, leading to bowel perforation secondary to overdistention with contrast material and the resultant shifted fluid [3]. MPS may be diagnosed prenatally by way of ultrasound. Samuel and colleagues [4] reported two cases in which ultrasound revealed progressive dilatation of the fetal intestine. Further evaluation with amniocentesis and subsequent amniography with diatrizoate meglumine plus diatrizoate sodium resulted in fetal passage of meconium, with a reduction in bowel diameter. At delivery, the neonate was noted to be free of obstruction. These investigators argued that given the risk/benefit profile of neonatal diatrizoate meglumine administration, amniography using diatrizoate meglumine plus diatrizoate sodium represents a reasonable alternative for cases of MPS diagnosed in utero; however, this practice has not been widely accepted and is not recommended by the authors.

MPS may be associated with several other conditions, and its diagnosis serves as an impetus to search for these related diseases. MPS is reported to be associated with Hirschsprung's disease [5–8], and some advocate the exclusion of Hirschsprung's disease in all neonates presenting with MPS [8,9]. Although MPS has been thought to be a separate entity from other meconium-related diseases, Rosenstein [9] described his experience with three neonates diagnosed with MPS who were later found to have CF. On further review, he found that 14% of patients who had CF were originally diagnosed with or had symptoms consistent with MPS [10]. Based on these findings, he and others have advocated that CF be excluded in patients who have MPS [8,11,12].

Meconium ileus

Meconium ileus (MI) refers to terminal ileal obstruction secondary to inspissated meconium. The condition can be further categorized into simple and complicated varieties, with simple referring to mechanical obstruction of the bowel and complicated denoting the additional findings of intestinal atresia, volvulus, antenatal perforation (meconium peritonitis), or giant cystic meconium peritonitis. MI is the presenting symptom in 6% to 20% of infants who have CF, and its presence mandates CF testing. The classic presentation is that of a newborn who has distention, vomiting, and failure to pass meconium. Plain radiographs demonstrate characteristic dilated intestine and a soap bubble or ground glass appearance in the right lower quadrant. Complicated MI includes the findings of air-fluid levels and calcifications, with intraperitoneal calcifications suggestive for CF [13]. Again, a diatrizoate meglumine enema is helpful in the diagnosis and treatment of MI, with the hallmark findings of a small colon accompanied by meconium pellets in the distal ileum and dilated small bowel. The study may prove therapeutic, but if the meconium does not clear with the initial enema, a repeat enema may be performed. Various solutions have been evaluated for clearing inspissated meconium. Burke and colleagues [14] recently described the use of various enemas in constipated mice, including perflubron, surfactant, polysorbate 80, diatrizoate meglumine, polyethylene glycol 3350 plus electrolytes, Dnase, N-acetylcysteine, pancrelipase, and normal saline. These investigators found all of these substances to be equally benign to intestinal mucosa, but diatrizoate meglumine and surfactant were superior at relieving the obstruction. Operative management is required in cases of enema failure. For simple MI, the bowel is irrigated by way of the ileum or an appendiceal stump, with subsequent closure of the enterotomy or formation of a stoma. A number of ostomies have been advocated for postoperative bowel irrigation, including Mikulicz, Bishop-Koop, or Santulli and Blanc. Recently, some investigators have recommended a T tube enterostomy for access for postoperative bowel irrigation [15]. A retrospective review at Texas Children's Hospital evaluated T tube enterostomy for MI and found that over 80% of children required no additional surgery, had the tube removed within 8 weeks, and suffered no complications during an average follow-up of 11.5 years [16]. In cases in which enemas or enterotomy with irrigation fails, resection of the affected segment of bowel with anastomosis may be required.

In complicated MI, the contrast enema may demonstrate findings consistent with a volvulus or atresia. Surgical intervention in complicated MI depends on the pathology encountered, but with volvulus or atresia, bowel resection and anastomosis is preferred; in cases of perforation and giant cystic meconium peritonitis, enterostomy is favored. Rescorla and colleagues [17] reviewed 51 neonates who had MI and found that half had complicated MI on presentation but were successfully managed with resection and anastomosis or enterostomy. Other investigators have noted that neonates who have complicated MI tend to have more long-term surgical complications, especially those who were treated with resection or enterostomy compared with those who merely underwent enterotomy and bowel irrigation [18]. In a separate study, Mushtaq and colleagues [19] reviewed their experience with MI in neonates who failed conservative management. These investigators reported that the children who were treated with resection and anastomosis had a shorter initial hospital stay compared with those who had enterostomy with simple bowel irrigation.

Meconium ileus equivalent (distal intestinal obstruction syndrome)

MI equivalent, or distal intestinal obstruction syndrome (DIOS), is seen in adolescent and adult patients who have CF. It is characterized by the presence of thick, inspissated stool in the distal ileum resulting in obstruction. The diagnosis may be difficult to make due to nonspecific findings consisting of abdominal pain, nausea and vomiting, constipation, anorexia, and possibly a palpable right lower quadrant mass. A number of risk factors for the development of DIOS have been evaluated, but few are predictive. Age is a generally agreed-on risk factor, with most cases occurring in adolescence or adulthood. Rosenstein and Langbaum [20] found that there was no relationship between DIOS and disease severity, pulmonary exacerbations, prior history of MI, or dose or type of pancreatic enzyme replacement. Proesmans and De Boeck [21] postulated that the high-calorie and high-fat diet employed by CF patients to meet increased energy requirements might compromise fiber intake, predisposing these patients to the development of DIOS. In a series of 40 patients, however, these investigators noted that patients who had DIOS tended to have a higher fiber intake than those who did not.

Plain abdominal films that reveal a granular appearance in the region of the terminal ileum may aid in the diagnosis of DIOS. CT scanning is of questionable value in distinguishing between different etiologies of right lower quadrant pain in CF patients. Shields and colleagues [22] reviewed a series of nine CF patients who had CF and appendicitis and reported that the diagnosis of appendicitis was delayed in most of these patients and that CT scan did not help distinguish between appendicitis and DIOS. Given the improvement in CT imaging technology since that report and the lack of a large review of imaging methods in this population, a re-evaluation of this issue may be beneficial. As in MPS and MI, administration of a contrast enema may be helpful in diagnosis and treatment, but unlike MPS and MI, oral therapies are often used for treatment of DIOS. Lillibridge and coworkers [23] first described the use of N-acetylcysteine as a prophylactic and therapeutic entity. Subsequently, O'Halloran and colleagues [24] reported good success with oral diatrizoate meglumine in DIOS, adding that the management could be done on an outpatient basis. Various investigators have proposed that polyethylene glycol 3350 plus electrolytes [25,26] and prokinetic agents may be of some benefit [27]. Recently, IV neostigmine has been used successfully in refractory DIOS [28]. Colonoscopy also is suggested as a potential diagnostic and therapeutic modality. Shidrawi and colleagues [29] presented their data of DIOS managed by way of colonoscopy and direct instillation of diatrizoate meglumine, showing clinical and radiographic improvement in 14 of 16 episodes. Surgical intervention for DIOS is reserved for cases refractory to other forms of management and uses many of the same techniques employed in complicated MI. Additional interventions have been proposed, including an intestinal button for bowel irrigation or a Chait cecostomy/appendicostomy [30,31].

Gastroesophageal reflux

GER is a common condition seen in children who have CF. Bendig and colleagues [32] first noted a relationship between the two entities, and since then, a myriad of associated complications have been identified [33]. Although advanced complications of GER are typically thought of as affecting adults, Hassall and colleagues [34] recently reported the finding of Barrett's esophagus in children who have CF and advocated endoscopic evaluation in the presence of symptoms of GER or abnormal pH probes. Postural drainage is one risk factor for the development of GER that has received attention. Although some investigators have found a significant increase in the number of reflux episodes in CF infants and children treated with head-down-tilt chest physiotherapy [35], others have failed to correlate positioning during physiotherapy with GER [36]. The initial management of GER associated with CF is conservative, using positioning, histamine blockers, and prokinetic agents, with surgery reserved for cases of failed medical management or those associated with apneic or "near-death" episodes. The use of fundoplication has been evaluated in lung transplant patients—an area of obvious interest in CF. Palmer and colleagues [37] reported their experience with a lung transplant recipient who had bronchiolitis obliterans syndrome (BOS). Work-up demonstrated GER, and fundoplication resulted in resolution of symptoms and improved pulmonary function, leading the investigators to hypothesize that GER was a potential cause of BOS and allograft dysfunction in lung transplantation. In a subsequent review of lung transplantation patients, Davis and coworkers [38] found 73% to have abnormal pH probes and reported an increase in survival in those who underwent fundoplication. In a separate study, Cantu and colleagues [39] evaluated the incidence of BOS and survival in lung transplant patients and found a significant decrease in BOS and an increase in 1- and 3-year survival in patients undergoing early fundoplication compared with those undergoing the procedure later, suggesting that early fundoplication should be considered in lung transplant recipients. Finally, O'Halloran and colleagues [40] evaluated a series of patients undergoing laparoscopic fundoplication and reported that patients who had undergone previous lung transplantation tended to have longer hospital stays and more frequent readmissions but that the overall surgical complication rate was similar to other patients. These investigators concluded that the laparoscopic approach may be used after lung transplantation.

Fibrosing colonopathy

Since first being reported by Smyth and colleagues [41] in 1994, FC has been the subject of significant debate. The condition is marked by nonspecific symptoms including abdominal pain, anorexia, nausea, and vomiting. Plain films add little to the diagnosis, and a contrast enema is generally undertaken for clarification. Classic enema findings have been reported, including shortening of the colon, strictures, and an abnormal haustral pattern [42]. Management in symptomatic patients is surgical, with resection of affected bowel [43].

The major debates are related to etiology, surveillance, and prevention. A number of investigators have suggested that high-dose pancreatic enzymes are responsible for the development of FC [44–46]; however, the finding of FC in patients on low-dose and, in two case reports, no pancreatic enzyme supplementation has challenged this theory [47,48]. Evaluation of

methacrylic acid copolymer, a component of pancreatic enzyme preparations, has provided another source of debate. Van Velzen and coworkers
[49] found that cecal gavage with methacrylic acid copolymer in pigs results
in colonic findings similar to those found in humans who have FC. A retrospective assessment of enzyme supplementation in patients who have FC
found that FC was limited to those patients who received formulations containing methacrylic acid copolymer [50]. Ramsden and colleagues [51] challenged this relationship when they evaluated 86 patients who had CF using
sonography, noting only one case in which a patient exposed to methacrylic
acid copolymer showed an early colonic stricture, with the remainder demonstrating no sign of damage. There have also been arguments regarding the
biologic mechanisms involved in the development of FC. In a longitudinal
study of patients who had CF that looked at IgG levels before and after
the initiation of pancreatic enzymes, Lee and coworkers [52] found that
peak IgG concentrations coincided with prior reports of duration of onset
of FC, proposing a possible immunologic mechanism. Smyth and colleagues
[53] performed gut lavage to evaluate inflammatory mediators as an etiology
for FC. Although they found increased levels of inflammatory mediators in
patients who had CF compared with control subjects, there was no significant difference between the levels obtained in CF patients who did or did not
have FC. Numerous methods for surveillance of FC, including ultrasound
and MRI, are under investigation. Haber and colleagues [54] and Dialer
and coworkers [55] found that patients who had CF had increased bowel
wall thickness compared with control subjects but did not find a correlation
between bowel wall thickness and increased pancreatic enzyme doses or clinical features of FC. Almberger and colleagues [56] looked at the utility of
MRI in patients who had CF on pancreatic enzyme supplementation.
They found that most of these children demonstrated acute bowel wall
thickening. After pancreatic enzyme doses were decreased, a subsequent improvement in clinical symptoms and bowel wall thickness on follow-up MRI
were noted. Finally, methods to prevent FC progression are being sought.
Schwarzenberg and colleagues [57] outlined a management plan for FC
that included supplemental parenteral nutrition, a low-fat formula for
oral intake, and discontinuation of pancreatic enzyme supplements. Their
patients eventually showed resolution of colitis, regeneration of colonic epithelium, resolution of small bowel narrowing, and weight gain. Although
the study included only a small number of patients and the regime required
months of therapy for improvement, it provides an interesting therapeutic
option for patients who have FC and potentially represents a means of
avoiding surgery.

Hepatobiliary disease

Hepatic disease occurs in about 4% of patients who have CF [58]. The
onset is generally insidious, with hepatomegaly, splenomegaly, and growth

failure being nonspecific clues. Later findings include a loss of hepatic synthetic function and cirrhosis, portal hypertension, bleeding varices, and ascites. Histologically, the condition is marked by focal fibrosis with subsequent multilobular cirrhosis [59]. Surveillance for the condition has been difficult, as there is no definitive association of hepatobiliary disease with abnormal hepatic function studies [58,60]. History of MI, DIOS, pancreatic insufficiency, and the presence of an abnormal biliary tract on ultrasound have been inconsistently associated with clinically significant liver disease and are not considered reliable precursor conditions for its development [60–63]. A recent report shows a link between glutathione-S-transferase polymorphism and the development of hepatic disease [64] and, although it is not widely used, it may provide a means of early identification of at-risk patients. Ultrasound is used to detect hepatobiliary disease in many CF patients. In one study, including 725 patients over a 9-year period, routine surveillance ultrasound was able to identify patients who had liver changes despite normal hepatic function studies [65]. In another study of 106 children, changes on ultrasound were found to be predictive of later liver disease [60]. Early identification of this problem may allow for treatment with ursodeoxycholic acid (UDCA). A 2-year prospective study examining UDCA treatment of CF-associated liver disease demonstrated an improvement in liver function studies and histology [66]. Similarly, another study showed that UDCA administration to patients who had hepatic involvement resulted in improved ultrasound, biochemical, and clinical findings [67]. In those who have advanced liver disease, first-line intervention for portal hypertension includes endoscopic sclerotherapy and variceal ligation. In refractory cases, a transjugular intrahepatic portosystemic shunt or surgical decompression should be considered [68,69]. With long-term prognosis being generally poor in patients who have hepatic failure, liver transplantation provides the potential for a more lasting solution. Several studies have documented the effectiveness of liver transplantation, with a 1-year survival rate of about 75% to 80%, although this prognosis tends to be poorer in patients requiring transplantation for liver and lung disease simultaneously [70,71].

Biliary tract disease is also common in patients who have CF. Gallstones have been reported to be present in 6% to 24% of patients, with symptomatic disease in about 4% [72]. Other biliary abnormalities associated with CF include microgallbladder, a contracted gallbladder, and an atretic cystic duct [73,74]. Clinical findings are similar to those with cholecystitis in the general population. The diagnosis is primarily clinical, but given the numerous conditions in the CF population that present with similar findings, delays in diagnosis are commonplace. Ultrasound is the diagnostic modality of choice. A contracted gallbladder, sometimes seen in CF, may lead to a false-positive hepatobiliary scan, leading to confusion in the diagnosis of cholecystitis [75]. Some investigators advocate using endoscopic retrograde cholangiopancreatography and UDCA in patients who have especially poor pulmonary function [76]; however, most recommend cholecystectomy for cholecystitis or symptomatic cholelithiasis [77,78]. To date, no study has compared the effectiveness or safety of laparoscopic versus open cholecystectomy in CF patients, but the authors recommend the laparoscopic approach unless there are other attenuating associations such as portal hypertension and significant adhesions from multiple prior operations. Although there are valid concerns about laparoscopy for patients who have underlying pulmonary compromise, in general, the use of laparoscopy minimizes postoperative pain and more likely diminishes pulmonary morbidity after an abdominal operation.

Perioperative considerations in the patient who has cystic fibrosis

CF is associated with a number of disease entities that may require operative intervention. In past years, the complication rates were extremely high, with a reported mortality rate of 30% in one series [79]. More recent series estimate the incidence of complications to be on the order of 10% to 12%, with mortality rates of 1% to 5% [80]. Given the underlying disease and the risks for complication, careful preoperative evaluation and optimization, intraoperative management, and postoperative care are warranted [81]. Particular attention should be focused on pulmonary care and nutritional status. Recommendations include preoperative pulmonary evaluation with pulmonary function testing, blood gas measurement, and chest films. Patients are managed with pneumatic vest or manual drainage, β-agonist and mucolytic nebulizer treatments, and individually tailored antibiotic therapy. This management is then extended through the postoperative period with enteral or parenteral nutritional supplementation. In cases in which an immediate operation is required, it is recommended that the patient undergo at least one session with pneumatic vest or manual drainage combined with beta-agonist and mucolytic nebulizer. Using this approach, Saltzman and colleagues [80] reported no significant unexpected decrement in growth or pulmonary status in CF patients undergoing surgical procedures.

References

[1] Clatworthy HW Jr, Howard WH, Lloyd J. The meconium plug syndrome. Surgery 1956; 39(1):131–42.

[2] Noblett HR. Treatment of uncomplicated meconium ileus by Gastrografin enema: a preliminary report. J Pediatr Surg 1969;4(2):190–7.

[3] Rescorla FJ, Grosfeld JL. Contemporary management of meconium ileus. World J Surg 1993;17(3):318–25.

[4] Samuel N, Dicker D, Landman J, et al. Early diagnosis and intrauterine therapy of meconium plug syndrome in the fetus: risks and benefits. J Ultrasound Med 1986;5(8):425–8.

[5] Gillis DA, Grantmyre EB. The meconium-plug syndrome and Hirschsprung's disease. Can Med Assoc J 1965;92:225–7.

[6] Van Leeuwen G, Glenn L, Woodruff C, et al. Meconium plug syndrome with aganglionosis. Pediatrics 1967;40(4):665–6.

[7] Berdon WE, Slovis TL, Campbell JB, et al. Neonatal small left colon syndrome: its relationship to aganglionosis and meconium plug syndrome. Radiology 1977;125(2):457–62.

[8] Burge D, Drewett M. Meconium plug obstruction. Pediatr Surg Int 2004;20(2):108–10.

[9] Rosenstein BJ. Cystic fibrosis presenting with the meconium plug syndrome. Am J Dis Child 1978;132(2):167–9.

[10] Rosenstein BJ, Langbaum TS. Incidence of meconium abnormalities in newborn infants with cystic fibrosis. Am J Dis Child 1980;134(1):72–3.

[11] Olsen MM, Luck SR, Lloyd-Still J. The spectrum of meconium disease in infancy. J Pediatr Surg 1982;17(5):479–81.

[12] Casaccia G, Trucchi A, Nahom A, et al. The impact of cystic fibrosis on neonatal intestinal obstruction: the need for prenatal/neonatal screening. Pediatr Surg Int 2003;19(1–2):75–8.

[13] Finkel LI, Slovis TL. Meconium peritonitis, intraperitoneal calcifications and cystic fibrosis. Pediatr Radiol 1982;12(2):92–3.

[14] Burke MS, Ragi JM, Karamanoukian HL. New strategies in nonoperative management of meconium ileus. J Pediatr Surg 2002;37(5):760–4.

[15] Steiner Z, Mogilner J, Siplovich L, et al. T-tubes in the management of meconium ileus. Pediatr Surg Int 1997;12(2–3):140–1.

[16] Mak GZ, Harberg FJ, Hiatt P, et al. T-tube ileostomy for meconium ileus: four decades of experience. J Pediatr Surg 2000;35(2):349–52.

[17] Rescorla FJ, Grosfeld JL, West KJ. Changing patterns of treatment and survival in neonates with meconium ileus. Arch Surg 1989;124(7):837–40.

[18] Fuchs JR, Langer JC. Long-term outcome after neonatal meconium obstruction. Pediatrics 1998;101(4):E7.

[19] Mushtaq I, Wright VM, Drake DP, et al. Meconium ileus secondary to cystic fibrosis. The East London experience. Pediatr Surg Int 1998;13(5–6):365–9.

[20] Rosenstein BJ, Langbaum TS. Incidence of distal intestinal obstruction syndrome in cystic fibrosis. J Pediatr Gastroenterol Nutr 1983;2(2):299–301.

[21] Proesmans M, De Boeck K. Evaluation of dietary fiber intake in Belgian children with cystic fibrosis: is there a link with gastrointestinal complaints? J Pediatr Gastroenterol Nutr 2002; 35(5):610–4.

[22] Shields MD, Levison H, Reisman JJ, et al. Appendicitis in cystic fibrosis. Arch Dis Child 1991;66(3):307–10.

[23] Lillibridge CB, Docter JM, Eidelman S. Oral administration of N-acetyl cysteine in the prophylaxis of "meconium ileus equivalent." J Pediatr 1967;71(6):887–9.

[24] O'Halloran SM, Gilbert J, McKendrick OM, et al. Gastrografin in acute meconium ileus equivalent. Arch Dis Child 1986;61(11):1128–30.

[25] Koletzko S, Stringer DA, Cleghorn GJ, et al. Lavage treatment of distal intestinal obstruction syndrome in children with cystic fibrosis. Pediatrics 1989;83(5):727–33.

[26] Cleghorn GJ, Stringer DA, Forstner GG, et al. Treatment of distal intestinal obstruction syndrome in cystic fibrosis with a balanced intestinal lavage solution. Lancet 1986; 1(8471):8–11.

[27] Koletzko S, Corey M, Ellis L, et al. Effects of cisapride in patients with cystic fibrosis and distal intestinal obstruction syndrome. J Pediatr 1990;117(5):815–22.

[28] Kurtzman TL, Borowitz SM. Successful use of neostigmine in a patient with refractory distal intestinal obstruction syndrome. J Pediatr Gastroenterol Nutr 2002;35(5):700–3.

[29] Shidrawi RG, Murugan N, Westaby D, et al. Emergency colonoscopy for distal intestinal obstruction syndrome in cystic fibrosis patients. Gut 2002;51(2):285–6.

[30] Redel CA, Motil KJ, Bloss RS, et al. Intestinal button implantation for obstipation and fecal impaction in children. J Pediatr Surg 1992;27(5):654–6.

[31] Stanton MP, Shin YM, Hutson JM. Laparoscopic placement of the Chait cecostomy device via appendicostomy. J Pediatr Surg 2002;37(12):1766–7.

[32] Bendig DW, Seilheimer DK, Wagner ML, et al. Complications of gastroesophageal reflux in patients with cystic fibrosis. J Pediatr 1982;100(4):536–40.

[33] Hallberg K, Fandriks L, Strandvik B. Duodenogastric bile reflux is common in cystic fibrosis. J Pediatr Gastroenterol Nutr 2004;38(3):312–6.

[34] Hassall E, Israel DM, Davidson AG, et al. Barrett's esophagus in children with cystic fibrosis: not a coincidental association. Am J Gastroenterol 1993;88(11):1934–8.

[35] Button BM, Heine RG, Catto-Smith AG, et al. Chest physiotherapy, gastro-oesophageal reflux, and arousal in infants with cystic fibrosis. Arch Dis Child 2004;89(5):435–9.

[36] Phillips GE, Pike SE, Rosenthal M, et al. Holding the baby: head downwards positioning for physiotherapy does not cause gastro-oesophageal reflux. Eur Respir J 1998;12(4):954–7.

[37] Palmer SM, Miralles AP, Howell DN, et al. Gastroesophageal reflux as a reversible cause of allograft dysfunction after lung transplantation. Chest 2000;118(4):1214–7.

[38] Davis RD Jr, Lau CL, Eubanks S, et al. Improved lung allograft function after fundoplication in patients with gastroesophageal reflux disease undergoing lung transplantation. J Thorac Cardiovasc Surg 2003;125(3):533–42.

[39] Cantu E III, Appel JZ III, Hartwig MG, et al. J. Maxwell Chamberlain Memorial Paper. Early fundoplication prevents chronic allograft dysfunction in patients with gastroesophageal reflux disease. Ann Thorac Surg 2004;78(4):1142–51 [discussion: 1142–51].

[40] O'Halloran EK, Reynolds JD, Lau CL, et al. Laparoscopic Nissen fundoplication for treating reflux in lung transplant recipients. J Gastrointest Surg 2004;8(1):132–7.

[41] Smyth RL, van Velzen D, Smyth AR, et al. Strictures of ascending colon in cystic fibrosis and high-strength pancreatic enzymes. Lancet 1994;343(8889):85–6.

[42] Crisci KL, Greenberg SB, Wolfson BJ, et al. Contrast enema findings of fibrosing colonopathy. Pediatr Radiol 1997;27(4):315–6.

[43] Reichard KW, Vinocur CD, Franco M, et al. Fibrosing colonopathy in children with cystic fibrosis. J Pediatr Surg 1997;32(2):237–41 [discussion: 241–2].

[44] Smyth RL, Ashby D, O'Hea U, et al. Fibrosing colonopathy in cystic fibrosis: results of a case-control study. Lancet 1995;346(8985):1247–51.

[45] Freiman JP, FitzSimmons SC. Colonic strictures in patients with cystic fibrosis: results of a survey of 114 cystic fibrosis care centers in the United States. J Pediatr Gastroenterol Nutr 1996;22(2):153–6.

[46] FitzSimmons SC, Burkhart GA, Borowitz D, et al. High-dose pancreatic-enzyme supplements and fibrosing colonopathy in children with cystic fibrosis. N Engl J Med 1997;336(18):1283–9.

[47] Jones R, Franklin K, Spicer R, Berry J. Colonic strictures in children with cystic fibrosis on low-strength pancreatic enzymes. Lancet 1995;346(8973):499.

[48] Serban DE, Florescu P, Miu N. Fibrosing colonopathy revealing cystic fibrosis in a neonate before any pancreatic enzyme supplementation. J Pediatr Gastroenterol Nutr 2002;35(3):356–9.

[49] van Velzen D, Ball LM, Dezfulian AR. Comparative and experimental pathology of fibrosing colonopathy. Postgrad Med J 1996;72(Suppl 2):S39–48 [discussion: S49–51].

[50] Bakowski MT, Prescott P. Patterns of use of pancreatic enzyme supplements in fibrosing colonopathy: implications for pathogenesis. Pharmacoepidemiol Drug Saf 1997;6(5):347–58.

[51] Ramsden WH, Moya EF, Littlewood JM. Colonic wall thickness, pancreatic enzyme dose and type of preparation in cystic fibrosis. Arch Dis Child 1998;79(4):339–43.

[52] Lee J, Ip W, Durie P. Is fibrosing colonopathy an immune mediated disease? Arch Dis Child 1997;77(1):66–70.

[53] Smyth RL, Croft NM, O'Hea U, et al. Intestinal inflammation in cystic fibrosis. Arch Dis Child 2000;82(5):394–9.

[54] Haber HP, Benda N, Fitzke G, et al. Colonic wall thickness measured by ultrasound: striking differences in patients with cystic fibrosis versus healthy controls. Gut 1997;40(3):406–11.

[55] Dialer I, Hundt C, Bertele-Harms RM, et al. Sonographic evaluation of bowel wall thickness in patients with cystic fibrosis. J Clin Gastroenterol 2003;37(1):55–60.

[56] Almberger M, Iannicelli E, Antonelli M, et al. The role of MRI in the intestinal complications in cystic fibrosis. Clin Imaging 2001;25(5):344–8.

[57] Schwarzenberg SJ, Wielinski CL, Shamieh I, et al. Cystic fibrosis-associated colitis and fibrosing colonopathy. J Pediatr 1995;127(4):565–70.

[58] Scott-Jupp R, Lama M, Tanner MS. Prevalence of liver disease in cystic fibrosis. Arch Dis Child 1991;66(6):698–701.

[59] Colombo C, Battezzati PM. Hepatobiliary manifestations of cystic fibrosis. Eur J Gastroenterol Hepatol 1996;8(8):748–54.

[60] Lenaerts C, Lapierre C, Patriquin H, et al. Surveillance for cystic fibrosis-associated hepatobiliary disease: early ultrasound changes and predisposing factors. J Pediatr 2003;143(3):343–50.

[61] Colombo C, Apostolo MG, Ferrari M, et al. Analysis of risk factors for the development of liver disease associated with cystic fibrosis. J Pediatr 1994;124(3):393–9.

[62] Waters DL, Dorney SF, Gruca MA, et al. Hepatobiliary disease in cystic fibrosis patients with pancreatic sufficiency. Hepatology 1995;21(4):963–9.

[63] Lindblad A, Strandvik B, Hjelte L. Incidence of liver disease in patients with cystic fibrosis and meconium ileus. J Pediatr 1995;126(1):155–6.

[64] Henrion-Caude A, Flamant C, Roussey M, et al. Liver disease in pediatric patients with cystic fibrosis is associated with glutathione S-transferase P1 polymorphism. Hepatology 2002; 36(4 Pt 1):913–7.

[65] Williams SM, Goodman R, Thomson A, et al. Ultrasound evaluation of liver disease in cystic fibrosis as part of an annual assessment clinic: a 9-year review. Clin Radiol 2002;57(5): 365–70.

[66] Lindblad A, Glaumann H, Strandvik B. A two-year prospective study of the effect of ursodeoxycholic acid on urinary bile acid excretion and liver morphology in cystic fibrosis-associated liver disease. Hepatology 1998;27(1):166–74.

[67] Nousia-Arvanitakis S, Fotoulaki M, Economou H, et al. Long-term prospective study of the effect of ursodeoxycholic acid on cystic fibrosis-related liver disease. J Clin Gastroenterol 2001;32(4):324–8.

[68] Shun A, Delaney DP, Martin HC, et al. Portosystemic shunting for paediatric portal hypertension. J Pediatr Surg 1997;32(3):489–93.

[69] Debray D, Lykavieris P, Gauthier F, et al. Outcome of cystic fibrosis-associated liver cirrhosis: management of portal hypertension. J Hepatol 1999;31(1):77–83.

[70] Noble-Jamieson G, Valente J, Barnes ND, et al. Liver transplantation for hepatic cirrhosis in cystic fibrosis. Arch Dis Child 1994;71(4):349–52.

[71] Milkiewicz P, Skiba G, Kelly D, et al. Transplantation for cystic fibrosis: outcome following early liver transplantation. J Gastroenterol Hepatol 2002;17(2):208–13.

[72] Stern RC, Rothstein FC, Doershuk CF. Treatment and prognosis of symptomatic gallbladder disease in patients with cystic fibrosis. J Pediatr Gastroenterol Nutr 1986;5(1):35–40.

[73] Rovsing H, Sloth K. Micro-gallbladder and biliary calculi in mucoviscidosis. Acta Radiol Diagn (Stockh) 1973;14(5):588–92.

[74] Roy CC, Weber AM, Morin CL, et al. Hepatobiliary disease in cystic fibrosis: a survey of current issues and concepts. J Pediatr Gastroenterol Nutr 1982;1(4):469–78.

[75] Giuliano V, Dadparvar S, Savit R, et al. Contracted gallbladder: a cause of false-positive hepatobiliary scan in patients with cystic fibrosis. Eur J Nucl Med 1996;23(5):595–7.

[76] Shen GK, Tsen AC, Hunter GC, et al. Surgical treatment of symptomatic biliary stones in patients with cystic fibrosis. Am Surg 1995;61(9):814–9.

[77] Snyder CL, Ferrell KL, Saltzman DA, et al. Operative therapy of gallbladder disease in patients with cystic fibrosis. Am J Surg 1989;157(6):557–61.

[78] Anagnostopoulos D, Tsagari N, Noussia-Arvanitaki S, et al. Gallbladder disease in patients with cystic fibrosis. Eur J Pediatr Surg 1993;3(6):348–51.

[79] Smith RM. Anesthetic management of patients with cystic fibrosis. Anesth Analg 1965;44:143–6.

[80] Saltzman DA, Johnson EM, Feltis BA, et al. Surgical experience in patients with cystic fibrosis: A 25-year perspective. Pediatr Pulmonol 2002;33:106–10.

[81] Warwick WJ. Guidebook for cystic fibrosis. 4th edition. Minneapolis (MN): University of Minnesota Press; 1983.

ELSEVIER
SAUNDERS

SURGICAL
CLINICS OF
NORTH AMERICA

Surg Clin N Am 86 (2006) 329–352

Congenital Diaphragmatic Hernia and Neonatal Lung Lesions

David W. Kays, MD

Division of Pediatric Surgery, University of Florida College of Medicine,
1600 SW Archer Road, Gainesville, FL 32610, USA

Increasingly, the diagnoses of chest lesions in infants are made not by symptoms of respiratory distress but by prenatal imaging. Because the availability and quality of prenatal imaging have increased, so has the frequency of prenatal diagnoses that include symptomatic and asymptomatic lesions. Early prenatal diagnosis of life-threatening lesions, such as congenital diaphragmatic hernia (CDH) and congenital cystic adenomatoid malformation (CAM or CCAM), allows detailed evaluation and subspecialty referral but may lead to decisions for pregnancy termination. It is imperative that counseling physicians have accurate and up-to-date information about prognosis in these difficult situations. Improved prenatal imaging also identifies lesions that may resolve spontaneously or may otherwise remain asymptomatic. As we gain in understanding of the natural history of these lesions, the advisability of routine surgical resection of asymptomatic lesions can be evaluated better.

This article discusses the embryologic development, diagnosis, treatment, and outcome of CDH and lung lesions of infancy. The focus is primarily on recent developments in the last decade and addresses areas of evolving controversy. Earlier writings are cited as needed to illustrate important historical points, identify concept development, and re-evaluate outdated thinking.

Embryology and animal models of lung and diaphragm development

Recent work in animal models has advanced our understanding of lung and diaphragm embryology. Although starting from different pathways and anlages, diaphragm and lung development are interrelated. Lung and

E-mail address: kaysdw@surgery.ufl.edu

airway epithelium first arise as two small buds of endodermally derived foregut cells, whereas the rest of the foregut separates longitudinally into esophagus and trachea [1]. Extralobar pulmonary sequestration is thought to arise when collections of cells with respiratory potential arise from the primitive foregut distal to the lung buds, which gives rise to systemic blood supply and often systemic venous drainage. CCAM arises secondary to abnormalities in the signaling pathways between the developing terminal bronchioles and the supporting mesenchyme. Congenital lobar emphysema results from partial or complete obstruction of a lobar feeding bronchus, seemingly related to deficient cartilaginous support of that bronchus. Complete pulmonary agenesis, although a rare occurrence, is frequently associated with other foregut abnormalities, including tracheoesophageal anomalies [2–6], other VACTERL associations [7,8], and ipsilateral radial ray anomalies [9].

The diaphragm forms from the fusion of the septum transversum, the paired pleuroperitoneal membranes, the mesenchyme that arises adjacent to the esophagus, and the ingrowth of muscles from the body wall [10–12]. Defects in fusion of these components were believed to give rise to the various diaphragmatic defects encountered. Babiuk et al used immunohistochemical markers of muscle precursors in conjunction with mutant mice to examine phrenic-diaphragm embryogenesis [13]. They found that myogenic cells and axons coalesce within the pleuroperitoneal fold and, contrary to previous explanations, they expand to form the neuromuscular component of the diaphragm. They found no contributions to the diaphragm from the lateral body wall, septum transversum, or paraesophageal mesenchyme. CDH in the rat model resulted solely from defects in the formation of this mesenchymal substratum in the pleuroperitoneal fold.

The relationship between the developing diaphragm and lung has been the subject of intense laboratory effort. In CDH, the question involves which comes first, the diaphragmatic defect or the lung hypoplasia. The most studied and cited model of CDH is the nitrofen rat model. Nitrofen (2,4 dichlorophenyl-p-nitorphenyl ether) exerts a teratogenic effect when given to pregnant rats between 9 and 11 days' gestation and results in a high incidence of CDH in offspring. In this model, pulmonary hypoplasia occurs earlier in development than would be expected by compression from the CDH contents alone, and from this finding has arisen the postulate that lung hypoplasia is the primary event in the development of CDH. Keijzer and colleagues [12] have shown that nitrofen exerts a direct negative effect on the developing lung because it interferes with branching morphogenesis and attenuates epithelial cell differentiation and proliferation in exposed lungs. This effect is additional to and separate from the mass effect exerted by abdominal contents on the developing lung after defective development of the diaphragm. Babiuk and colleagues [13] elegantly showed that CDH in the nitrofen model occurs in the amuscular mesenchymal component of the primordial diaphragm and is not related to abnormal muscle formation. More importantly, the diaphragm defect is not secondary to a defect of lung formation and occurs independently of abnormal lung development. These data support the finding that in the nitrofen rat model of CDH, the diaphragm defect is a primary event and does not arise secondary to lung hypoplasia. This finding is consistent with commonly held thought regarding CDH in humans. In comparing the rat model and the human condition, it is important to remember that a teratogen causes CDH in this rat model, and no teratogen has been implicated in human CDH.

CDH also can be induced in rats by providing a vitamin A–deficient diet [14]. The retinoid hypothesis in the development of CDH is supported by many experimental observations, including the development of CDH in mutant mice that are deficient in cellular retinoid receptors. The incidence of CDH in the nitrofen rat model can be decreased by the specific administration of vitamin A [15,16]. Vitamin A also attenuates the lung hypoplasia seen in this model by blocking the development of lung hypoplasia early in gestation [16]. In humans, a single study showed that markers of vitamin A status were decreased in infants who had CDH compared with controls [17], but these findings have yet to be duplicated. A review of the experimental evidence regarding lung and diaphragm development is presented in more detail by Rottier and Tibboel [18].

Congenital diaphragmatic hernia in humans: genetics

The cause of CDH in humans is not known. Although genetic influences are clearly important, specific information is limited. Structural chromosomal abnormalities are common in prenatally diagnosed CDH, and they occurred in 10% and 34% of prenatally diagnosed patients in two reviews [19,20]. CDH has been associated with abnormalities on nearly every chromosome, but it most commonly occurs with chromosomal duplications or deletions, including Turner syndrome (monosomy X), Down syndrome (trisomy 21), Edward syndrome (trisomy 18), and Patau syndrome (trisomy 13) [19–21]. Pallister-Killian syndrome (tetrasomy 12p) also is frequently encountered [22,23]. CDH can occur as part of a syndrome caused by a known gene, as in Denys-Drash syndrome (WT1) [19], Simpson-Golabi-Behmel syndrome (GPC3) [24], craniofrontonasal syndrome (EPNB 1) [25], neonatal Marfan syndrome (FBN1) [26], and spondylocostal dysostosis (DLL3) [27]. Most cases of CDH, however, occur as isolated nonsyndromic presentations. Familial occurrences have been described, and the risk of a second occurrence with an otherwise negative family history is estimated to be 2% [28,29]. The existing knowledge on this subject recently was reviewed by Slavotinek [21].

Prenatal diagnosis and markers of severity

The severity of CDH is a wide spectrum, and an understanding of the correlation between prenatal findings and clinical prognosis is vital for counseling families accurately. Unfortunately, there is variable congruence between the prenatal imaging and resultant clinical picture, and differences in treatment and outcome at different centers blur the validity of prognostic variables. It is clear, however, that improved imaging has led to an increase in prenatal diagnosis of this disorder. Accurate prenatal imaging is important to identify associated anomalies and assess anatomic severity. Two-dimensional ultrasound continues to evolve, and three-dimensional ultrasound and MRI have been added to the diagnostic armamentarium [30–34]. Associated anomalies are present in a high percentage of fetuses, approaching 40% in two separate studies [35,36]. Such anomalies have been thought to compromise survival [35], but it is increasingly clear that most associated anomalies, such as atrial septal defect (ASD), malrotation, Meckel's diverticulum, and unilateral kidney, should have little effect on survival. Chromosomal anomalies and serious heart defects are exceptions and negatively affect survival. Graziano [37] reviewed the experience of the CDH Study Group and found that of 2636 patients reported, 280 (10.6%) had significant heart defects, of which ventricular septal defect (VSD) was the most common (42.2%) (Fig. 1). Overall survival rate for CDH was 67% but dropped to 41% in the heart defect group (Fig. 2). Patients with univentricle anatomy and CDH had only a 5% survival rate.

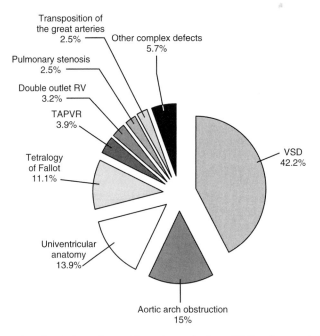

Fig. 1. Types of cardiac defects observed in patients who have CDH and congenital heart disease (*n* = 280). (*From* Graziano JN. Cardiac anomalies in patients with congenital diaphragmatic hernia and their prognosis: a report from the Congenital Diaphragmatic Hernia Study Group. J Pediatr Surg 2005;40(6):1046; with permission.)

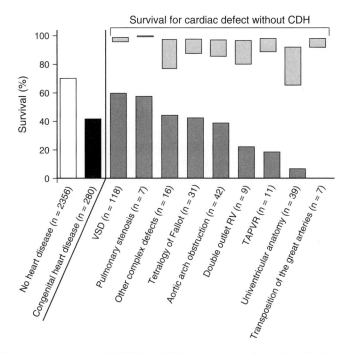

Fig. 2. Survival for patients with CDH, stratified by type of cardiac defect. The shaded bars at the top of the graph provide reference ranges of survival for each cardiac defect in patients without CDH. *P < 0.001, compared with CDH without congenital heart disease. **P < 0.001 compared with CDH with biventricular heart disease. ***P = 0.03 compared with CDH with all other heart diseases. TAPVR, total anomalous pulmonary venous return. (*From* Graziano JN. Cardiac anomalies in patients with congenital diaphragmatic hernia and their prognosis: a report from the Congenital Diaphragmatic Hernia Study Group. J Pediatr Surg 2005; 40(6):1047; with permission.)

Numerous attempts have been made to correlate prenatal imaging with postnatal outcome in patients without associated life-threatening anomalies, but with mixed results. The lung-to-head ratio (LHR), first described by Metkus and Harrison in 1996 [51], is an attempt to report two-dimensional lung size in the fetus relative to a growth standard (head circumference) and correlate the finding with outcome. In their initial prospective report of 15 patients, LHR was measured at 24 to 26 weeks. No patient with an LHR less than 1 survived (n = 3). All patients with LHR more than 1.4 survived, and survival rate was 38% when the LHR was 1.0 to 1.4. Overall survival rate in the 15 patients was 47%. LHR seemed to be validated by Laudy and colleagues [38] in a review of 26 patients, which showed 100% survival rate if the LHR was more than 1.4, regardless of gestational age at testing. Survival rate for the series was 50%. Heling and colleagues [39] were unable to correlate LHR with survival.

MRI and three-dimensional ultrasound have been used to calculate three-dimensional lung volumes in fetal CDH, and researchers have compared the validity of these measurements to two-dimensional LHR. Ruano and colleagues [40] showed good correlation between MRI and three-dimensional ultrasound measurements of lung volume in CDH and demonstrated that patients who died of CDH had a lower range of measured lung volumes than survivors [30]. As expected, MRI was useful for diagnosing fetal CCAM, chylothorax, and esophageal atresia [41].

Liver position on prenatal imaging, either entirely abdominal or partly intrathoracic, also has been described as a measure of severity [42]. Data from the CDH Study Group demonstrate that 75% of all patients who have CDH have some portion of liver in their chest [43], which suggests that this is not a sufficiently discriminating observation. Perhaps the volume or fraction of liver in the chest may be a more specific predictor of outcome.

Other risk factors that have been variably shown to predict poor outcome include the antenatal factors of prenatal diagnosis, polyhydramnios, and right-sided defect [44–46]. Similarly, postnatal factors, such as poor aeration on chest radiograph [47], also have been shown to correlate with poor outcome. Each of these factors has failed validation when tested in later studies, however [48–50], even when re-evaluated at the same center [51]. Great caution should be used in citing and interpreting these risk factors during counseling of families with a fetal diagnosis of CDH.

Two studies have correlated successfully early postnatal physiologic measurements with outcome. The Congenital Diaphragmatic Hernia Study Group developed an equation for predicting survival based on birth weight and 5-minute Apgar score [52], and the Canadian Neonatal Network validated the SNAP-II score as predictive of mortality in CDH in their population of 88 patients [53]. These objective evaluations allow better stratification of illness severity in series and have been used to provide evidence of improved survival with evolving treatment strategies [5].

Treatment and outcome

Infants born with CDH face fundamental physiologic problems, including pulmonary hypoplasia and pulmonary hypertension. Historically, efforts to improve survival have focused primarily on one or the other of these aspects.

Prenatal interventions

Because of the low CDH survival rates of only 20% to 42% experienced in the late 1980s and early 1990s [44,54], Harrison and others [55,56] pursued in utero surgical interventions to promote lung growth. After initial animal studies, the first open human fetal repair of CDH was performed by Harrison in 1990. Eventually 21 fetuses underwent open fetal repair but only 5 survived [57,58]. Some fetuses showed evidence of lung growth, but technical complications and premature labor resulted in poor outcomes for most patients. Open fetal repair for CDH was abandoned.

After the failure of open fetal repair to improve survival, surgical fetal interventions for CDH took a new direction. Congenital laryngeal atresia was recognized to cause large fetal lungs. Based on this and other observations, Wilson and colleagues [59] and DiFiore and colleagues [60] demonstrated that fetal tracheal occlusion prevented fetal pulmonary hypoplasia in a fetal lamb nephrectomy model and resulted in increased lung growth in the fetal lamb CDH model. Harrison and colleagues [61] applied this concept to human fetuses with CDH in an attempt to promote lung growth and improve survival. Three approaches eventually were used, including open fetal tracheal ligation, fetoscopic tracheal clipping, and fetoscopic tracheal occlusion by a detachable balloon. Open fetal tracheal ligation was met with poor survival, and fetoscopic tracheal ligation showed better survival but with significant tracheal morbidity, including several patients with bilateral recurrent laryngeal nerve injuries. Fetoscopic tracheal occlusion showed the most promise [62], and in 2003, Harrison and colleagues [63] reported the results from a National Institutes of Health–sponsored trial that compared fetoscopic tracheal occlusion with standard postnatal care. Entry criteria included left CDH with some degree of liver herniation into the chest and LHR less than 1.4. Twenty-four patients were randomized, but the trial was stopped before completion. Eight of 11 treated fetuses survived (73%), but because of continued improvement in standard postnatal care, 10 of 13 (77%) control patients also survived. Despite a great deal of effort, fetal surgical interventions for CDH failed to show an improvement in survival and cannot be recommended at this time.

Postnatal management

The last decade of postnatal CDH management has shown an ongoing search for a magic bullet. As with prenatal interventions, early excitement about the use of extracorporeal membrane oxygenation (ECMO) [64,65], delayed surgery [66–68], surfactant [69], nitric oxide [70], and even sildenafil [71,72] has been tempered by subsequent reports that cast doubt as to the survival benefit of these therapies. Despite several studies that showed dramatic improvements in survival with changed therapeutic strategy [48,73], other reports discount those claims [74,75]. Survival reported by the CDH study group has continued to improve from 63% reported in 1998 [76] to 67% reported in 2005 [37].

Postnatal outcome of CDH treatment varies from center to center, even in the same facility over time as treatment strategy evolves. Reickert and colleagues [77] showed in 1997 that of 411 patients who had CDH and were treated at 16 different level-III neonatal intensive care with ECMO, survival rate to discharge varied from 39% to 92%, and ECMO use varied from 32% to 60%. No effort was made to stratify the severity of CDH encountered at these centers, but it seems unlikely that this alone would account for the large differences in survival encountered. The CDH literature shows wide variation in treatment approaches at different centers, and differences in outcome are likely caused, at least in part, to differences in therapy. There remains a paucity of randomized and properly controlled trials in the CDH literature [78], which makes it difficult to compare differences in therapy. Much of current therapeutic strategies arise from an accumulation of observational data.

Delayed surgery

Repair of CDH was once a surgical emergency at birth, but stabilization and delay of surgical repair to 24 hours and beyond have been embraced enthusiastically. Pulmonary gas exchange often improves in the first 24 hours after birth, and respiratory compliance improves with preoperative stabilization [79]. Although there is no evidence that delayed repair is harmful, there is also no convincing evidence that such delay improves survival or decreases risk of pulmonary hypertension [80–83]. Because delay in surgery is not harmful, there is no compelling reason to perform emergent surgery at birth, and our practice is to delay operative repair of the CDH.

Surfactant

Although the lamb and rat models of CDH suggest surfactant deficiency [84–87], this is controversial in humans. Evaluation of bronchoalveolar lavage fluid analyzed for components of surfactant in infants with CDH showed no differences when compared with age-matched controls, which suggests that a primary surfactant deficiency is unlikely [88]. Surfactant kinetic studies in human infants with CDH compared with control infants found no differences in surfactant phosphatidylcholine pool size or half-life [89,90].

The Congenital Diaphragmatic Hernia Study Group is a multicenter international cooperative organization of tertiary referral centers that cares for patients who have CDH and shares their data through a voluntary database. Started in 1995, this database currently holds more than 2500 patients and has provided important information about CDH care and outcome, including surfactant use in term, preterm, and ECMO patients who have CDH [91–93]. Logistic regression or multivariate analyses were performed to adjust for differences in severity of illness between patients who receive surfactant and those who do not. Conclusions from these individual reports are as follows: (1) In term infants with CDH, the use of ECMO and development of chronic lung disease was higher and survival was lower in the surfactant-treated group of patients (Fig. 3). After adjusted logistic regression, the odds ratios generated showed no benefit to surfactant

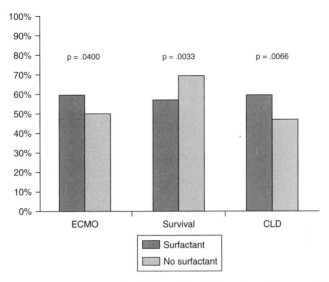

Fig. 3. Survival, need for ECMO, and incidence of chronic lung disease in prenatally diagnosed cohort treated with surfactant ($n = 192$) compared with infants who were not treated with surfactant ($n = 330$). (*From* Van Meurs K. Is surfactant therapy beneficial in the treatment of the term newborn infant with congenital diaphragmatic hernia? J Pediatr 2004;145(3):314; with permission.)

therapy with regard to survival, need for ECMO, or development of chronic lung disease [91]. (2) In preterm infants, patients who received surfactant (209 patients) had a higher odds ratio of dying than those who did not receive surfactant (215 patients). Multivariate analysis to adjust for severity of illness did not change this result [92]. (3) In patients who had CDH and were on ECMO support, surfactant administration did not improve survival, shorten the ECMO run, or decrease the need for oxygen at 30 days compared with patients who did not receive surfactant [93]. Taken individually and together, these studies show no benefit to surfactant administration in patients with CDH, and there was potential for worse outcome in surfactant-treated patients.

Nitric oxide

As a powerful, relatively nontoxic therapeutic agent delivered by inhalation directly to the target organ, nitric oxide was expected to have a dramatic effect on pulmonary hypertension in CDH. Despite a rapid and sometimes dramatic effect on oxygenation when given to a patient with a pulmonary hypertensive crisis, inhaled nitric oxide has not been shown to improve survival or decrease the need for ECMO in a controlled trial of nitric oxide treatment in CDH [94]. Hyperventilation was used in most patients in this multicenter trial, and ventilator-induced lung injury could have masked a beneficial effect of nitric oxide. This outcome was different from that for newborns from a separate arm of the same study who did not have CDH and who experienced a decreased need for ECMO when treated with nitric oxide [95]. Other investigators have reported good results using nitric oxide combined with high-frequency oscillatory ventilation in CDH but without adequate controls [96–98]. A Cochrane review in 2001 found no clear data to support the use of inhaled nitric oxide in infants who have CDH [99].

Sildenafil

Sildenafil is a specific phosphdiesterase-5 inhibitor shown to decrease pulmonary vascular resistance [100]. In a piglet model of meconium aspiration it was significantly more effective in ameliorating pulmonary hypertension than inhaled nitric oxide [101]. Oral sildenafil has been used in isolated, uncontrolled cases to treat neonatal pulmonary hypertension [102]. In patients who have CDH, oral [72] and intravenous [71] sildenafil has been used to treat pulmonary hypertension that is refractory to inhaled nitric oxide. Two patients had objective response, but only one recovered and survived. This medication may be of some unique benefit, but insufficient data exist currently. Study of this drug in a prospective, randomized fashion is indicated.

Extracorporeal membrane oxygenation

ECMO originally was used as rescue therapy in patients who had CDH with pulmonary hypertension after corrective surgery. Retrospective review of 730 neonates from the CDH Study Group treated from 1995 to 1997 showed that ECMO use was associated with improved survival when used in patients who had CDH and had a predicted mortality of $\geq 80\%$ [103]. This benefit was not evident when ECMO was used in patients with less severe disease. As therapies have evolved, the timing of ECMO support has changed. In 1995, 20% of ECMO use in patients who had CDH was postoperative, but by 2001 this use had declined to only 5% [104], which illustrated the trend to preoperative stabilization with ECMO rather than postoperative rescue. By 2002, there were 2077 patients in the CDH registry, and 770 had been treated with ECMO (37%). Despite widespread acceptance and use, however, a Cochrane review concluded that ECMO offers short-term benefits for babies with diaphragmatic hernia, but the overall effect of using ECMO in this group remains unclear [105].

The mode of ECMO support for CDH patients also has been evaluated. Dimmitt reviewed the ELSO registry for the 1990s and reported in 2001 that veno-arterial (VA) ECMO was used in 86% of patients who had CDH compared with only 14% who received veno-venous (VV) support [106]. The pre-ECMO status was similar in the groups, although the VV group received more pressors and more frequent use of surfactant and nitric oxide. Survival was not different (58% for VV ECMO and 52% for VA; $P = 0.57$) but seizures were more common in the VA group (12.3% versus 6.7%;

$P = 0.0024$), as was cerebral infarction (10.5% versus 6.7%; $P = 0.03$). Sixty-four patients were converted from VV to VA (17%) and the survival rate was less (43.8%) but not significantly so. The authors concluded that VV ECMO for CDH had similar survival rates to VA ECMO but with less neurologic morbidity, and they saw no disadvantage to VV ECMO as the initial mode of ECMO support in CDH. These findings mirrored those of Schmidt and colleagues [107] and Kugelman and colleagues [108] in their single institution reviews.

Despite ongoing, widespread use of ECMO in CDH, there are reports of centers using ECMO significantly less frequently in their populations while still achieving high survival rates. Some centers report ECMO use in less than 15% of patients who have CDH [50,109]. These centers exclude a small proportion of severely ill infants from ECMO who meet institutional criteria for lethal pulmonary hypoplasia. They also have significant outborn populations, which exerts a selection bias, because the most severe outborn patients do not survive transfer into the accepting center. These centers' excellent survival rates, while using ECMO sparingly, again raise the question of benefit of ECMO in patients who have CDH.

Lung distension in congenital diaphragmatic hernia

Liquid perfluorocarbons possess unique physical properties, including high density, ability to carry oxygen and carbon dioxide, and low surface tension, which may prove useful in the ventilation of patients who have CDH and other forms of respiratory failure. A report in 2001 showed that distension of CDH lungs with perfluorocarbon on ECMO seemed to accelerate lung growth in five patients who had CDH and were on ECMO and improved subsequent gas exchange off ECMO [110]. A prospective, randomized pilot study of this therapy was published in 2003 in which eight patients who had CDH and were on ECMO were treated with perfluorocarbon instillation into their lungs to 5 to 8 cm of water compared with standard conventional ventilation on ECMO [111]. Study subjects realized nonstatistically significant improvements in time on ECMO, ventilator-free days, and survival compared with controls. A more definitive trial of this novel intervention is warranted and may hold the most promise for patients who have severe pulmonary hypoplasia.

Ventilation

Hyperventilation and induced alkalosis to decrease pulmonary hypertension and control ductal shunting were common therapeutic strategies in the late 1980s and 1990s and still are used in many centers. These therapies never showed improved survival, and studies of CDH mortality showed that pulmonary barotrauma, as evidenced by diffuse alveolar damage, hyaline membrane formation, pneumothorax, pulmonary hemorrhage, and occasionally even interstitial fibrosis, was the dominant finding at postmortem examination [73,112]. Iatrogenic barotrauma represented a potentially avoidable cause of mortality in patients who had CDH and was postulated to contribute to 25% of CDH deaths [73].

The single most significant advance in the management of patients who have CDH in the last 20 years has been the development and propagation of a neonatal ventilation strategy that significantly limits inflation pressure, allows tolerance of hypercapnia and relative postductal hypoxemia, and eliminates hyperventilation. The gentle ventilation strategy was pioneered by Wung and colleagues [114], first in neonates with pulmonary hypertension who did not have CDH [113] and then in neonates who had CDH. This strategy, especially the tolerance of hypercarbia in pulmonary hypertension, ran counter to conventional wisdom and was not quickly accepted into practice [115]. Validation of concept and results were reported by Wilson [73] and Kays, however [48]. Detailed ventilation analysis of 89 patients showed that pneumothorax rates plummeted (from 43% to 2%) and survival rates improved dramatically (from 50%–89% in treated patients) with the introduction of a lung protective strategy that avoided hyperventilation and limited inflation pressures to ≤25 cm of water [48]. Other researchers have reported similar series [5,50,116], and survival rates of more than 80% in patients with isolated CDH have been achieved in several centers using gentle ventilation.

High-frequency oscillatory ventilation

High survival rates in CDH have been achieved by some investigators using high-frequency oscillatory ventilation [97,98,117], but others report no improvement in outcome compared with management with conventional ventilators [118–120]. The question of whether high-frequency oscillatory ventilation is best used as rescue if conventional ventilation fails or should be a primary mode of ventilation is not clear. It is clear, however, that barotrauma, which most frequently presents as pneumothorax but manifests in other aspects of lung failure, is associated with decreased survival in CDH [48,121,122]. Lung protective ventilation, whether by conventional mechanical ventilation or high-frequency oscillatory ventilation, must be provided to optimize CDH survival. A clear and unwavering treatment strategy that protects every alveolus with which patients who have CDH are born, is the closest we can come to a magic bullet in CDH.

Outcomes

An improved understanding of CDH pathophysiology and expanded application of lung protective treatment strategies has led to an improved

CDH survival rate. Infants who survive CDH are at risk of brain injury, [123] neurodevelopmental disability [124], hearing loss [125,126], feeding difficulties [127], gastroesophageal reflux [128,129], lung disease [130], scoliosis [131], pectus excavatum [131], and recurrence of their diaphragmatic hernia. Some of these outcome issues are anatomic and unavoidable. Other outcome issues reflect potential toxic effects of treatment strategies and may be avoided or eliminated in the future.

Although most infants who have CDH survive without major neurologic sequelae, newborns who have more severe CDH have small lungs and are at risk for periods of hypoxemia, acidosis, poor perfusion, and need for ECMO. These more severely affected infants are at high risk for hypoxic-ischemic brain injury and other secondary neurologic effects of severe illness. A review of 31 patients who had CDH who also required ECMO showed that 35% had central nervous system abnormalities on CT scan, which manifested primarily as enlarged ventricles, focal and diffuse brain atrophy, and intracranial hemorrhage. At 2 years, these patients showed mild cognitive and physical delay [124]. MRI at discharge showed evidence of brain injury in eight of eight CDH survivors, including some with relatively mild CDH [132]. In three separate series, 44% to 55% of CDH survivors required hearing amplification because of hearing loss [133–135]. It is important to note that many of these survivors came from the era of hyperventilation.

Neonatal lung anomalies

Fetal lung lesions may cause significant mass effect, result in nonimmune hydrops, and lead to fetal or infant demise. Therapeutic options for these severely affected infants are evolving. The abundant use of prenatal imaging also has led to the identification of small fetal lung lesions that may be asymptomatic at birth and beyond. Management of these lesions is not clear.

Prenatal diagnosis and interventions

Prenatal diagnosis of CCAM , pulmonary sequestrations, and congenital lobar emphysema are the subject of an evolving literature. Ultrafast fetal MRI after initial identification of a chest lesion by two-dimensional ultrasound is reported to be a useful and important adjunct. MRI has been shown to confirm ultrasound diagnosis, provide more detailed anatomic information, and achieve greater diagnostic accuracy than ultrasound alone [41,136,137]. Three-dimensional ultrasound also offers more detailed imaging and was tested in eight cases of hyperechogenic fetal lung lesions, correctly identifying the abnormal feeding vessel in all three cases of pulmonary sequestration and showing no such vessel in the five CAMs [138]. Postnatally, CT and MR angiography have been used to identify anomalous systemic feeding vessels in pulmonary sequestrations with high accuracy [32,139–141], and these imaging advances obviate the need for more invasive angiography.

Fetal lung lesions can lead to nonimmune hydrops. Of 175 prenatally diagnosed lung lesions reported by Adzick and colleagues [142], 134 were CCAMs. All of the fetuses without hydrops survived, whereas all 25 with hydrops who did not undergo some type of fetal intervention died. Thirteen women with hydropic fetuses underwent open fetal surgery; eight fetuses survivors. Six fetuses with a large unilocular pulmonary cyst had percutaneous placement of a thoracoamniotic shunt, and five survived.

Forty-one of the 175 lesions were extralobar pulmonary sequestrations. Twenty-eight of these regressed dramatically on prenatal studies, were asymptomatic at birth, and were later identifiable only by CT or MRI. None of these was resected. Of the remaining 13 fetuses with extralobar sequestrations, 2 aborted electively, 1 developed hydrops and died, 3 had hydrothorax treated with prenatal drainage procedures, and 7 were symptomatic postnatally and underwent resection.

The size and follow-up of this study warrants attention. The authors stressed the poor prognosis in patients with nonimmune hydrops secondary to fetal lung lesions when only followed expectantly. Survival with fetal intervention was superior in patients who had CCAM and nonimmune hydrops. Of note, the details of postnatal ventilatory support in the children who died were not provided.

An expanded experience with thoracoamniotic shunting for fetal pleural effusion and CCAM was reported in 2004 [143]. This procedure seems to play a beneficial role for the fetus with a large CCAM or sequestration with associated large hydrothorax and secondary nonimmune hydrops but may be complicated by preterm delivery [144].

Although the development of nonimmune hydrops with prenatal CCAM is clearly a marker of severity, others have not found the association universally fatal, even without fetal therapy. Ierullo reported [145] 34 cases of prenatal CCAM, and 76% improved or resolved during prenatal monitoring, including resolution of hydrops in 3 of 6 cases. Illanes reported [123] 48 cases of prenatal lung lesions, with hydrops in 9. Of these fetuses, three survived, whereas six progressed and resulted in fetal or infant demise. The Fetal Therapy group at the University of California at San Francisco reported three prenatally diagnosed fetuses with CCAM and hydrops who were treated with maternal steroids in the second trimester. All three patients enjoyed resolution of the hydrops and delivery at term without respiratory distress [146].

Postnatal management

Symptomatic lung lesions in infants and children warrant resection. Lobectomy is the procedure most frequently used and results are excellent, with minimal morbidity and mortality in experienced hands [147,148].

Symptomatic lesions are resected when indicated, either at presentation or after a period of treatment (ie, antibiotics for infection).

Management of asymptomatic lung lesions in infants and children remains controversial. Authors who favor resection of prenatally diagnosed but asymptomatic lung lesions favor resection before 1 year of age [81,149,150]. Adzick recommends resection after 1 month of age, whereas Laberge recommends no later than 3 to 6 months to maximize potential for compensatory lung growth [149,150]. Thoracoscopic techniques are also used for anatomic pulmonary resections, even in infants [151,152], and their applicability is likely related to the experience level of the surgeon.

Cystic adenomatoid malformation

The natural history of the asymptomatic CCAM found by prenatal imaging is not clear. Although most authors favor resection of symptomatic and asymptomatic CCAM [148–150,153], there is an increase in the number of series reporting careful follow-up and expectant management in asymptomatic lesions. Series that favor resection cite that CCAM eventually becomes infected in most cases [149] and has an associated risk of malignancy, including rhabdomyosarcoma [154,155], pleuropulmonary blastoma [156], and bronchoalveolar carcinoma [157]. Series that favor observation of asymptomatic lesions cite that malignancy is rare, the true incidence of infection in asymptomatic lesions is not known, and a single incidence of previous infection does not result in an increase in operative complications [81]. Reports of apparent spontaneous resolution of CCAM during gestation and postnatally add support to the nonoperative strategy. Prenatally diagnosed CCAM resolved spontaneously during gestation at a rate of 15% to 30% in recent representative series [158,159]. Plain chest radiography is not sufficiently sensitive to define this, and postnatal CT is required to confirm resolution of the CCAM. Postnatal resolution of CCAMs also occurs but much less commonly, and it occurred in only 2 of 56 cases (4%) reported by Butterworth and Blair [160].

Two recent studies reported observation alone of asymptomatic CCAM. Van Leeuwen and colleagues reported 14 cases in 1999 [161]. Four patients were symptomatic at birth and underwent resection and 10 were asymptomatic. Five received or were due for elective resection (based on surgeon preference), whereas 5 others were observed for 36±15 months without adverse sequelae. Aziz and Langer [81] reported on 35 asymptomatic patients who had CCAM. Fifteen asymptomatic patients underwent elective resection—6 patients before and 9 patients after 6 months. Three patients developed symptomatic infection between 6 and 12 months and underwent resection. Seventeen remained asymptomatic without resection at a median follow-up of 3 years. These data suggest that nonoperative management of CCAM remains controversial even in centers that practice it, with a significant proportion of asymptomatic patients receiving elective resection.

Infection that led to resection developed in 10% of asymptomatic children during observation [81].

Pulmonary sequestration and congenital lobar emphysema

These lesions have a highly favorable prognosis when diagnosed prenatally compared with CCAM, and survival is excellent [142,162]. Hydrops occasionally can result. Both lesions may resolve during gestation and the postnatal period. Congenital lobar emphysema may improve with bronchial development. Although symptomatic lesions warrant aggressive surgical management, observation of asymptomatic patients is more commonly practiced in these lesions than CCAM [149,150].

Summary

CDH and neonatal lung lesions are increasingly diagnosed during fetal life, and expanded use of three-dimensional ultrasound and fetal MRI have improved diagnostic detail and accuracy. Chromosomal abnormalities and severe congenital heart lesions negatively impact CDH outcome, but survival at several centers that have abandoned hyperventilation in favor of strict lung protective strategies exceeds 80% in patients who have isolated CDH. Congenital lung lesions range from small, asymptomatic imaging abnormalities to large, space-occupying lesions that cause fetal hydrops. Symptomatic lesions should be resected during infancy, and resection remains the standard for most asymptomatic lesions. Increasing numbers of reports indicate that small, asymptomatic lesions are being treated with observation and follow-up alone, and maturation of this literature is expected in the years to come.

References

[1] Cardoso WV. Lung morphogenesis revisited: old facts, current ideas. Dev Dyn 2000;219(2): 121–30.
[2] Kukoski R, Blonigen B, Macri E, et al. p27 and cyclin E/D2 associations in testicular germ cell tumors: implications for tumorigenesis. Appl Immunohistochem Mol Morphol 2003; 11(2):138–43.
[3] Knowles S, Thomas RM, Lindenbaum RH, et al. Pulmonary agenesis as part of the VAC-TERL sequence. Arch Dis Child 1988;63(7 Spec No):723–6.
[4] Matsushima H, Takayanagi N, Satoh M, et al. Congenital bronchial atresia: radiologic findings in nine patients. J Comput Assist Tomogr 2002;26(5):860–4.
[5] Downard CD, Kim HB, Laningham F, et al. Esophageal atresia, duodenal atresia, and unilateral lung agenesis: a case report. J Pediatr Surg 2004;39(8):1283–5.
[6] Noorily MJ, Farmer DL, Flake AW. The association of complete laryngotracheoesophageal cleft with left lung agenesis: pathophysiological clues provided by an experiment of nature. J Pediatr Surg 1998;33(10):1546–9.
[7] Steadland KM, Langham MR Jr, Greene MA, et al. Unilateral pulmonary agenesis, esophageal atresia, and distal tracheoesophageal fistula. Ann Thorac Surg 1995;59(2):511–3.

[8] Walford N, Htun K, Chen J, et al. Intralobar sequestration of the lung is a congenital anomaly: anatomopathological analysis of four cases diagnosed in fetal life. Pediatr Dev Pathol 2003;6(4):314–21.

[9] Cunningham ML, Mann N. Pulmonary agenesis: a predictor of ipsilateral malformations. Am J Med Genet 1997;70(4):391–8.

[10] Wells L. Development of the human diaphragm and pleural sacs. Contr Embryol Carneg Instn 1954;35:107–37.

[11] de Lorimier A. Diaphragmatic hernia. In: Ashcraft KW, Holder TM, editors. Pediatric surgery. 2nd edition. Philadelphia: WB Saunders; 1993. p. 204–5.

[12] Keijzer R, Liu J, Deimling J, et al. Dual-hit hypothesis explains pulmonary hypoplasia in the nitrofen model of congenital diaphragmatic hernia. Am J Pathol 2000;156(4): 1299–306.

[13] Babiuk RP, Zhang W, Clugston R, et al. Embryological origins and development of the rat diaphragm. J Comp Neurol 2003;455(4):477–87.

[14] Anderson D. Incidence of congenital diaphragmatic hernia in the young of rats bred on a diet deficient in vitamin A. Am J Dis Child 1941;62:888–9.

[15] Babiuk RP, Thebaud B, Greer JJ. Reductions in the incidence of nitrofen-induced diaphragmatic hernia by vitamin A and retinoic acid. Am J Physiol Lung Cell Mol Physiol 2004;286(5):L970–3.

[16] Correia-Pinto J, Baptista MJ, Estevao-Costa J, et al. Heart-related indices in experimental diaphragmatic hernia. J Pediatr Surg 2000;35(10):1449–52.

[17] Major D, Cadenas M, Fournier L, et al. Retinol status of newborn infants with congenital diaphragmatic hernia. Pediatr Surg Int 1998;13(8):547–9.

[18] Rottier R, Tibboel D. Fetal lung and diaphragm development in congenital diaphragmatic hernia. Semin Perinatol 2005;29(2):86–93.

[19] Witters I, Devriendt K, Moerman P, et al. Bilateral tibial agenesis with ectrodactyly (OMIM 119100): further evidence for autosomal recessive inheritance. Am J Med Genet 2001;104(3):209–13.

[20] Howe DT, Kilby MD, Sirry H, et al. Structural chromosome anomalies in congenital diaphragmatic hernia. Prenat Diagn 1996;16(11):1003–9.

[21] Slavotinek AM. Fryns syndrome: a review of the phenotype and diagnostic guidelines. Am J Med Genet 2004;124(4):427–33.

[22] Chiesa J, Hoffet M, Rousseau O, et al. Pallister-Killian syndrome [i(12p)]: first pre-natal diagnosis using cordocentesis in the second trimester confirmed by in situ hybridization. Clin Genet 1998;54(4):294–302.

[23] Wilson RD, Harrison K, Clarke LA, et al. Tetrasomy 12p (Pallister-Killian syndrome): ultrasound indicators and confirmation by interphase fish. Prenat Diagn 1994;14(9): 787–92.

[24] Li M, Shuman C, Fei YL, et al. GPC3 mutation analysis in a spectrum of patients with overgrowth expands the phenotype of Simpson-Golabi-Behmel syndrome. Am J Med Genet 2001;102(2):161–8.

[25] Twigg SR, Kan R, Babbs C, et al. Mutations of ephrin-B1 (EFNB1), a marker of tissue boundary formation, cause craniofrontonasal syndrome. Proc Natl Acad Sci U S A 2004;101(23):8652–7.

[26] Jacobs AM, Toudjarska I, Racine A, et al. A recurring FBN1 gene mutation in neonatal Marfan syndrome. Arch Pediatr Adolesc Med 2002;156(11):1081–5.

[27] Bulman MP, Kusumi K, Frayling TM, et al. Mutations in the human delta homologue, DLL3, cause axial skeletal defects in spondylocostal dysostosis. Nat Genet 2000;24(4): 438–41.

[28] Austin-Ward ED, Taucher SC. Familial congenital diaphragmatic hernia: is an imprinting mechanism involved? J Med Genet 1999;36(7):578–9.

[29] Norio R, Kaariainen H, Rapola J, et al. Familial congenital diaphragmatic defects: aspects of etiology, prenatal diagnosis, and treatment. Am J Med Genet 1984;17(2):471–83.

[30] Ruano R, Joubin L, Sonigo P, et al. Fetal lung volume estimated by 3-dimensional ultra-sonography and magnetic resonance imaging in cases with isolated congenital diaphragmatic hernia. J Ultrasound Med 2004;23(3):353–8.

[31] Hubbard AM, Crombleholme TM, Adzick NS, et al. Prenatal MRI evaluation of congenital diaphragmatic hernia. Am J Perinatol 1999;16(8):407–13.

[32] Xu H, Jiang D, Kong X, et al. Pulmonary sequestration: three dimensional dynamic contrast-enhanced MR angiography and MRI. J Tongji Med Univ 2001;21(4):345–8.

[33] Leung JW, Coakley FV, Hricak H, et al. Prenatal MR imaging of congenital diaphragmatic hernia. AJR Am J Roentgenol 2000;174(6):1607–12.

[34] Coakley FVT. MRI: role of magnetic resonance imaging in fetal surgery. Top Magn Reson Imaging 2001;12(1):39–51.

[35] Fauza DO, Wilson JM. Congenital diaphragmatic hernia and associated anomalies: their incidence, identification, and impact on prognosis. J Pediatr Surg 1994;29(8):1113–7.

[36] Kaiser L, Vizer M, Arany A, et al. Correlation of prenatal clinical findings with those observed in fetal autopsies: pathological approach. Prenat Diagn 2000;20(12):970–5.

[37] Graziano JN. Cardiac anomalies in patients with congenital diaphragmatic hernia and their prognosis: a report from the Congenital Diaphragmatic Hernia Study Group. J Pediatr Surg 2005;40(6):1045–9 [discussion: 1049–50].

[38] Laudy JA, Van Gucht M, Van Dooren MF, et al. Congenital diaphragmatic hernia: an evaluation of the prognostic value of the lung-to-head ratio and other prenatal parameters. Prenat Diagn 2003;23(8):634–9.

[39] Heling KS, Wauer RR, Hammer H, et al. Reliability of the lung-to-head ratio in predicting outcome and neonatal ventilation parameters in fetuses with congenital diaphragmatic hernia. Ultrasound Obstet Gynecol 2005;25(2):112–8.

[40] Ruano R, Benachi A, Joubin L, et al. Three-dimensional ultrasonographic assessment of fetal lung volume as prognostic factor in isolated congenital diaphragmatic hernia. BJOG 2004;111(5):423–9.

[41] Matsuoka S, Takeuchi K, Yamanaka Y, et al. Comparison of magnetic resonance imaging and ultrasonography in the prenatal diagnosis of congenital thoracic abnormalities. Fetal Diagn Ther 2003;18(6):447–53.

[42] Albanese CT, Lopoo J, Goldstein RB, et al. Fetal liver position and perinatal outcome for congenital diaphragmatic hernia. Prenat Diagn 1998;18(11):1138–42.

[43] Doyle NM, Lally KP. The CDH Study Group and advances in the clinical care of the patient with congenital diaphragmatic hernia. Semin Perinatol 2004;28(3):174–84.

[44] Adzick NS, Harrison MR, Glick PL, et al. Diaphragmatic hernia in the fetus: prenatal diagnosis and outcome in 94 cases. J Pediatr Surg 1985;20(4):357–61.

[45] Adzick NS, Vacanti JP, Lillehei CW, et al. Fetal diaphragmatic hernia: ultrasound diagnosis and clinical outcome in 38 cases. J Pediatr Surg 1989;24(7):654–7 [discussion: 657–8].

[46] Geary MP, Chitty LS, Morrison JJ, et al. Perinatal outcome and prognostic factors in prenatally diagnosed congenital diaphragmatic hernia. Ultrasound Obstet Gynecol 1998;12(2):107–11.

[47] Donnelly LF, Sakurai M, Klosterman LA, et al. Correlation between findings on chest radiography and survival in neonates with congenital diaphragmatic hernia. AJR Am J Roentgenol 1999;173(6):1589–93.

[48] Kays DW, Langham MR Jr, Ledbetter DJ, Talbert JL. Detrimental effects of standard medical therapy in congenital diaphragmatic hernia. Ann Surg 1999;230(3):340–8 [discussion: 348–51].

[49] Holt PD, Arkovitz MS, Berdon WE, et al. Newborns with diaphragmatic hernia: initial chest radiography does not have a role in predicting clinical outcome. Pediatr Radiol 2004;34(6):462–4.

[50] Boloker J, Bateman DA, Wung JT, et al. Congenital diaphragmatic hernia in 120 infants treated consecutively with permissive hypercapnea/spontaneous respiration/elective repair. J Pediatr Surg 2002;37(3):357–66.

[51] Metkus AP, Filly RA, Stringer MD, et al. Sonographic predictors of survival in fetal diaphragmatic hernia. J Pediatr Surg 1996;31(1):148–51 [discussion: 151–2].

[52] The Congenital Diaphragmatic Hernia Study Group. Estimating disease severity of congenital diaphragmatic hernia in the first 5 minutes of life. J Pediatr Surg 2001;36(1):141–5.

[53] Skarsgard ED, Blair GK, Lee SK. Toward evidence-based best practices in neonatal surgical care-I: the Canadian NICU Network. J Pediatr Surg 2003;38(5):672–7.

[54] Harrison MR, Adzick NS, Estes JM, et al. A prospective study of the outcome for fetuses with diaphragmatic hernia. JAMA 1994;271(5):382–4.

[55] Harrison MR, Langer JC, Adzick NS, et al. Correction of congenital diaphragmatic hernia in utero, V. Initial clinical experience. J Pediatr Surg 1990;25(1):47–55 [discussion: 56–47].

[56] Harrison MR, Adzick NS, Longaker MT, et al. Successful repair in utero of a fetal diaphragmatic hernia after removal of herniated viscera from the left thorax. N Engl J Med 1990;322(22):1582–4.

[57] Harrison MR, Adzick NS, Flake AW, et al. Correction of congenital diaphragmatic hernia in utero: VI. Hard-earned lessons. J Pediatr Surg 1993;28(10):1411–7 [discussion: 1417–8].

[58] Harrison MR, Adzick NS, Flake AW, et al. The CDH two-step: a dance of necessity. J Pediatr Surg 1993;28(6):813–6.

[59] Wilson JM, DiFiore JW, Peters CA. Experimental fetal tracheal ligation prevents the pulmonary hypoplasia associated with fetal nephrectomy: possible application for congenital diaphragmatic hernia. J Pediatr Surg 1993;28(11):1433–9 [discussion: 1439–40].

[60] DiFiore JW, Fauza DO, Slavin R, et al. Experimental fetal tracheal ligation reverses the structural and physiological effects of pulmonary hypoplasia in congenital diaphragmatic hernia. J Pediatr Surg 1994;29(2):248–56 [discussion: 256–7].

[61] Harrison MR, Mychaliska GB, Albanese CT, et al. Correction of congenital diaphragmatic hernia in utero IX: fetuses with poor prognosis (liver herniation and low lung-to-head ratio) can be saved by fetoscopic temporary tracheal occlusion. J Pediatr Surg 1998;33(7):1017–22 [discussion: 1022–3].

[62] Harrison MR, Sydorak RM, Farrell JA, et al. Fetoscopic temporary tracheal occlusion for congenital diaphragmatic hernia: prelude to a randomized, controlled trial. J Pediatr Surg 2003;38(7):1012–20.

[63] Harrison MR, Keller RL, Hawgood SB, et al. A randomized trial of fetal endoscopic tracheal occlusion for severe fetal congenital diaphragmatic hernia. N Engl J Med 2003; 349(20):1916–24.

[64] Hardesty RL, Griffith BP, Debski RF, et al. Extracorporeal membrane oxygenation: successful treatment of persistent fetal circulation following repair of congenital diaphragmatic hernia. J Thorac Cardiovasc Surg 1981;81(4):556–63.

[65] Langham MR Jr, Krummel TM, Greenfield LJ, et al. Extracorporeal membrane oxygenation following repair of congenital diaphragmatic hernias. Ann Thorac Surg 1987;44(3): 247–52.

[66] Tibboel D, Bos AP, Pattenier JW, et al. Pre-operative stabilisation with delayed repair in congenital diaphragmatic hernia. Z Kinderchir 1989;44(3):139–43.

[67] West KW, Bengston K, Rescorla FJ, et al. Delayed surgical repair and ECMO improves survival in congenital diaphragmatic hernia. Ann Surg 1992;216(4):454–60 [discussion: 460–2].

[68] Breaux CW Jr, Rouse TM, Cain WS, et al. Improvement in survival of patients with congenital diaphragmatic hernia utilizing a strategy of delayed repair after medical and/or extracorporeal membrane oxygenation stabilization. J Pediatr Surg 1991;26(3):333–6 [discussion: 336–8].

[69] Glick PL, Leach CL, Besner GE, et al. Pathophysiology of congenital diaphragmatic hernia. III: Exogenous surfactant therapy for the high-risk neonate with CDH. J Pediatr Surg 1992;27(7):866–9.

[70] Kluth D, Nestoris S, Tander B, et al. Inhaled nitric oxide increases survival rates in newborn rats with congenital diaphragmatic hernia. Eur J Pediatr Surg 1997;7(2):90–2.

[71] Harris K. Extralobar sequestration with congenital diaphragmatic hernia: a complicated case study. Neonatal Netw 2004;23(6):7–24.

[72] Keller TM, Rake A, Michel SC, et al. MR assessment of fetal lung development using lung volumes and signal intensities. European Radiology 2004;14(6):984–9.

[73] Wilson JM, Lund DP, Lillehei CW, et al. Congenital diaphragmatic hernia: a tale of two cities. The Boston experience. J Pediatr Surg 1997;32(3):401–5.

[74] Stege G, Fenton A, Jaffray B. Nihilism in the 1990s: the true mortality of congenital diaphragmatic hernia. Pediatrics 2003;112(3 Pt 1):532–5.

[75] Scott L, Cameron B, Bass J, et al. Apparent truth about congenital diaphragmatic hernia: a population-based database is needed to establish benchmarking for clinical outcomes for CDH. J Pediatr Surg 2004;39(5):661–5.

[76] Clark RH, Hardin WD Jr, Hirschl RB, et al. Current surgical management of congenital diaphragmatic hernia: a report from the Congenital Diaphragmatic Hernia Study Group. J Pediatr Surg 1998;33(7):1004–9.

[77] Reickert CA, Hirschl RB, Atkinson JB, et al. Congenital diaphragmatic hernia survival and use of extracorporeal life support at selected level III nurseries with multimodality support. Surgery 1998;123(3):305–10.

[78] Moya FR, Lally KP. Evidence-based management of infants with congenital diaphragmatic hernia. Semin Perinatol 2005;29(2):112–7.

[79] Nakayama DK, Motoyama EK, Tagge EM. Effect of preoperative stabilization on respiratory system compliance and outcome in newborn infants with congenital diaphragmatic hernia. J Pediatr 1991;118(5):793–9.

[80] Moyer V, Moya F, Tibboel R, et al. Late versus early surgical correction for congenital diaphragmatic hernia in newborn infants. Cochrane Database Syst Rev 2000;3: CD001695.

[81] Aziz D, Langer JC, Tuuha SE, et al. Perinatally diagnosed asymptomatic congenital cystic adenomatoid malformation: to resect or not? J Pediatr Surg 2004;39(3):329–34.

[82] Wilson JM, Lund DP, Lillehei CW, et al. Delayed repair and preoperative ECMO does not improve survival in high-risk congenital diaphragmatic hernia. J Pediatr Surg 1992;27(3): 368–72 [discussion: 373–5].

[83] Moyer V, Moya F, Tibboel R, et al. Late versus early surgical correction for congenital diaphragmatic hernia in newborn infants. Cochrane Database Syst Rev 2002;3:CD001695.

[84] Glick PL, Stannard VA, Leach CL, et al. Pathophysiology of congenital diaphragmatic hernia II: the fetal lamb CDH model is surfactant deficient. J Pediatr Surg 1992;27(3):382–7 [discussion: 387–8].

[85] Kitterman JA. Fetal lambs with surgically produced congenital diaphragmatic hernia (CDH) are deficient in pulmonary surfactant. J Pediatr Surg 1993;28(9):1218–9.

[86] Mysore MR, Margraf LR, Jaramillo MA, et al. Surfactant protein A is decreased in a rat model of congenital diaphragmatic hernia. Am J Respir Crit Care Med 1998;157(2):654–7.

[87] Alfanso LF, Arnaiz A, Alvarez FJ, et al. Lung hypoplasia and surfactant system immaturity induced in the fetal rat by prenatal exposure to nitrofen. Biol Neonate 1996;69(2): 94–100.

[88] Zimmermann LJ, Bunt JE, de Jongste JC, et al. Prospective evaluation of surfactant composition in bronchoalveolar lavage fluid of infants with congenital diaphragmatic hernia and of age-matched controls. Crit Care Med 1998;26(3):573–80.

[89] Janssen DJ, Tibboel D, Carnielli VP, et al. Surfactant phosphatidylcholine pool size in human neonates with congenital diaphragmatic hernia requiring ECMO. J Pediatr 2003; 142(3):247–52.

[90] Cogo PE, Zimmermann LJ, Meneghini L, et al. Pulmonary surfactant disaturated-phosphatidylcholine (DSPC) turnover and pool size in newborn infants with congenital diaphragmatic hernia (CDH). Pediatr Res 2003;54(5):653–8.

[91] Van Meurs K. Is surfactant therapy beneficial in the treatment of the term newborn infant with congenital diaphragmatic hernia? J Pediatr 2004;145(3):312–6.

[92] Neville HL, Jaksic T, Wilson JM, et al. Bilateral congenital diaphragmatic hernia. J Pediatr Surg 2003;38(3):522–4.

[93] Colby CE, Lally KP, Hintz SR, et al. Surfactant replacement therapy on ECMO does not improve outcome in neonates with congenital diaphragmatic hernia. J Pediatr Surg 2004; 39(11):1632–7.

[94] The Neonatal Inhaled Nitric Oxide Study Group (NINOS). Inhaled nitric oxide and hypoxic respiratory failure in infants with congenital diaphragmatic hernia. Pediatrics 1997; 99(6):838–45.

[95] The Neonatal Inhaled Nitric Oxide Study Group (NINOS). Inhaled nitric oxide in term and near-term infants: neurodevelopmental follow-up. J Pediatr 2000;136(5):611–7.

[96] Okuyama H, Kubota A, Oue T, et al. Inhaled nitric oxide with early surgery improves the outcome of antenatally diagnosed congenital diaphragmatic hernia. J Pediatr Surg 2002; 37(8):1188–90.

[97] Serrano P, Reyes G, Lugo-Vicente H. Congenital diaphragmatic hernia: mortality determinants in a Hispanic population. P R Health Sci J 1998;17(4):317–21.

[98] Somaschini M, Bellan C, Chinaglia D, et al. Congenital misalignment of pulmonary vessels and alveolar capillary dysplasia: how to manage a neonatal irreversible lung disease? J Perinatol 2000;20(3):189–92.

[99] Finer NN, Barrington KJ. Nitric oxide for respiratory failure in infants born at or near term. Cochrane Database Syst Rev 2001;4:CD000399.

[100] Travadi JN, Patole SK. Phosphodiesterase inhibitors for persistent pulmonary hypertension of the newborn: a review. Pediatr Pulmonol 2003;36(6):529–35.

[101] Schulze-Neick I, Li J, Reader JA, et al. The endothelin antagonist BQ123 reduces pulmonary vascular resistance after surgical intervention for congenital heart disease. J Thorac Cardiovasc Surg 2002;124(3):435–41.

[102] Juliana AE, Abbad FC. Severe persistent pulmonary hypertension of the newborn in a setting where limited resources exclude the use of inhaled nitric oxide: successful treatment with sildenafil. Eur J Pediatr 2005;164(10):626–9.

[103] The Congenital Diaphragmatic Hernia Study Group. Does extracorporeal membrane oxygenation improve survival in neonates with congenital diaphragmatic hernia? J Pediatr Surg 1999;34(5):720–4 [discussion: 724–5].

[104] Khan AM, Lally KP. The role of extracorporeal membrane oxygenation in the management of infants with congenital diaphragmatic hernia. Semin Perinatol 2005;29(2): 118–22.

[105] Elbourne D, Field D, Mugford M. Extracorporeal membrane oxygenation for severe respiratory failure in newborn infants. Cochrane Database Syst Rev 2002;1:CD001340.

[106] Dimmitt RA, Moss RL, Rhine WD, et al. Venoarterial versus venovenous extracorporeal membrane oxygenation in congenital diaphragmatic hernia: the extracorporeal life support organization registry, 1990–1999. J Pediatr Surg 2001;36(8):1199–1204.

[107] Schmidt M, Theissen P, Deutsch HJ, et al. Magnetic resonance imaging of ductus arteriosus Botalli apertus in adulthood. Int J Cardiol 1999;68(2):225–9.

[108] Kugelman A, Gangitano E, Pincros J, et al. Venovenous versus venoarterial extracorporeal membrane oxygenation in congenital diaphragmatic hernia. J Pediatr Surg 2003;38(8): 1131–6.

[109] Sokol J, Bohn D, Lacro RV, et al. Fetal pulmonary artery diameters and their association with lung hypoplasia and postnatal outcome in congenital diaphragmatic hernia. Am J Obstet Gynecol 2002;186(5):1085–90.

[110] Fauza DO, Hirschl RB, Wilson JM. Continuous intrapulmonary distension with perfluorocarbon accelerates lung growth in infants with congenital diaphragmatic hernia: initial experience. J Pediatr Surg 2001;36(8):1237–40.

[111] Hirschl RB, Philip WF, Glick L, et al. A prospective, randomized pilot trial of perfluorocarbon-induced lung growth in newborns with congenital diaphragmatic hernia. J Pediatr Surg 2003;38(3):283–9.

[112] Sakurai Y, Azarow K, Cutz E, et al. Pulmonary barotrauma in congenital diaphragmatic hernia: a clinicopathological correlation. J Pediatr Surg 1999;34(12):1813–7.

[113] Wung JT, James LS, Kilchevsky E, et al. Management of infants with severe respiratory failure and persistence of the fetal circulation, without hyperventilation. Pediatrics 1985; 76(4):488–94.

[114] Wung JT, Sahni R, Moffitt ST, et al. Congenital diaphragmatic hernia: survival treated with very delayed surgery, spontaneous respiration, and no chest tube. J Pediatr Surg 1995;30(3): 406–9.

[115] Walsh-Sukys MC, Cornell DJ, Houston LN, et al. Treatment of persistent pulmonary hypertension of the newborn without hyperventilation: an assessment of diffusion of innovation. Pediatrics 1994;94(3):303–6.

[116] Bagolan P, Casaccia G, Crescenzi F, et al. Impact of a current treatment protocol on outcome of high-risk congenital diaphragmatic hernia. J Pediatr Surg 2004;39(3): 313–8.

[117] Desfrere L, Jarreau PH, Dommergues M, et al. Impact of delayed repair and elective high-frequency oscillatory ventilation on survival of antenatally diagnosed congenital diaphragmatic hernia: first application of these strategies in the more "severe" subgroup of antenatally diagnosed newborns. Intensive Care Med 2000;26(7):934–41.

[118] Kamata S, Usui N, Ishikawa S, et al. Prolonged preoperative stabilization using high-frequency oscillatory ventilation does not improve the outcome in neonates with congenital diaphragmatic hernia. Pediatr Surg Int 1998;13(8):542–6.

[119] Kinsella JP, Truog WE, Walsh WF, et al. Randomized, multicenter trial of inhaled nitric oxide and high-frequency oscillatory ventilation in severe, persistent pulmonary hypertension of the newborn. J Pediatr 1997;131(1 Pt 1):55–62.

[120] Azarow K, Messineo A, Pearl R, et al. Congenital diaphragmatic hernia: a tale of two cities. The Toronto experience. J Pediatr Surg 1997;32(3):395–400.

[121] Chou HC, Tang JR, Lai HS, et al. Prognostic indicators of survival in infants with congenital diaphragmatic hernia. J Formos Med Assoc 2001;100(3):173–5.

[122] Saifuddin A, Arthur RJ. Congenital diaphragmatic hernia: a review of pre- and postoperative chest radiology. Clin Radiol 1993;47(2):104–10.

[123] Illanes S, Hunter A, Evans M, et al. Prenatal diagnosis of echogenic lung: evolution and outcome. Ultrasound Obstet Gynecol 2005;26(2):145–9.

[124] Ahmad A, Gangitano E, Odell RM, et al. Survival, intracranial lesions, and neurodevelopmental outcome in infants with congenital diaphragmatic hernia treated with extracorporeal membrane oxygenation. J Perinatol 1999;19(6 Pt 1):436–40.

[125] Georgeson KE, Robertson DJSP. Minimally invasive surgery in the neonate: review of current evidence. Semin Perinatol 2004;28(3):212–20.

[126] Fligor BJ, Neault MW, Mullen CH, et al. Factors associated with sensorineural hearing loss among survivors of extracorporeal membrane oxygenation therapy. Pediatrics 2005;115(6): 1519–28.

[127] Muratore CS, Utter S, Jaksic T, et al. Nutritional morbidity in survivors of congenital diaphragmatic hernia. J Pediatr Surg 2001;36(8):1171–6.

[128] Kieffer J, Sapin E, Berg A, et al. Gastroesophageal reflux after repair of congenital diaphragmatic hernia. J Pediatr Surg 1995;30(9):1330–3.

[129] Kamiyama M, Kawahara H, Okuyama H, et al. Gastroesophageal reflux after repair of congenital diaphragmatic hernia. J Pediatr Surg 2002;37(12):1681–4.

[130] Trachsel D, Selvadurai H, Bohn D, et al. Long-term pulmonary morbidity in survivors of congenital diaphragmatic hernia. Pediatr Pulmonol 2005;39(5):433–9.

[131] Vanamo K, Peltonen J, Rintala R, et al. Chest wall and spinal deformities in adults with congenital diaphragmatic defects. J Pediatr Surg 1996;31(6):851–4.

[132] Hunt RW, Kean MJ, Stewart MJ, et al. Patterns of cerebral injury in a series of infants with congenital diaphragmatic hernia utilizing magnetic resonance imaging. J Pediatr Surg 2004; 39(1):31–6.

[133] Cortes RA, Keller RL, Townsend T, et al. Survival of severe congenital diaphragmatic hernia has morbid consequences. J Pediatr Surg 2005;40(1):36–45.

[134] Rasheed A, Tindall S, Cueny DL, et al. Neurodevelopmental outcome after congenital diaphragmatic hernia: extracorporeal membrane oxygenation before and after surgery. J Pediatr Surg 2001;36(4):539–44.

[135] Robertson CM, Cheung PY, Haluschak MM, et al. High prevalence of sensorineural hearing loss among survivors of neonatal congenital diaphragmatic hernia: Western Canadian ECMO Follow-up Group. Am J Otol 1998;19(6):730–6.

[136] Quinn TM, Hubbard AM, Adzick NS. Prenatal magnetic resonance imaging enhances fetal diagnosis. J Pediatr Surg 1998;33(4):553–8.

[137] Breysem L, Bosmans H, Dymarkowski S, et al. The value of fast MR imaging as an adjunct to ultrasound in prenatal diagnosis. Eur Radiol 2003;13(7):1538–48.

[138] Ruano R, Benachi A, Aubry MC, et al. Prenatal diagnosis of pulmonary sequestration using three-dimensional power Doppler ultrasound. Ultrasound Obstet Gynecol 2005;25(2):128–33.

[139] Franco J, Aliaga R, Domingo ML, et al. Diagnosis of pulmonary sequestration by spiral CT angiography. Thorax 1998;53(12):1089–92.

[140] Au VW, Chan JK, Chan FL. Pulmonary sequestration diagnosed by contrast enhanced three-dimensional MR angiography. Br J Radiol 1999;72(859):709–11.

[141] Wassia HL, Hussein H, Binyaheb S, et al. CT scan diagnosis of extralobar pulmonary sequestration: angiography not required. Saudi Medical Journal 2003;24(5 Suppl):S35.

[142] Adzick NS, Harrison MR, Crombleholme TM, et al. Fetal lung lesions: management and outcome. Am J Obstet Gynecol 1998;179(4):884–9.

[143] Wilson RD, Baxter JK, Johnson MP, et al. Thoracoamniotic shunts: fetal treatment of pleural effusions and congenital cystic adenomatoid malformations. Fetal Dign Ther 2004;19(5):413–20.

[144] Picone O, Benachi A, Mandelbrot L, et al. Thoracoamniotic shunting for fetal pleural effusions with hydrops. Am J Obstet Gynecol 2004;191(6):2047–50.

[145] Ierullo AM, Ganapathy R, Crowley S, et al. Neonatal outcome of antenatally diagnosed congenital cystic adenomatoid malformations. Ultrasound Obstet Gynecol 2005;26(2):150–3.

[146] Tsao K, Hawgood S, Vu L, et al. Resolution of hydrops fetalis in congenital cystic adenomatoid malformation after prenatal steroid therapy. J Pediatr Surg 2003;38(3):508–10.

[147] Schwartz MZ, Ramachandran P. Congenital malformations of the lung and mediastinum: a quarter century of experience from a single institution. J Pediatr Surg 1997;32(1):44–7.

[148] Shanmugam G, MacArthur K, Pollock J. Congenital lung malformations: antenatal and postnatal evaluation and management. Eur J Cardiothorac Surg 2005;27(1):45–52.

[149] Laberge JM, Puligandla P, Flageole H. Asymptomatic congenital lung malformations. Semin Pediatr Surg 2005;14(1):16–33.

[150] Adzick NS. Management of fetal lung lesions. Clin Perinatol 2003;30(3):481–92.

[151] Rothenberg S. Experience with thoracoscopic lobectomy in infants and children. J Pediatr Surg 2003;38(1):102–4.

[152] Koontz CS, Oliva V, Gow KW, et al. Video-assisted thoracoscopic surgical excision of cystic lung disease in children. J Pediatr Surg 2005;40(5):835–7.

[153] Khosa JK, Leong SL, Borzi PA. Congenital cystic adenomatoid malformation of the lung: indications and timing of surgery. Pediatr Surg Int 2004;20(7):505–8.

[154] Pai S, Eng HL, Lee SY, et al. Rhabdomyosarcoma arising within congenital cystic adenomatoid malformation. Pediatr Blood Cancer 2005;45(6):841–5.

[155] Ozcan C, Celik A, Ural Z, et al. Primary pulmonary rhabdomyosarcoma arising within cystic adenomatoid malformation: a case report and review of the literature. J Pediatr Surg 2001;36(7):1062–5.

[156] Hill D. USCAP specialty conference: case 1-type I pleuropulmonary blastoma. Pediatr Dev Pathol 2005;8(1):77–84.

[157] Granata C, Gambini C, Balducci T, et al. Bronchioloalveolar carcinoma arising in congenital cystic adenomatoid malformation in a child: a case report and review on malignancies originating in congenital cystic adenomatoid malformation. Pediatr Pulmonol 1998;25(1): 62–6.

[158] Gornall AS, Budd JL, Draper ES, et al. Congenital cystic adenomatoid malformation: accuracy of prenatal diagnosis, prevalence and outcome in a general population. Prenat Diagn 2003;23(12):997–1002.

[159] Pumberger W, Hormann M, Deutinger J, et al. Longitudinal observation of antenatally detected congenital lung malformations (CLM): natural history, clinical outcome and long-term follow-up. Eur J Cardiothorac Surg 2003;24(5):703–11.

[160] Butterworth SA, Blair G. Postnatal spontaneous resolution of congenital cystic adenomatoid malformations. J Pediatr Surg 2005;40(5):832–4.

[161] van Leeuwen K, Teitelbaum DH, Hirschl RB, et al. Prenatal diagnosis of congenital cystic adenomatoid malformation and its postnatal presentation, surgical indications, and natural history. J Pediatr Surg 1999;34(5):794–8 [discussion 798–9].

[162] Lopoo JB, Goldstein RB, Lipshutz GS, et al. Fetal pulmonary sequestration: a favorable congenital lung lesion. Obstet Gynecol 1999;94(4):567–71.

ELSEVIER
SAUNDERS

SURGICAL
CLINICS OF
NORTH AMERICA

Surg Clin N Am 86 (2006) 353–370

Congenital Chest Wall Defects

Rebecca M. McGuigan, MD[a],
Kenneth S. Azarow, MD[a,b,*]

[a]Department of Surgery, Madigan Army Medical Center, Tacoma, WA 98431, USA
[b]Department of Surgery, Uniformed Services University of Health Sciences,
Bethesda, MD USA

This article reviews congenital anterior chest wall deformities, namely pectus excavatum (PE), pectus carinatum (PC), and cleft sternum. Although the origin of these disorders was once debated in the literature, it is generally agreed that PE and carinatum deformities are a result of dysmorphic growth of costal cartilage that results in an abnormal position/rotation of the sternum [1]. Sternal cleft is an embryologic phenomenon caused by failure of lateral mesodermal plates to fuse during the first weeks in utero. These deformities usually present in isolation and are not typically part of any syndrome.

Pectus excavatum

Background

This depression defect of the anterior chest wall is the most prevalent of the anterior chest wall deformities and the most extensively studied and reported. It also has been called funnel chest or trichterbrust. The prevalence is approximately 1:400 live births [2]. There is no known genetic link, but 40% of patients who have PE report that a family member has a chest wall deformity [3]. It is more common in men, with a male to female ratio of approximately 5:1 [3]. The depression of the sternum usually can be detected in infancy and progresses, often markedly, during the growth phase of puberty. There is no known chromosomal abnormality associated with PE, but it has been reported in conjunction with Marfan's syndrome,

* Corresponding author.
E-mail address: Kenneth.azarow@us.army.mil (K.S. Azarow).

0039-6109/06/$ - see front matter © 2006 Elsevier Inc. All rights reserved.
doi:10.1016/j.suc.2005.12.012
surgical.theclinics.com

Ehlers-Danlos syndrome, osteogenesis imperfecta, syndactylism, club foot, and Klippel-Fiel syndrome [1]. It is rarely associated with congenital cardiac anomalies [4]. Many patients who have PE also have scoliosis.

Pathophysiology

Half a century ago there were several theories regarding the mechanism of the sternal depression seen in PE. Brodkin [5] and Chin and Adler [6] wrote that the anterior portion of the diaphragm is replaced with fibrous tissue and applies abnormal force to the posterior aspect of the sternum. Brown [7] contended that a substernal ligament pulled on the sternum and caused the deformity. Ravitch and others, however, were convinced that the sternum and diaphragm were normal and the defect was caused by overgrowth of the ribs pushing the sternum into a posterior position [8,9]. Currently it is widely agreed that the latter theory is correct.

Although there is little disagreement that PE is a significant cosmetic deformity with consequential psychological effects on young people, there is ongoing debate regarding its physiologic effects. The anteroposterior diameter of the chest is diminished to varying degrees in PE, and the heart is often displaced in the left chest on imaging. Subjectively, patients complain of dyspnea with exertion, diminished exercise capacity in comparison to their peers, chest pain, palpitations, frequent upper respiratory infections, and wheezing. A disproportional number of patients are diagnosed with exercise-induced asthma. Several papers in the last two decades have compared patients who have PE with normal control subjects. Pulmonary function tests in patients who have PE reveal a mild restrictive pattern, with total lung capacity, forced vital capacity, and vital capacity in the low-to-normal range [10,11]. The severity of the pectus deformity correlates roughly with the reduction in vital capacity and total lung capacity [12]. Forced expiratory volume in 1 second (FEV_1) to forced vital capacity ratio is normal, which indicates absence of obstructive disease [11]. Some patients have abnormalities on the electrocardiogram, namely right bundle block and right axis deviation [13]. There is a known association between PE and mitral valve prolapse [14].

Many patients who have PE complain of subjective exercise limitation, and results of exercise testing have been somewhat varied. Quiqley and colleagues [11] found that upon exercise testing on a treadmill, there were no objective differences in cardiorespiratory function or aerobic capacity between patients who had PE and control subjects. Some researchers believe the subjective exercise intolerance to be the result of physical deconditioning. Others have challenged this idea. Malek and colleagues [12] controlled for level of conditioning in a recent study and found the maximum oxygen uptake (VO_2max) to be 75% of predicted in patients who had, which suggested mild but not marked impairment. Malek and colleagues [12] also noted that the oxygen pulse, a surrogate for stroke volume, was diminished in patients who had, which is consistent with several other studies. Perhaps the right atrium and ventricle are compressed by the sternum when upright, causing decreased filling and subsequent inability to increase stroke volume and oxygen delivery during exercise. If this theory is true, perhaps patients' exercise ability would be positional, because sternal compression of the heart may be affected by body position. Compression and reduced filling have been documented in several studies [15,16]. Zhao and associates [17] recently readdressed this issue. Patients who had PE and control subjects performed sitting and supine cycling while undergoing echocardiography for stroke volume measurements. They found that in patients who had PE, the oxygen uptake (VO_2) plateau in the supine position was higher than in the sitting position. Supine exercise stroke volume also was higher than sitting exercise stroke volume. The supine stroke volume was the same as in control subjects. It is likely that patients who have PE have a real exercise limitation that is cardiac in origin. Discrepancy among studies is probably related to differences in conditioning, differences in the severity of disease, and difficulty obtaining true exercise capacity independent of patient effort. Whether the situation is improved by operative correction remains to be seen and is discussed later in this article.

Evaluation

History and physical examination are the only two essential components in the evaluation of patients for PE. One should obtain a history of the duration and progression of the sternal depression, family history, any other medical conditions, and a thorough review of systems, especially focused on cardiac and pulmonary symptoms and disease. Diagnosis is easily made on physical examination, with a prominent depression deformity of the sternum (Fig. 1). One should note carefully the presence or absence of scoliosis or a heart murmur. The gross appearance of PE may be classified as originally described by Chin [18]. A type I defect is localized and symmetric. Type II is diffuse and symmetric. Type III is asymmetric, either localized or diffuse. One group uses Moire photographs to define further the contour of pectus defects [19].

The deformity may be characterized further by posteroanterior/lateral chest radiograph or CT of the chest. One may derive a "Welch index" or a fronto-sagittal thoracic index from the chest film [17,20]. More recently, several other pectus severity indices were described. The most commonly used index is also known by some as the "Haller index," which is derived from a CT image through the deepest part of the pectus deformity (Fig. 2). The transverse diameter of the chest is divided by the anteroposterior diameter at this level. In Haller's original report, patients who had operative correction of PE had an index more than 3.25 [21]. Derveaux and colleagues [22] pointed out that

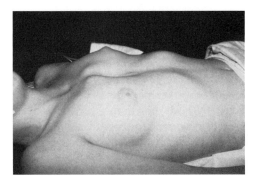

Fig. 1. Pectus excavatum.

this simple index may not portray accurately the severity and complexity of many pectus deformities. They used three indices obtained from the lateral chest radiograph. The lower vertebral index portrays the depth of the thorax at the xiphisternal junction and the upper vertebral index at the sternomanubrial junction. The configuration index is a ratio of the upper to lower sternovertebral distances. Preoperative chest radiograph is mandatory, and the use of CT scan depends on individual practice. It rarely affects management, and some researchers argue that it exposes children to unnecessary radiation. Some experts view it as an important tool in preoperative decision making and planning and postoperative follow-up.

Further evaluation may include pulmonary function tests (resting spirometry), exercise testing, and echocardiography. Some physicians order these tests as a matter of routine, whereas others selectively obtain them if a patient complains of significant respiratory symptoms or if a heart murmur is detected on physical examination.

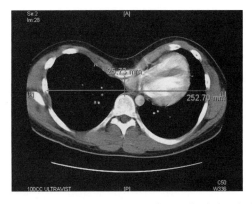

Fig. 2. Chest CT of patient with pectus excavatum. The "Haller index" is demonstrated along with displacement of the heart into the left chest.

Management

The modern treatment of PE began with Ravitch's description of repair in 1949 [23]. Most modern open operations are modifications of his original technique. Options for therapy include

1. Physiotherapy/exercise programs
2. Open costochondroplasty (also known as the modified Ravitch repair)
3. Minimally invasive repair of PE (MIRPE) with a stainless steel retrosternal bar (with or without videoendoscopy)
4. Sternal turnover
5. Endoscopic costochondroplasty
6. Compressive orthotic therapy
7. Subcutaneous implant

Physiotherapy and exercise programs are mentioned in passing because they are included in some treatment pathways, although they are not effective [24]. For 50 years after Ravitch's paper in 1949, most centers exclusively performed variations of his technique [3,19]. The procedure is usually performed through a transverse inframammary incision (one also may use a vertical incision in the midline of the sternum, if necessary, for exposure in severe defects). Skin flaps are raised, followed by subpectoralis flaps superiorly and laterally to expose the deformed cartilage. The deformed cartilage is resected subperichondrially, using care to leave some cartilage and the entire perichondrium in place. This procedure must be done bilaterally and symmetrically, even if only one side appears deformed. The retrosternal space is mobilized bluntly. A wedge-shaped transverse osteotomy is made on the anterior sternum at the superior aspect of the depression and carried down to the posterior table, which is then fractured. Some surgeons advocate the use of a retrosternal bar, first made popular by Rehbein and Wernicke [25] and Adkins and Blades [26], whereas others oppose this technique. This splint or strut eventually must be removed (usually after 6 months) and has been known to dislodge and migrate [27]. Some use a Marlex mesh "hammock" under the sternum instead [28], and others have used a polytetrafluoroethylene (PTFE) bar [29]. The sternal osteotomy is then closed with heavy nonabsorbable suture; some surgeons place a wedge of cartilage or bone in the osteotomy to obtain a better contour [30]. Subcutaneous or pleural drains (if the pleura is entered) are placed. The pectoralis muscles are closed in the midline and approximated to the rectus abduminus muscle inferiorly.

In 1998, Nuss and colleagues [24] reported a new technique, MIRPE. They noted that many deformities in children, such as clubfoot and scoliosis, are treated by various casting and bracing devices. The chest wall is malleable in childhood, and we should be able to mold it in a similar fashion. They developed the following technique. Over a 9-year period, they treated 42 children by placing a convex steel bar under the sternum through small bilateral thoracic incisions. It was placed at the deepest point of deformity from midaxillary to midaxillary line (Fig. 3). The bar was removed after 2 years. The average age of the patients in this study was approximately 4 years. Since then the technique has been modified and performed in older patients. Initially the bar was placed blindly through a substernal tunnel, but after one report of myocardial injury, many physicians currently perform the procedure using videothoracoscopy or with a third subxiphoid incision to guide the bar manually. Lateral stabilizers are used to fix the bar and prevent displacement. Bar removal is performed after 2 to 3 years as an outpatient procedure [31]. This procedure is growing in popularity, with many patients asking for the "Nuss bar" by name after reading about it on the Internet. A survey of pediatric surgeons was published in 2000, just 2 years after Nuss' first paper. Forty-two percent of responders were using MIRPE as their procedure of choice [32]. Others are also performing this procedure in adults [33]. Some surgeons remain skeptical of this method, however, and there seems to be a learning curve involved in its application [34].

The sternal turnover was developed by Wada and colleagues in Japan [35]. This technique involves separating the sternum from the muscle and ribs, creating several transverse osteotomies in the deformed part of the sternum to flatten it, and turning it over on its longitudinal axis. Heavy suture is then used to sew the body of the sternum to the superior stump and the xiphoid process [36]. Some surgeons have used a vascular pedicle to preserve blood supply to the graft [37], but Wada and colleagues have not found this to be necessary in more than 1300 procedures. Despite their success with this operation, it has not gained popularity in the United States. There is concern over the possibility of osteomyelitis, and some have reported difficulty with an anterior hump postoperatively [38].

Other researchers have described the use of compressive orthotics, silicone, and other implants to "fill" the defect [39,40] and endoscopic costochondroplasty [41]. None of these methods has gained widespread use.

Although there is some variation in practice in terms of method of repair, there is also some difference of opinion regarding the optimal age of repair of PE. There have been several reports of constrictive pulmonary disease, coined "acquired asphyxiating thoracic dystrophy," after PE repair at an

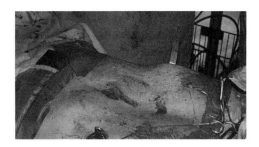

Fig. 3. Intraoperative photograph of Nuss bar placement in a teenage boy. The bar is placed in this direction and then flipped. Also note the subxiphoid incision used to guide the bar.

early age [42–44]. The reported cases all involved children who had extensive repairs before age 4. Many surgeons avoid repair before age 4, although some argue that the problem with acquired asphyxiating thoracic dystrophy lies not in the timing of the repairs but in the overaggressive resection of cartilage [27]. Many surgeons agree that age 6 to 12 years is the ideal time to perform repair from a physiologic standpoint, although repair at a later age is effective and safe [45]. Because early repair is not mandatory, waiting until a patient is older may give him or her a chance to mature and participate in the decision to operate.

Outcome

This discussion focuses on the open modified Ravitch repair and the MIRPE. In the short-term, the morbidity of pectus repair is fairly low and there is almost no mortality. The reported hospital stay for open repair is 3 to 6 days, and average blood loss is reported to be minimal or less than 100 mL [3,30]. Complications are uncommon in large series. They include somewhat minor problems, such as wound infection and seroma, and rare postoperative pneumothorax, hemothorax, hemopericardium, pneumonia, and dislodgment/migration of posterior struts when used. For the MIRPE, reported hospital stay is 4 to 5 days, and blood loss is minimal [31,34]. Complications include flipping or dislodgment of the bar (2.8%–11%) [31,34,46], pericarditis, pleural effusion, pneumothorax, and infection. There was one report of cardiac perforation with passage of the bar (the patient survived) [31].

The medium- to long-term results may be looked at in terms of cosmetic and functional outcome. Satisfactory cosmetic results are achieved in 84% to 97% of patients after open repair [3,19,47], although sternal depression may recur to some degree during puberty [48]. Excellent cosmetic result is reported in 85% of patients after MIRPE [31]. Because it is a relatively new technique, however, the durability of this result remains to be seen.

Functional outcome after pectus repair is more intensely debated in the literature. Patients who have PE have mild restrictive lung disease and diminished exercise tolerance, probably because of sternal compression of the right atrium and ventricle. Patients subjectively feel that their dyspnea, exercise tolerance, and chest pain improve after operation. It is not clear whether this is a psychological or a physical phenomenon, however. Several papers have compared cardiopulmonary parameters before and after operation. Most studies have found that pulmonary function tests worsen after open repair, with a decrease in total lung capacity, residual volume, functional residual capacity, and FEV_1 [22,49]. This decrease is likely caused by a limitation of thoracic cage expansion and decreased chest wall compliance after operation [50]. Others have reported that pulmonary function did not worsen in patients postoperatively, perhaps because they performed a less extensive operation [11].

Although pulmonary function clearly does not improve with open pectus repair, several investigators have found that exercise time, VO_2max, and stroke volume do increase after operation [12,13,45,49]. One group's result did not agree with these findings [51]. Most evidence seems to indicate that patients improve physiologically after pectus repair, not because of improvement in lung function but because of an increase in stroke volume during exercise.

The cardiopulmonary effects of MIRPE have not been studied extensively. Nuss' group reported that pulmonary function tests were stable or improved in 72% with the bar in place. Mitral valve prolapse resolved in 54% of affected patients [31]. One report of 11 patients indicated that pulmonary function test (PFTs) were worse and exercise stroke volume increased 3 months after placement of the bar [52]. It is likely that the bar causes some restriction with time as a patient grows. Studies of patients after bar removal will be more informative. A preliminary report of 45 patients studied after bar removal revealed a small improvement in resting spirometry, especially in older patients who had lower preoperative values [53].

Experts continue to study and debate the physiologic effects of correcting PE. None argues the cosmetic improvement and subsequent positive psychological effects on these young patients, however. Lately there has been an effort to document this finding objectively. A pilot study administered quality-of-life questionnaires to parents and children before and after pectus repair. Both groups noted significant improvement in body image satisfaction and feelings of frustration, sadness, and isolation [54]. Many researchers believe that psychosocial development is actually the strongest indication for repair. This issue also factors into the timing of operation, and perhaps patients should be of sufficient age to assess the personal impact of the deformity. Many people who have PE never seek surgical care and lead normal and successful lives.

An ongoing multicenter trial is comparing outcomes after Ravitch and Nuss procedures. This study, which is part of the American Pediatric Surgical Association Outcomes and Clinical Trials Center, is a prospective observational study that will assess objective change in the deformity and quality of life and pre- and postoperative cardiopulmonary function.

Pectus carinatum

Background

PC is a congenital protrusion deformity of the chest and is the second most common congenital defect of the anterior chest wall. It has been called pigeon breast, chicken breast, and pyramidal chest. It is approximately five to six times less common than PE [55,56]. The male to female ratio is approximately 4:1 [57]. It often is not diagnosed until after age 10, perhaps because it is simply not noticed as readily in younger children with more protuberant abdomens [57,58]. There is no known chromosomal link with PC and it usually presents as an isolated deformity. By some reports, as many as 10% of patients have a coexisting cardiac anomaly [59]. As with PE, several patients—26% in one report—have a family history of some type of chest wall defect [60]. In the study, 12% of patients also had scoliosis.

Pathophysiology

The pathogenesis of PC is widely believed to be the same as PE. Abnormal overgrowth of the costal cartilage during childhood and adolescence causes the sternum to be pushed outward [61]. Although PC is clearly a cosmetic deformity with psychological effects on young people, the physiologic effects of this disorder are not well understood and not as well studied as PE. Many patients complain of chest pain, dyspnea with mild exertion, and poor endurance [56]. It has been hypothesized that the fixed anteroposterior diameter of the chest leads to decreased respiratory excursion of the thorax, which might result in tachypnea and diaphragmatic breathing, especially during exercise [56,62].

Evaluation

Thorough history and physical examination are essential in the evaluation, just as with PE. A prominent protrusion of the sternum is noted on physical examination (Fig. 4). One of several patterns may be noticed and are classified as follows. Type I or chondrogladiolar deformities, also known as keel chest, involve protrusion of the gladiolus and inferior cartilages. Type II or chondromanubrial deformities are much less common and are called pouter pigeon breast. This type is described as prominence of the manubrium and protrusion of the superior costal cartilages. Type III or lateral PC deformities are asymmetric deformities notable for unilateral protrusion or rotation of the sternum [55,56]. In addition to physical examination, chest

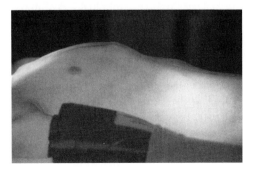

Fig. 4. Pectus carinatum (chondrogladiolar type).

radiograph or CT scan may be helpful to characterize the defect further. A pectus severity index may be calculated and is usually 1.2 to 2 in patients who require repair (pectus severity index in normal subjects is 2.56) [57]. Moire photographs also may be used to evaluate the contour of the chest [60]. Spirometry and echocardiogram are probably unnecessary in most patients, unless symptoms of dyspnea are significant or if a heart murmur is detected.

Management

Ravitch [63] first advocated surgical correction of PC in 1952. Lester [64] reported two methods involving resection of the sternum, and Chin and Brodkin described a procedure called xiphosternopexy [18,65]. The repair performed most often in modern times is modeled after Ravitch's approach. Options for therapy that are used currently include

1. Physiotherapy/exercise programs
2. Compressive orthotic therapy
3. Open costochondroplasty (modified Ravitch repair)
4. Endoscopic costochondroplasty

Although some surgeons have called physiotherapy useless [66], it is often included as part of a stepwise approach to management. Many experts also dismiss compressive orthotics as ineffective. Proponents argue, however, that compression molds cartilage and bone into a more normal shape and avoids possible interruption of sternal and costal growth plates [67]. Several different custom-fitting braces are available for this purpose, recent reports have noted success with their use [67,68]. Compliance with these devices can be a problem, however, and the durability of the changes is uncertain. The emergence of the Nuss bar has renewed interest in this type of therapy. A recent study of use of an orthotic brace in 25 children found results to be favorable (88% had resolution of the carinatum deformity) [69].

Most surgeons perform an open repair that is similar to that described for the repair of PE and varies somewhat based on the type of deformity (ie, keel chest, pigeon breast, or lateral/asymmetric). A transverse submammary incision is made and subcutaneous and subpectoralis flaps are raised. A wedge-shaped anterior sternal osteotomy is created at the superior aspect of the abnormal forward curve. Abnormal cartilage is removed subperichondrially, using care to leave all of the perichondrium behind. Robicsek and colleagues [56] advocated resecting 2 to 6 cm of the distal sternum and sewing the xiphoid to the cut edge of the sternum. Pigeon breast often requires two sternal osteotomies. Pieces of costal cartilage may be placed into the osteotomy or into the open perichondrial sheaths [2,55]. As with PE, some use sternal support, either in the form of a steel strut [55] or Marlex mesh [56]. In lateral or asymmetric deformities, it is important to resect the cartilage on both sides of the sternum to correct the angle of the sternum adequately [58]. A subcutaneous or pleural drain is usually placed and removed before patient discharge.

To avoid the large incision in this largely cosmetic operation, some surgeons attempt to perform this procedure through several smaller incisions with the use of an endoscope [70]. This is a longer operation, involves considerable skill with endoscopic surgery, and has not gained widespread popularity.

In terms of timing of operation for PC, the same argument of avoiding extensive and early cartilage resection applies to this condition. Because PC usually does not present before age 4, however, concern over asphyxiating thoracic dystrophy is not usually an issue. Some recommend waiting until the teenage years to repair PC to allow full growth and development and prevent possible recurrence of the defect during puberty [71]. Other physicians believe that the repair should be made when the deformity becomes obvious and that waiting for full growth is unnecessary [60].

Outcome

Once again the discussion focuses on outcome after open repair of PC. Large series report no mortality and minimal morbidity from this operation. Mean hospital stay ranges from 2.5 to 5.8 days. Complications are uncommon and include wound infection, wound seroma, pneumothorax, and persistent mild defects [56,57,60]. Outcome is largely measured subjectively in terms of cosmetic success. Most patients have good to excellent appearance with long-term follow-up [56,57,60,71]. Most unsatisfactory results are probably the result of inadequate cartilage resection (ie, leaving behind knobby cartilages) rather than recurrence and respond well to operative revision [56,60].

Few papers have discussed functional outcome after PC repair. Patients note a subjective improvement in chest discomfort, dyspnea, and stamina. One report documented a slight improvement in vital capacity by spirometry 6 months postoperatively [55]. A study of pre- and postoperative cardiorespiratory performance in five patients who underwent PC repair found no change in pulmonary function tests or progressive exercise performance [62].

Sternal cleft

Background

Congenital sternal cleft is a rare disorder in which there is a gap in the midline of the anterior chest wall between the two halves of the sternum (Fig. 5). Typically the contour of the mediastinal structures can be seen beneath the skin. It is rare and the exact incidence is not known. In one series of 5182 chest wall defects, 0.15% were sternal clefts. Seventy-five percent of these patients were female [72]. Isolated sternal cleft is a separate entity from

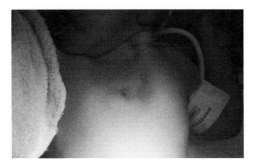

Fig. 5. Sternal cleft (superior U type).

ectopia cordis and other midline fusion deformities. It may be seen in association with craniofacial hemangiomas or rarely with other vascular malformations, such as aneurysm of the ascending aorta or obliteration of the right innominate artery [73,74]. There is no known causal gene, teratogen, or nutritional deficiency. Most reports consist of small series and single cases.

Pathophysiology

During embryologic development, mesodermal cells from the lateral plate mesoderm migrate ventrally to form two parallel mesenchymal bands. By the tenth gestational week, these bands fuse in a craniocaudal direction. Sternal cleft is thought to result from failure of these bands to fuse properly [75,76]. Some researchers find this explanation implausible, given that fusion is said to occur craniocaudally and the most common defect is a gap in the superior aspect of the sternum. Other possible causes include primary absence of the cephalic single element and secondary splitting of the sternum [77]. Although most patients are asymptomatic [78], cardiopulmonary effects of cleft sternum may result from altered respiratory dynamics, because there is paradoxical motion of the anterior chest. Some physicians have reported cyanosis, dyspnea, and recurrent pneumonia [79,80].

Evaluation

Sternal cleft is always obvious at birth, but occasionally presentation to a surgeon is delayed (Fig. 5). On physical examination, the heart can be seen beating in the midline of the anterior chest wall just beneath the skin. The skin and mediastinal structures retract during inspiration and protrude during expiration, Valsalva maneuver, coughing, or crying. Sometimes there is ulcerated skin or a draining sinus tract from the pericardium [81]. Three types of sternal cleft may be noted on examination. Superior cleft sternum is most common. It is an incomplete defect that involves the upper sternum or manubrium. The inferior aspect of the sternum is fused, which creates a U- or V-type deformity. In the V deformity there is often only a narrow bridge at the xiphoid process, which is sometimes referred to as a subtotal sternal cleft. Patients who have this abnormality also may have a midline raphe or band-like scar that extends to the umbilicus [72]. Some surgeons refer to superior cleft sternum as a partial ectopia cordis, but the heart is actually in a normal anatomic position. Complete cleft sternum, also called bifid sternum or sternal fissure, is the rarest type, and the sternal bars are completely separate. There may also be diastasis of the rectus muscles. Inferior cleft sternum is also an incomplete defect: the upper sternum is fused but there is a gap inferiorly. This type may be associated with other abnormalities of midline fusion [80,82,83]. A chest radiograph should be obtained to evaluate further the status of the sternum/sternal bars. Echocardiogram also should be obtained.

Management

Sternal cleft should be repaired for three reasons: to provide bony protection of the heart and great vessels, to improve respiratory dynamics, and to improve the appearance of the chest wall [77]. Most authors advocate repair of sternal cleft in the early neonatal period, at which time the chest wall is compliant and primary closure is usually possible. After 4 weeks of life, primary repair becomes difficult to impossible, and complex reconstruction of the chest wall must be performed. Described methods include the use of sliding chondrotomies, autologous grafts, and prosthetic implants.

The primary repair procedure varies somewhat based on the type of sternal cleft. Vertical midline incision is made and the skin and sternal bands are dissected away from the pericardium and pleura. Any midline skin ulceration, sinus tract, or raphe should be excised. In complete cleft sternum, the bands usually may be brought together as one closes a midline sternotomy, approximating the lateral bands with interrupted suture. Superior cleft sternum requires separation of the inferior bridge, often excising a wedge of cartilage and converting the defect to a complete one, and then approximating the two bands [77,84,85]. Some surgeons describe switching or crossing over the medial attachments of the sternocleidomastoid muscle or approximating the strap muscles in the midline to avoid cervical lung herniation [77,83]. Division of the sternoclavicular joints also may facilitate primary repair. Diastasis recti should be corrected if present. The pectoralis muscles are then united and closed in the midline. It is important to assess hemodynamic status after approximation of the bands and before completing the closure [77].

Defects that present later require more complex repairs. Young patients may be repaired by creating sliding lateral chondrotomies followed by approximation of the sternal bands [75,78]. A more complex version of this idea involves dividing the costochondral cartilages of several ribs medially and uniting them laterally with the underlying rib, gaining distance on either side to allow closure of the sternal bands [81]. If it is not possible to approximate the sternum by mobilizing and advancing ribs, several other techniques have been described. One may create a periosteal bed by incising, elevating, and suturing together the periosteum of each sternal band. This bed bridges the gap between the bars and is filled with autologous chondral or rib graft and kept in position with sternal wire [78,86]. In cases in which the pectoralis muscle does not come together in the midline, a sheet of Marlex mesh is sometimes used [78]. Others reported two cases in which they inserted a lateral rib homograft between the sternal edges and then covered the defect with mesh [72]. Another group described a 2-day-old with sternal bars that were atrophic and could not be approximated. Pectoralis major flaps were created and closed in the midline [87]. Other described methods of repair have included use of autogenous periosteal graft from the tibia [88] and acrylic plaque [89].

Outcome

The outcome after repair of sternal cleft is generally good. One center reported its experiences with eight patients. Two patients died shortly after birth. One presented as an adult with a minor deformity. Five others had operations as babies, four of whom had long-term follow-up (ages 16–28). They had good quality of life without any significant pulmonary symptoms [84]. Another group reported their short- and long-term cosmetic results in eight patients who ranged in age from 15 days to 5 years as excellent. One of the eight patients required reoperation with subsequent success [72]. A third group also reported on eight patients, all of whom had good aesthetic and structural results after mean follow-up of 7 years [78].

Summary

The three major congenital chest wall deformities are PE, PC, and sternal cleft. They tend to be isolated defects with cosmetic, psychological, and physiologic consequences for young people. Treatment of all three deformities is primarily surgical. PE and PC are different in appearance but similar in etiology; until recently, correction consisted primarily of variations on the original procedures described by Ravitch more than a half century ago. With the introduction of the substernal Nuss bar, treatment of chest wall defects is currently evolving. Along with this relatively new therapy will come a reanalysis of the indications, timing, extent, and success of intervention.

References

[1] Williams AM, Crabbe DC. Pectus deformities of the anterior chest wall. Paediatr Respir Rev 2003;4(3):237–42.

[2] Fonkalsrud EW, DeUgarte D, Choi E. Repair of pectus excavatum and carinatum deformities in 116 adults. Ann Surg 2002;236(3):304–12 [discussion: 312–4].

[3] Fonkalsrud EW. Current management of pectus excavatum. World J Surg 2003;27(5):502–8.

[4] Shamberger RC, Welch KJ, Castaneda AR, et al. Anterior chest wall deformities and congenital heart disease. J Thorac Cardiovasc Surg 1988;96(3):427–32.

[5] Brodkin HA. Congenital anterior chest wall deformities of diaphragmatic origin. Dis Chest 1953;24(3):259–77.

[6] Chin EF, Adler RH. The surgical treatment of pectus excavatum (funnel chest). BMJ 1954; 4870:1064–6.

[7] Brown AL. Pectus excavatum (funnel chest): anatomic basis, surgical treatment of the incipient stage in infancy, and correction of the deformity in the fully developed stage. J Thorac Surg 1939;9:164–84.

[8] Davis WC, Berley FV. Pectus excavatum and pectus carinatum: report on the surgical treatment of eleven patients. Am J Surg 1956;91(5):770–6.

[9] Ravitch MM. Operative treatment of congenital deformities of the chest. Am J Surg 1961; 101:588–97.

[10] Castile RG, Staats BA, Westbrook PR. Symptomatic pectus deformities of the chest. Am Rev Respir Dis 1982;126(3):564–8.

[11] Quigley PM, Haller JA Jr, Jelus KL, et al. Cardiorespiratory function before and after corrective surgery in pectus excavatum. J Pediatr 1996;128(5 Pt 1):638–43.

[12] Malek MH, Fonkalsrud EW, Cooper CB. Ventilatory and cardiovascular responses to exercise in patients with pectus excavatum. Chest 2003;124(3):870–82.

[13] Kowalewski J, Brocki M, Dryjanski T, et al. Pectus excavatum: increase of right ventricular systolic, diastolic, and stroke volumes after surgical repair. J Thorac Cardiovasc Surg 1999; 118(1):87–92 [discussion: 92–83].

[14] Shamberger RC, Welch KJ, Sanders SP. Mitral valve prolapse associated with pectus excavatum. J Pediatr 1987;111(3):404–7.

[15] Bevegard S, Holmgren A, Jonsson B. The effect of body position on the circulation at rest and during exercise, with special reference to the influence on the stroke volume. Acta Physiol Scand 1960;49:279–98.

[16] Howard R. Funnel chest: its effect on cardiac function. Arch Dis Child 1959;34(173):5–7.

[17] Zhao L, Feinberg MS, Gaides M, et al. Why is exercise capacity reduced in subjects with pectus excavatum? J Pediatr 2000;136(2):163–7.

[18] Chin EF. Surgery of funnel chest and congenital sternal prominence. Br J Surg 1957;44(186): 360–76.

[19] Shamberger RC, Welch KJ. Surgical repair of pectus excavatum. J Pediatr Surg 1988;23(7): 615–22.

[20] Welch KJ. Satisfactory surgical correction of pectus excavatum deformity in childhood: a limited opportunity. J Thorac Surg 1958;36(5):697–713.

[21] Haller JA Jr, Kramer SS, Lietman SA. Use of CT scans in selection of patients for pectus excavatum surgery: a preliminary report. J Pediatr Surg 1987;22(10):904–6.

[22] Derveaux L, Clarysse I, Ivanoff I, et al. Preoperative and postoperative abnormalities in chest x-ray indices and in lung function in pectus deformities. Chest 1989;95(4): 850–6.

[23] Ravitch M. The operative treatment of pectus excavatum. Ann Surg 1949;129(4):429–44.

[24] Nuss D, Kelly RE Jr, Croitoru DP, et al. A 10-year review of a minimally invasive technique for the correction of pectus excavatum. J Pediatr Surg 1998;33(4):545–52.

[25] Rehbein F, Wernicke HH. The operative treatment of the funnel chest. Arch Dis Child 1957; 32(161):5–8.

[26] Adkins PC, Blades B. A stainless steel strut for correction of pectus escavatum. Suvr Med (Sofiia) 1961;113:111–3.

[27] Robicsek F. Surgical treatment of pectus excavatum. Chest Surg Clin N Am 2000;10(2): 277–96.

[28] Robicsek F, Fokin A. Surgical correction of pectus excavatum and carinatum. J Cardiovasc Surg (Torino) 1999;40(5):725–31.

[29] Genc A, Mutaf O. Polytetrafluoroethylene bars in stabilizing the reconstructed sternum for pectus excavatum operations in children. Plast Reconstr Surg 2002;110(1):54–7.

[30] Davis JT, Weinstein S. Repair of the pectus deformity: results of the Ravitch approach in the current era. Ann Thorac Surg 2004;78(2):421–6.

[31] Croitoru DP, Kelly RE Jr, Goretsky MJ, et al. Experience and modification update for the minimally invasive Nuss technique for pectus excavatum repair in 303 patients. J Pediatr Surg 2002;37(3):437–45.

[32] Hebra A, Swoveland B, Egbert M, et al. Outcome analysis of minimally invasive repair of pectus excavatum: review of 251 cases. J Pediatr Surg 2000;35(2):252–7 [discussion: 257–8].

[33] Coln D, Gunning T, Ramsay M, et al. Early experience with the Nuss minimally invasive correction of pectus excavatum in adults. World J Surg 2002;26(10):1217–21.

[34] Molik KA, Engum SA, Rescorla FJ, et al. Pectus excavatum repair: experience with standard and minimal invasive techniques. J Pediatr Surg 2001;36(2):324–8.

[35] Wada J, Ikeda K, Ishida T, et al. Results of 271 funnel chest operations. Ann Thorac Surg 1970;10(6):526–32.

[36] Wada J, Ade WR. Turnover procedure. Chest Surg Clin N Am 2000;10(2):317–28.

[37] Hawkins JA, Ehrenhaft JL, Doty DB. Repair of pectus excavatum by sternal eversion. Ann Thorac Surg 1984;38(4):368–73.

[38] Davis MV, Shah HH. Sternal turnover operation for pectus excavatum. Ann Thorac Surg 1974;17(3):268–72.

[39] Allen RG, Douglas M. Cosmetic improvement of thoracic wall defects using a rapid setting silastic mold: a special technique. J Pediatr Surg 1979;14(6):745–9.

[40] Johnson PE. Refining silicone implant correction of pectus excavatum through computed tomography. Plast Reconstr Surg 1996;97(2):445–9.

[41] Komuro Y, Masuda T, Kobayashi S, et al. Endoscopic correction of pectus excavatum. Ann Plast Surg 1999;43(3):232–8.

[42] Weber TR. Further experience with the operative management of asphyxiating thoracic dystrophy after pectus repair. J Pediatr Surg 2005;40(1):170–3 [discussion: 173].

[43] Weber TR, Kurkchubasche AG. Operative management of asphyxiating thoracic dystrophy after pectus repair. J Pediatr Surg 1998;33(2):262–5.

[44] Haller JA Jr, Colombani PM, Humphries CT, et al. Chest wall constriction after too extensive and too early operations for pectus excavatum. Ann Thorac Surg 1996;61(6):1618–24 [discussion: 1625].

[45] Haller JA Jr, Loughlin GM. Cardiorespiratory function is significantly improved following corrective surgery for severe pectus excavatum: proposed treatment guidelines. J Cardiovasc Surg (Torino) 2000;41(1):125–30.

[46] Wu PC, Knauer EM, McGowan GE, et al. Repair of pectus excavatum deformities in children: a new perspective of treatment using minimal access surgical technique. Arch Surg 2001;136(4):419–24.

[47] Lacquet LK, Morshuis WJ, Folgering HT. Long-term results after correction of anterior chest wall deformities. J Cardiovasc Surg (Torino) 1998;39(5):683–8.

[48] Kowalewski J, Brocki M, Zolynski K. Long-term observation in 68 patients operated on for pectus excavatum: surgical repair of funnel chest. Ann Thorac Surg 1999; 67(3):821–4.

[49] Morshuis WJ, Folgering HT, Barentsz JO, et al. Exercise cardiorespiratory function before and one year after operation for pectus excavatum. J Thorac Cardiovasc Surg 1994;107(6):1403–9.

[50] Derveaux L, Ivanoff I, Rochette F, et al. Mechanism of pulmonary function changes after surgical correction for funnel chest. Eur Respir J 1988;1(9):823–5.

[51] Wynn SR, Driscoll DJ, Ostrom NK, et al. Exercise cardiorespiratory function in adolescents with pectus excavatum: observations before and after operation. J Thorac Cardiovasc Surg 1990;99(1):41–7.

[52] Sigalet DL, Montgomery M, Harder J. Cardiopulmonary effects of closed repair of pectus excavatum. J Pediatr Surg 2003;38(3):380–5 [discussion: 380–5].

[53] Lawson ML, Mellins RB, Tabangin M, et al. Impact of pectus excavatum on pulmonary function before and after repair with the Nuss procedure. J Pediatr Surg 2005;40(1): 174–80 [discussion: 180].

[54] Lawson ML, Cash TF, Akers R, et al. A pilot study of the impact of surgical repair on disease-specific quality of life among patients with pectus excavatum. J Pediatr Surg 2003; 38(6):916–8.

[55] Fonkalsrud EW, Beanes S. Surgical management of pectus carinatum: 30 years' experience. World J Surg 2001;25(7):898–903.

[56] Robicsek F, Cook JW, Daugherty HK, et al. Pectus carinatum. J Thorac Cardiovasc Surg 1979;78(1):52–61.

[57] Fonkalsrud EW, Anselmo DM. Less extensive techniques for repair of pectus carinatum: the undertreated chest deformity. J Am Coll Surg 2004;198(6):898–905.

[58] Robicsek F. Surgical treatment of pectus carinatum. Chest Surg Clin N Am 2000;10(2): 357–76.

[59] Lees RF, Caldicott JH. Sternal anomalies and congenital heart disease. Am J Roentgenol Radium Ther Nucl Med 1975;124(3):423–7.

[60] Shamberger RC, Welch KJ. Surgical correction of pectus carinatum. J Pediatr Surg 1987; 22(1):48–53.

[61] Pena A, Perez L, Nurko S, et al. Pectus carinatum and pectus excavatum: are they the same disease? Am Surg 1981;47(5):215–8.

[62] Cahill JL, Lees GM, Robertson HT. A summary of preoperative and postoperative cardio-respiratory performance in patients undergoing pectus excavatum and carinatum repair. J Pediatr Surg 1984;19(4):430–3.

[63] Ravitch MM. Unusual sternal deformity with cardiac symptoms operative correction. J Thorac Surg 1952;23(2):138–44.

[64] Lester CW. Pigeon breast (pectus carinatum) and other protrusion deformities of the chest of developmental origin. Ann Surg 1953;137(4):482–9.

[65] Brodkin HA. Pigeon breast, congenital chondrosternal prominence, etiology and surgical treatment by xiphosternopexy. AMA Arch Surg 1958;77(2):261–70.

[66] Howard R. Pigeon chest (protrusion deformity of the sternum). Med J Aust 1958;45(20): 664–6.

[67] Haje SA, Bowen JR. Preliminary results of orthotic treatment of pectus deformities in children and adolescents. J Pediatr Orthop 1992;12(6):795–800.

[68] Egan JC, DuBois JJ, Morphy M, et al. Compressive orthotics in the treatment of asymmetric pectus carinatum: a preliminary report with an objective radiographic marker. J Pediatr Surg 2000;35(8):1183–6.

[69] Frey AS, Durrett G, Garcia VF, et al. Non-operative management of pectus carinatum. Presented at the 36th Meeting of the American Pediatric Surgical Association. Phoenix, Arizona, May 29–June 1, 2005.

[70] Kobayashi S, Yoza S, Komuro Y, et al. Correction of pectus excavatum and pectus carinatum assisted by the endoscope. Plast Reconstr Surg 1997;99(4):1037–45.

[71] Pickard LR, Tepas JJ, Shermeta DW, et al. Pectus carinatum: results of surgical therapy. J Pediatr Surg 1979;14(3):228–30.

[72] Acastello E, Majluf R, Garrido P, et al. Sternal cleft: a surgical opportunity. J Pediatr Surg 2003;38(2):178–83.

[73] Hersh JH, Waterfill D, Rutledge J, et al. Sternal malformation/vascular dysplasia association. Am J Med Genet 1985;21(1):177–86.

[74] Pasic M, Carrel T, Tonz M, et al. Sternal cleft associated with vascular anomalies and micrognathia. Ann Thorac Surg 1993;56(1):165–8.

[75] Eijgelaar A, Bijtel JH. Congenital cleft sternum. Thorax 1970;25(4):490–8.

[76] Sadler TW. Embryology of the sternum. Chest Surg Clin N Am 2000;10(2):237–44.

[77] Domini M, Cupaioli M, Rossi F, et al. Bifid sternum: neonatal surgical treatment. Ann Thorac Surg 2000;69(1):267–9.

[78] de Campos JR, Filomeno LT, Fernandez A, et al. Repair of congenital sternal cleft in infants and adolescents. Ann Thorac Surg 1998;66(4):1151–4.

[79] Mogilner J, Siplovich L, Bar-Ziv J, et al. Surgical management of the cleft sternum. J Pediatr Surg 1988;23(10):889–91.

[80] Firmin RK, Fragomeni LS, Lennox SC. Complete cleft sternum. Thorax 1980;35(4):303–6.

[81] Verska JJ. Surgical repair of total cleft sternum. J Thorac Cardiovasc Surg 1975;69(2):301–5.

[82] Samarrai AA, Charmockly HA, Attra AA. Complete cleft sternum: classification and surgical repair. Int Surg 1985;70(1):71–3.

[83] Fokin AA. Cleft sternum and sternal foramen. Chest Surg Clin N Am 2000;10(2):261–76.

[84] Daum R, Zachariou Z. Total and superior sternal clefts in newborns: a simple technique for surgical correction. J Pediatr Surg 1999;34(3):408–11.

[85] Salley RK, Stewart S. Superior sternal cleft: repair in the newborn. Ann Thorac Surg 1985; 39(6):582–3.

[86] Knox L, Tuggle D, Knott-Craig CJ. Repair of congenital sternal clefts in adolescence and infancy. J Pediatr Surg 1994;29(12):1513–6.

[87] Snyder BJ, Robbins RC, Ramos D. Primary repair of complete sternal cleft with pectoralis major muscle flaps. Ann Thorac Surg 1996;61(3):983–4.

[88] Valla JS, Bechraoui T, Belghith M, et al. Congenital sternal cleft: closed with a periosteal graft. Chir Pediatr 1989;30(5):219–21.

[89] Krontiris A, Tsironis A. Bifid sternum: successful repair by use of an acrylic plaque [report of a case]. J Int Coll Surg 1964;41:301–7.

ELSEVIER
SAUNDERS

SURGICAL
CLINICS OF
NORTH AMERICA

Surg Clin N Am 86 (2006) 371–381

Inguinal and Scrotal Disorders

Jeffrey H. Haynes, MD

Division of Pediatric Surgery, Department of Surgery,
Virginia Commonwealth University's Medical College of Virginia Hospitals,
P.O. Box 980015, Richmond, VA 23298-0015, USA

Inguinal and scrotal pathology compose a large percentage of a general pediatric surgeon's practice. This article reviews these conditions and their associated pathology, diagnosis, and treatment. Current controversy in management is highlighted. For brevity, an in-depth knowledge of embryology and pathophysiology is assumed and is beyond the scope of this monograph.

Inguinal hernia and hydrocele

Congenital inguinal hernia and hydrocele in children are a result of the failure of the processus vaginalis to obliterate. The end result is the same, with the provision for the extra-abdominal passage of peritoneal fluid (resulting in a hydrocele) or a viscus (resulting in a hernia). The processus vaginalis may obliterate at any point between the internal inguinal ring and the scrotum, or it may do so incompletely. These variations account for the diverse classification of hernias and hydroceles, including complete or scrotal hernias, communicating or noncommunicating hydroceles, hydroceles of the spermatic cord in males, and the canal of Nuck in girls.

Although the exact process is unclear, it is generally agreed that obliteration of the processus vaginalis occurs only after the seventh month of gestation [1], thus accounting for the higher incidence of inguinal hernias in the premature infant [2]. Also not clearly defined is a known heredity factor, with hernias occurring more frequently in twin gestations and in infants who have a family history of hernia [3].

The incidence of congenital inguinal hernia has been variously reported to be between 0.8% and 4% of live births [4]. Boys are 10 to 12 times more affected than girls. The risk of incarceration has been reported to be as high as 60% in the first 6 months of life, leading to the generally accepted recommendation for surgical repair of hernia at the earliest elective date

---

E-mail address: jhhaynes@hsc.vcu.edu

0039-6109/06/$ - see front matter © 2006 Elsevier Inc. All rights reserved.
doi:10.1016/j.suc.2005.12.005   *surgical.theclinics.com*

after diagnosis [5]. For hydroceles, elective repair is related to the presence or absence of communication. A clearly communicating hydrocele may be repaired electively. In the absence of communication, resolution of the hydrocele is the rule; however, persistence beyond age 1 year suggests communication, and elective exploration is recommended.

Femoral and direct hernias are uncommon in children relative to adults and usually diagnosed correctly in the operating room. Femoral hernias are more common in girls and, similar to direct hernias, are often found in children who have had a previous indirect herniorrhaphy.

The "gold standard" for repair of the pediatric indirect inguinal hernia remains high ligation of the processus vaginalis at the internal ring [6]. This ligation has been performed laparoscopically, but with short-term follow-up, no clear advantage over open repair is demonstrated [7]. The treatment of the unusual direct pediatric hernia is dictated by local findings at operation, with the end result being the reinforcement of the inguinal floor. Femoral hernias are probably best treated using a Cooper's ligament repair. In the adolescent with a larger direct hernia, consideration may be given to a laparoscopic preperitoneal tension-free mesh herniorraphy as opposed to direct groin exploration and repair [8].

For years, attempts to quantify the risk of a metachronous hernia have been made to objectively determine which patients should undergo contralateral inguinal exploration. For example, specific groups in the infant population have been assumed to have a higher risk of bilateral patent processus vaginalis. Their characteristics include prematurity, twin gestation, left-sided presentation, age less than 1 year, increased abdominal pressure, and female sex. These findings have led to the recommendation for routine bilateral groin exploration in these groups. Practice patterns have varied and are often a result of surgeon preference. Surveys of North American pediatric surgeons confirm this individualized treatment pattern and a lack of consensus [9,10]. Because of ongoing concern for unneeded contralateral exploration, potential vas deferens injury and scarring in the male patient, and possible wound infection, more objective measures to quantify the presence of a patent processus vaginalis have been developed.

Preoperative herniograms are of historical interest. Although they were judged effective, they were complicated and not practical [11]. Recently, intraoperative evaluation has received more attention. The Goldstein test, or intraoperative insufflation of the hernia sac, has been advocated; crepitance in the contralateral canal or scrotum indicates a positive test and exploration is undertaken [12]. More recently, this practice has been largely supplanted by the use of laparoscopy. Its advocates cite the high frequency of a patent processus vaginalis, which may lead to a hernia. In addition, they cite the excellent visualization and ease of the procedure [13–15] and the precision with which a patent processus may be identified. Critics cite cost, invasion of the peritoneal (violation) cavity by an instrument that does not need to be there, and trocar site morbidity [16]. Ultimately, it must be remembered while comparing the studies available that most patent processus do not become clinical inguinal hernias. Accordingly, it could be argued that the finding of a patent processus should not lead to groin exploration until it is better known which processus become hernias. Longer-term population studies are needed, possibly with laparoscopic documentation of the status of the contralateral side and then long-term observation, particularly of those found to be patent. In this way, the true risk is identified. Alternately, in this day of expert pediatric anesthesia in the otherwise well child, there may be little downside to repairing the contralateral hernia only if and when it becomes clinically apparent.

Varicocele

Varicocele may be defined as diffuse dilation of the pampiniform plexus (the venous drainage of the scrotum). Generally, the venous drainage of the scrotum begins with multiple scrotal veins that coalesce with the plexus. This drainage ascends along the cord structures and ultimately forms a single testicular vein, draining on the right into the vena cave and on the left into the left renal vein.

The etiology remains unclear. Most theories have as a common thread an increased venous backpressure with subsequent venous varicosity. These theories are based on valvular incompetence [17], anatomic angle of venous drainage [18], and external compression of the drainage system [19]. The vasoconstrictive effect of epinephrine from the left adrenal vein onto the subjacent left testicular vein has been postulated [20].

Varicocele usually first appears near midpuberty. Overall, varicoceles are estimated to occur in 15% of the population [21]. They are almost all left-sided and rarely bilateral. Right-sided varicocele has been reported with situs inversus, adding to the emphasis on anatomic etiology [22]. Most adolescents who have varicocele are asymptomatic and discovered on routine examination. There may be some mild discomfort. Although the mechanism is unclear, there is general agreement that larger varicoceles are more likely to result in testicular injury than smaller ones, and that this injury appears to be a function of increasing time [23]. Adolescents who have pain, large varicoceles, or loss of ipsilateral testicular volume over time should undergo surgical therapy. Prior surgical therapies focusing on mass ligation of the internal spermatic vessels have had good results, but a significant incidence of postoperative hydrocele is reported [24].

In this era of minimally invasive procedures, subinguinal microsurgical varicocelectomy, with preservation of the testicular and cremasteric arteries and lymphatics, offers excellent results with little morbidity [25,26].

The acute scrotum

The emergent evaluation of a painful swollen and red scrotum remains a diagnostic challenge because there are very few absolutes. Like most acute surgical problems, the best approach is a careful history and physical examination in conjunction with sound surgical judgment. Diagnostic tests are often helpful in this process, but despite recent refinements in technique, they remain diagnostic adjuncts only. The time taken to acquire these tests and the availability of those experienced to interpret them must also be cautiously taken into account.

Testicular torsion

The diagnosis to be ruled out is testicular torsion because testicular loss increases with ongoing ischemic time, and the cornerstone of therapy remains emergent surgical exploration. Testicular torsion occurs in a bimodal age distribution. It may occur in the neonatal period but more commonly affects adolescents [27]. In adolescents, there is the presumed bell-clapper deformity that predisposes the testes to torsion. Neonatal torsion is anatomically an extravaginal process and usually does not warrant intervention because the testis is most likely necrotic. The history is usually that of acute onset of scrotal pain that may radiate to the groin and may be accompanied by nausea and vomiting. Prior similar episodes that spontaneously resolved may represent a partial torsion and remain a strong historical clue [28]. Gradual onset of pain is often more consistent with epididymitis or testicular appendiceal torsion. Pain of longer duration, usually greater than 24 hours, may also point to a nonsurgical cause or to testicular torsion that has progressed to necrosis.

The physical examination may be difficult at best due to pain and distress. No pathognomonic physical findings of testicular torsion have been reported. Those signs that have been reported as being useful include a high riding gonad due to foreshortening of the spermatic cord by the torsion, a transverse testicular lie, absence of the cremate reflex, and anterior presentation of the epididymis [29]. Unless the examination provides focal findings such as localized epididymal tenderness, testicular torsion should remain the diagnosis to be excluded.

Diagnostic adjuncts

As mentioned, any test ordered in an attempt to refine a clinical suspicion of testicular torsion must be done under strict time constraints due to the possibility of progressive testicular ischemia and necrosis. Obtaining such tests may be more problematic at night due to lack of immediately available diagnostic staff. A delay exceeding 1 to 2 hours is probably not acceptable given the risk of gonadal loss if torsion is strongly suspected. The interpretive expertise of available diagnostic staff must also be considered when relying on such tests in the decision algorithm, and may be more of an issue in lower volume community hospitals as opposed to higher volume children's centers. Finally, the individual limitations of each test must be recognized and taken into account.

Duplex ultrasonography

This modality, although operator dependent, is very sensitive in detecting spermatic cord blood flow. It must be remembered, however, that the detection of such flow does not rule out torsion and should not preclude emergent exploration [30]. More recent studies have attempted to further refine ultrasonic predictive value using Doppler waveform spectral analysis and high-resolution ultrasound [31]. Specificity has not approached 100%. It may be that ultrasound is more useful in supporting a nonsurgical cause of the acute scrotum [29]. Consideration of a nonsurgical cause coupled with a supportive ultrasonographic finding such as an enlarged testicular appendage may lead to expectant observation.

Nuclear imaging

Technetium 99m scintigraphy offers detailed images of testicular anatomy and blood flow and has been reported to have 90% accuracy in diagnosis of torsion [32]. The significant downside is the time required to prepare the radioisotope, assemble technical staff, perform the scan, and obtain experienced interpretation. For these reasons, many physicians do not employ this test unless their strong suspicion is a nonsurgical etiology of the scrotal pain.

Urinalysis

Urinalysis is quick and should always be performed. Epididymitis may show pyuria, but not reliably so [33]. Testicular torsion often results in a normal urinalysis. Urethral discharge should be sought in the adolescent boy as a source of discovered pyuria.

Treatment

To reiterate, a clinical impression of testicular torsion should result in emergent operative exploration. Unless clinical findings dictate otherwise, such as a paratesticular mass, the approach should be trans-scrotal. The median raphe is incised and the testicle assessed after detorsion is completed. Normal testes with clearly restored blood flow and those of questionable viability after intraoperative observation should undergo fixation within the tunica. Clearly necrotic testes in most cases should be removed. The data supporting contralateral gonadal injury induced by a retained necrotic testis are not conclusive [34]. When a necrotic testis is left behind, however, the postoperative swelling, erythema, and pain are not inconsequential as the gonad atrophies and is resorbed. In addition, leaving behind an unknowingly necrotic testis in the hopes of in situ recovery risks scrotal abscess formation. At the end of the scrotal exploration, the contralateral gonad should undergo tunical fixation because the consequences of future gonadal loss are life changing and there is a higher potential of contralateral torsion secondary to an increased incidence of bilateral bell-clapper deformity.

Nonsurgical causes of the acute scrotum

Epididymitis appears to be a more frequent nonsurgical cause of the acute scrotum than testicular torsion [33]. The diagnosis of epididymitis is suggested classically by a gradual onset of pain and localized tenderness over the epididymis, and is supported by pyuria and, eventually, positive urine cultures. Treatment is with antibiotics and analgesics. Follow-up should include consideration of anatomic imaging to rule out associated genitourinary tract abnormalities, particularly in infants and young children.

There are a number of testicular and epididymal appendages that may undergo torsion and mimic an acute scrotum [35]; these are usually of the pedunculated variety. The onset of pain is more gradual, and examination may reveal more focal findings. In particular, the "blue dot" sign is a well-known and pathognomonic indicator of torsion of the appendix testis or the appendix epididymis. Treatment is symptomatic with analgesics, and rapid resolution is the rule. Occasionally scrotal exploration is warranted to resect the necrotic appendage that can significantly diminish the discomfort.

Other less common conditions that mimic the surgical scrotum include orchitis, undisclosed trauma to the scrotum, atypical paratesticular tumor presentation, and Henoch-Schönlein purpura, which may present with bilateral scrotal swelling and tenderness [36].

The undescended testis

Cryptorchidism occurs in approximately 3% of term male infants; the incidence rises with an increase in prematurity because testicular descent usually occurs in the seventh month of gestation [37]. Classification and terminology of the undescended testis is variable. The division into palpable and impalpable testes may offer the clearest categorization for management purposes.

Goals of treatment

Although the complex embryologic, hormonal, and mechanical etiologies of normal testicular descent are beyond the scope of this review, the rationale for the secure placement of the gonad into the scrotum is well defined. Orchidopexy avoids the known risk of torsion of the cryptorchid testis and reduces the risk of trauma to the testis lying in an ectopic position near or in the inguinal region. The psychosocial impact of monorchia or anorchia should not be underestimated. The exact relationship of fertility to cryptorchidism and subsequent orchidopexy is controversial. The cryptorchid testis has been shown to have a decreased number of germ cells at birth and the loss has been documented to be progressive; the etiology is unclear [38]. Pathologic evaluation of germ cell hypoplasia as a function of time has led to the surgical recommendation for orchidopexy by 1 year of age. A recent review of the available literature supports this recommendation [39].

The risk of testicular malignancy increases from approximately 0.5% in the normal testis to 3% to 5% in cryptorchidism [40]. Whether the risk of neoplasia is related to the physically undescended position of the testis or is a result of the same combination of factors responsible for its nondescent is debated [41]. Because early orchidopexy does not appear to abate the risk of malignancy, and a testicle contralateral to a cryptorchid one carries a higher risk of malignancy, a combination of factors is likely responsible for testicular nondescent and subsequent malignancy [42]. Although the argument to perform orchidopexy in prevention of malignancy may not be entirely solvent, fixation has been advocated to permit better surveillance and thus, it is hoped, earlier detection. It is unfortunate that evidence suggests this may not be the case. Studies have shown that tumor stage at diagnosis and disease-free survival is not significantly different between cryptorchid gonads and those following orchidopexy [43,44].

The palpable testis

Most infants and children referred for surgical evaluation of undescended testes are found to have a palpable gonad after a careful examination. Keys to success include a problem-focused examination in a calm child with a reassuring parent present. Ultimately, the found position of the palpable testis dictates management. Retractile testes are common and a result of the cremasteric muscle reflex. If the gonad can be brought down fully into the scrotum along anatomic lines, then nothing further need be done. Over time, cremaster muscle weakening, testicular mass increase, and the force of gravity overcome the initial retraction. Occasionally, the retractile testis remains so into early adolescence and results in atrophy. In these patients, orchidopexy may be warranted. An ectopic testicle is one that has descended outside of the usual anatomic path and is usually outside the external ring. Common locations include the perineal or femoral regions; treatment is orchidopexy. Trapped testis refers to a testicle that originally descended along normal anatomic lines but now has reascended. This situation is usually in response to scarring after inguinal exploration; however, it may occur as a primary process. Orchidopexy is curative.

The impalpable testis

Approximately 20% of undescended testes are impalpable [45]. The impalpable testis may be intracanalicular, intra-abdominal, or absent (in utero torsion). Congenital anorchia is unusual and is a diagnosis of exclusion. Thus, the most efficient and cost-effective method to locate the impalpable testis is desirable. Preoperative imaging may be reassuring if the gonad is localized, but in no instance should a negative study be interpreted as meaning the testis is not present. This is particularly true of ultrasound, which has a high rate of false positives and negatives [46]. Similarly, CT and MRI cannot uniformly demonstrate an intra-abdominal testis [47]. There is some specialized experience with nuclear scintigraphy and magnetic resonance angiography, but the data are limited and the techniques do not enjoy widespread application [48]. It has been stated correctly that because a false negative can occur in all of these tests, their usefulness is extremely limited in avoiding surgical exploration and localization of the impalpable testis. Alternately, obtaining these tests may be more useful as a preoperative "road map" in the event the testicle is imaged.

Although the traditional open exploration for the impalpable testis has long-term acceptance and efficacy, laparoscopic exploration has gained widespread popularity for its sensitivity and minimal morbidity [49]. The minimally invasive aspect of laparoscopy is well known. In a review of multiple studies of children undergoing laparoscopic exploration for impalpable testes, 22% to 58% of patients were shown to have vanishing testis syndrome (torsion) or agenesis as evidenced by a blind ending vas deferens and spermatic vessels [50]. These children were then spared an inguinal exploration that may have otherwise proceeded to a full retroperitoneal exploration in the search for the testis. In further support of laparoscopic exploration, studies have laparoscopically located testes that were previously declared absent after open groin exploration [51]. Cost has also become less of an issue with the recent demonstration that with all factors considered, laparoscopy with reusable components could cost less than open groin and retroperitoneal exploration [52].

Finally, laparoscopy does not limit the surgeon's choice of "next step" when the exploration is completed and the testis is located. For practiced laparoscopists, laparoscopic orchidopexy has been shown to be successful, allowing the minimally invasive approach to continue through the orchidopexy [53]. More traditionally, after the testis is identified laparoscopically, an "open" orchidopexy is performed, proceeding with the security of having identified the exact location of the testis. Laparoscopic experience with staged orchidopexy (Fowler-Stephens) for intra-abdominal testes has also been reported with good success [54].

References

[1] Skandalakis JE, Gray SW. The anterior body wall. In: Skandalakis JE, Gray SW, editors. Embryology for surgeons. 2nd edition. Baltimore (MD): Williams and Wilkins; 1994. p. 578–80.
[2] Rescorla F, Grosfeld J. Inguinal hernia repair in the perinatal period and early infancy—clinical considerations. J Pediatr Surg 1984;19(6):832–7.
[3] Czeizel A, Gardonyi J. A family study of congenital inguinal hernia. Am J Med Genet 1979; 4(3):247.

[4] Bronsther B. Inguinal hernia in children—a study of 1000 cases and review of the literature. J Am Womens Assoc 1972;27:524.

[5] Rowe M, Clatworthy H Jr. Incarcerated and strangulated hernias in children. A study of high risk factors. Arch Surg 1970;101(2):136–9.

[6] Gross RE. Inguinal hernia. The surgery of infancy and childhood. Philadelphia: WB Saunders; 1953.

[7] Becmeur F, Philippe P, Lemandat-Schultz A, et al. A continuous series of 96 laparoscopic inguinal hernia repairs in children by a new technique. Surg Endosc 2004;18(12): 1738–41.

[8] Quilici PJ, Greaney EM Jr, Quilici J, et al. Laparoscopic inguinal hernia repair: optimal technical variations and results in 1700 cases. Am Surg 2000;66(9):848–52.

[9] Antonoff MB, Kreykes NS, Salzman DA, et al. American Academy of Pediatrics section on surgery hernia survey revisited. J Pediatr Surg 2005;40(6):1009–14.

[10] Levitt MA, Ferraraccio D, Arbesman MC, et al. Variability of inguinal hernia surgical technique: a survey of North American pediatric surgeons. J Pediatr Surg 2002;37(5): 745–51.

[11] Ducharme JC, Bertrand R, Charar R. Is it possible to diagnose an inguinal hernia by X-ray? J Can Radiol Assoc 1967;18:44.

[12] Christenberry DP, Powell RW. Intraoperative diagnostic pneumoperitoneum (Goldstein test) in the infant and child with unilateral inguinal hernia. Am J Surg 1987;154(6):628.

[13] Rescorla FJ, West KW, Engum SA, et al. The "other side" of pediatric hernias: the role of laparoscopy. Am Surg 1997;63(8):690–3.

[14] Chan KL, Hui WC, Tam PK. Prospective randomized single center, single blind comparison of laparoscopic vs open repair of pediatric inguinal hernia. Surg Endosc 2005;19(7): 927–32.

[15] Bhatia Am, Gow KW, Heiss KF, et al. Is the use of laparoscopy to determine presence of contralateral patent processus vaginalis justified in children greater than 2 years of age? J Pediatr Surg 2004;39:778–81.

[16] Backman T, Arnbjornsson F, Kullendorff CM. Omentum herniation at a 2-mm trocar site. J Laparoendosc Adv Surg Tech A 2005;15(1):87–8.

[17] Ahlberg NE, Bartley O, Chidekel N, et al. Right and left gonadal veins: an anatomical and statistical study. Acta Radiol 1966;4:593–601.

[18] Saypol DC, Howards SS, Turner TT, et al. Influence of surgically induced varicocele on testicular blood flow, temperature and histology in adult rats and dogs. J Clin Invest 1981;68: 39–45.

[19] Williams PL, Warwick R, Dyson M, et al. Gray's anatomy. 37th edition. Edinburgh, UK: Churchill Livingstone; 1989.

[20] Basmajian JV. Grant's method of anatomy. 8th edition. Baltimore (MD): Williams and Wilkins; 1971.

[21] Yarborough MA, Burns JR, Keller FS. Incidence and clinical significance of subclinical varicoceles. J Urol 1989;141:1372–4.

[22] Wilms G, Oyen R, Casselman J, et al. Solitary or predominantly right sided varicocele, a possible sign for situs inversus. Urol Radiol 1988;9:243–6.

[23] Haans LC, Laven JS, Mali WP, et al. Testis volumes, semen quality and hormonal patters in adolescents with and without a varicocele. Fertil Steril 1991;56(4):731–6.

[24] Abdulmaaboud MR, Shokeir AA, Farage Y, et al. Treatment of varicocele: a comparative study of conventional open surgery, percutaneous retrograde slerotherapy and laparoscopy. Urology 1998;52:294–300.

[25] Kocvara R, Dvoracek J, Sedlacek J, et al. Lymphatic sparing laparoscopic varicocelectomy: a microsurgical repair. J Urol 2005;173(5):1751–4.

[26] Schiff J, Kelly C, Goldstein M, et al. Managing varicoceles in children: results with microsurgical varicocelectomy. Br J Urol Int 2005;95(3):399–402.

[27] Colodny AH. Acute urologic conditions. Peds Ann 1994;23:207–10.

[28] Kadish HA, Bolte RG. A retrospective review of pediatric patients with epididymitis, testicular torsion, and torsion of testicular appendages. Pediatrics 1998;102:73–6.

[29] Ciftci AO, Senocak ME, Tanyel FC, et al. Clinical predictors for differential diagnosis of acute scrotum. Eur J Pediatr Surg 2004;14(5):333–8.

[30] Karmazyn B, Steinberg R, Kornreich L, et al. Clinical and sonographic criteria of the acute scrotum in children: a retrospective study of 172 boys. Pediatr Radiol 2005;35(3): 302–10.

[31] Dogra VS, Rubens DJ, Gottlieb RH, et al. Torsion and beyond: new twists in spectral Doppler evaluation of the scrotum. J Ultrasound Med 2004;23(8):1077–85.

[32] Melloul M, Paz A, Lask D, et al. The value of radionuclide scrotal imaging in the diagnosis of acute testicular torsion. Br J Urol 1995;72:628–31.

[33] Haecker FM, Hauri-hohl A, Von Schweinintz D. Acute epididymitis in children: a 4 year retrospective study. Eur J Pediatr Surg 2005;15(3):180–6.

[34] Husman D. Urologic emergencies. In: Belman A, King L, Kramer S, editors. Clinical pediatric urology. 4th edition. London: Martin Dunitz; 2002. p. 1104–9.

[35] Skandalakis JE, Gray SW. Male reproductive tract. In: Skandalakis JE, Gray SW, editors. Embryology for surgeons. 2nd edition. Baltimore (MD): Williams and Wilkins; 1994. p. 777–80.

[36] Huang LH, Yeung CY, Shyur SD, et al. Diagnosis of Henoch Schonlein purpura by sonography and radionuclear scanning in a child presenting with bilateral acute scrotum. J Microbiol Immunol Infect 2004;37(3):192–5.

[37] Cortes D. Cryptorchidism: aspects of pathogenesis, histology and treatment. Scand J Urol Nephrol 1998;32:9–54.

[38] Hadziselimovic F, Herzog B. Treatment with leutinizing hormone releasing hormone analogues after successful orchiopexy markedly improves the chance of fertility later in life. J Urol 1997;158:1193–5.

[39] Lee PA. Fertility after cryptorchidism: epidemiology and other outcome studies. Urology 2005;66(2):427–31.

[40] Silver R, Docimo S. Cryptorchidism. In: Gonzales E, Bauer S, editors. Pediatric urology practice. Philadelphia: Lippincott, Williams and Wilkins; 1999. p. 499–522.

[41] Prener A, Engholm G, Jensen O. Genital anomalies and risk for testicular cancer in Danish men. Epidemiology 1995;7:14–7.

[42] Swerdlow A, Higgins C, Pike M. risk of testicular cancer in cohort of boys with cryptorchidism. BMJ 1997;314:1507–11.

[43] Raina V, Shukla N, Chen C, et al. Germ cell tumors in uncorrected cryptorchid testis at Institute Rotary, Cancer Hospitak, New Delhi. Br J Cancer 1995;71:380–2.

[44] Jones B. Influence of prior orchidopexy on stage and prognosis of testicular cancer. Eur Urol 1991;19:201–3.

[45] Levitt SB, Kogan SJ, Engel RM, et al. The impalpable testis: a rational approach to management. J Urol 1978;120:515–20.

[46] Cain MP, Garra B, Gibbons MD. Scrotal-inguinal ultrasonography: a technique for identifying the non-palpable inguinal testis without laparoscopy. J Urol 1996;33:791–4.

[47] Hrebinko R, Bellinger M. The limited role of imaging techniques in managing children with undescended testes. J Urol 1993;150:458–60.

[48] Lam WW, Tam PK, Ai VH, et al. Gadolinium infusion magnetic resonance angiogram: a new non-invasive and accurate method of preoperative localization of impalpable undescended testis. J Pediatr Surg 1998;33:123–6.

[49] Peters CA. Laparoscopy in pediatric urology. Curr Opin Urol 2004;14(2):67–73.

[50] Franco I. Evaluation and management of impalpable testes. In: Belman AB, King LR, Kramer SA, editors. Clinical pediatric urology. London: Martin Dunitz; 2002. p. 1155–72.

[51] Lakhoo K, Thomas DF, Najmaldin AS. Is inguinal exploration for impalpable testis an outdated operation? Br J Urol 1996;77:452–4.

[52] Lorenzo AJ, Samuelson ML, Docimo SG, et al. Cost analysis of laparoscopic versus open orchiopexy in the management of unilateral nonpalpable testicles. J Urol 2004;172(2): 712–6.
[53] Radmayr C, Oswald J, Schwentner C, et al. Long term outcome of laparoscopically managed nonpalpable testes. J Urol 2003;170(6 Pt 1):2409–11.
[54] Ben-Meir D, Hutson JM. Successful outpatient management of the nonpalpable intra-abdominal testis with staged Fowler-Stephens orchiopexy. J Urol 2004;172(6 Pt 1):2399–402.

ELSEVIER
SAUNDERS

SURGICAL
CLINICS OF
NORTH AMERICA

Surg Clin N Am 86 (2006) 383–392

Congenital Neck Lesions

Eitan Gross, MD[a],*, Jean-Yves Sichel, MD[b]

[a]Department of Pediatric Surgery, The Hebrew University-Hadassah Medical School,
Hadassah Medical Center, PO Box 12000, Jerusalem, Israel 91120
[b]Department of Otolaryngology/Head and Neck Surgery,
The Hebrew University-Hadassah Medical School, Hadassah Medical Center,
PO Box 12000, Jerusalem, Israel 91120

The thyroid gland begins to develop during the third week of pregnancy as a median outgrowth from the floor of the primitive pharynx at the level of the foramen cecum. It descends along the midline of the neck and reaches its final position by the seventh week of gestation. During this migration the thyroid is connected to the tongue by the thyroglossal duct, which normally involutes by the eighth week of fetal life. At the same time, the hyoid bone is developing from the second and third branchial arches. This simultaneous development permits the thyroglossal duct to become connected intimately with the hyoid at the anterior, posterior, or central portion. The inferior part of the thyroglossal duct becomes the pyramidal lobe of the adult thyroid gland [1].

Thyroglossal duct cyst

Embryology and clinical presentation

Failure of any part of the duct to involute results in cyst formation from the secreting epithelial lining of the duct. Most of the thyroglossal duct cyst (TDC) (approximately 80%) is found at the level of the hyoid bone or just below it, and few cysts are located above it.

TDC accounts for approximately 70% of congenital neck masses. Approximately half of patients present before 20 years of age [2,3]. It usually manifests as a painless midline or near midline mass. Anterior cervical infection or draining sinus also might be the presenting symptom. In Telander and Deane's report, 35% of patients had a previous history of infection [3].

---

* Corresponding author.
E-mail address: eitangr@hadassah.org.il (E. Gross).

Diagnosis and treatment

The differential diagnoses of this midline mass in a child include lymphadenopathy, hemangioma, lipoma, ectopic thyroid, and dermoid or sebaceous cyst. Evaluation may be aided by a cervical sonography, which reveals whether the mass is cystic or solid and if thyroid tissue is seen in its normal location. When a normally located thyroid is found, a thyroid scan is unnecessary to exclude ectopic thyroid in the TDC [4]. CT and MRI are infrequently needed for evaluation in children.

Infected TDCs are treated with antibiotics and incision and drainage when indicated. The Sistrunk operation, first described in 1920, is the recommended surgical treatment for TDC [5]. This operation includes excision of the cyst, the central portion of the hyoid bone, and a cylinder of tissue above it following the presumed embryologic course of the TDC, toward the base of the tongue (Fig. 1). There is no need to identify exactly the duct above the hyoid or to approximate the cut edges of the bone. The recurrence rate reported after the Sistrunk procedure is up to 5% [6], which is much lower than the 38% recurrence rate reported when simple excision of the cyst is performed [2].

TDCs are lined by squamous or ciliated columnar epithelium and may include thyroid elements [3]. Approximately 1% of TDCs are associated with malignancy [2]. The primary tumor reported has been papillary

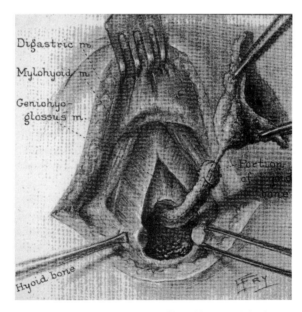

Fig. 1. The Sistrunk operation. The TDC, center of hyoid bone, and the tissues around the duct are dissected out. (*From* Sistrunk WE. The surgical treatment of cysts of the thyroglossal tract. Ann Surg 1920;71:122–3).

carcinoma [6,7], but every type of thyroid malignancy, with the possible exception of medullary carcinoma, has been found in TDC [4,5,7]. This finding further emphasizes the need for TDC resection during childhood. The recommended treatment for these carcinomas is controversial, ranging from only the Sistrunk operation followed by thyroid hormone as suppressant therapy, to neck dissection when lymph nodes are involved, to total thyroidectomy followed by iodine ablation therapy, to thyroid supplements [6,8]. Therapy should be tailored to the individual child based on the histology, invasiveness of the tumor, and lymph node involvement.

Branchial cleft cyst and fistula

Embryology and clinical presentation

The branchial apparatus is positioned at the cranial part of the primitive foregut [1]. It includes arches, clefts, and pouches and is first noticed by the end of the fourth week of gestation. It plays an important role in the formation of the head and neck of the embryo. Most (95%) branchial cleft anomalies arise from the second cleft [2]. Normally, the second branchial pouch gives rise to the palatine fossa and tonsils. Branchial cleft anomalies may manifest as sinus, fistula, cyst or skin tags, and cartilage. Any combination of these anomalies may occur. A fistula of the second branchial cleft represents an abnormal communication between the skin of the neck and the tonsillar fossa. An isolated cyst may be present and has no connection to the skin or the pharynx. The classic location of a branchial cyst is anterior and deep to the sternocleidomastoid muscle at the level of the carotid bifurcation [3]. It can occur anywhere along the line from the tonsillar fossa to the supraclavicular area of the neck, however [2]. Clinically, these cysts usually appear as painless masses along the anterior border of the sternocleidomastoid muscle. When infected, the area becomes red, tender, and painful. Recurrent infection in this region should make a physician consider the possibility of an underlying pathologic condition, such as branchial cleft cyst.

Although cystic anomalies are more common in adolescents and adults, fistulas are seen mainly during the first decade of life [3]. A branchial cleft fistula manifests as a tiny, often draining, opening at the medial border of the sternocleidomastoid muscle. In 2% to 3% of affected children it might be bilateral, which is often familial [2].

Diagnosis and treatment

Fig. 2 depicts the tract of a second cleft fistula. It can be delineated preoperatively by injection of contrast material to the external opening; however, when the diagnosis is made clinically there is no need for such preoperative evaluation. Surgical excision of the entire fistula's tract or cyst is the recommended therapy. Indications are secondary infection and

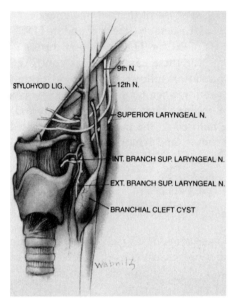

Fig. 2. Second branchial cleft fistula tract. (*From* Lore JM Jr, Medina JE. Atlas of head and neck surgery. 4th edition. Philadelphia: Elsevier Saunders; 2005. p. 839.)

reported malignancy found in the remnants that persist into adulthood [9]. Branchial fistulas and cysts are lined by squamous, columnar, or ciliated epithelium [2].

Excision of a second branchial cleft fistula begins with an elliptical incision around the fistula's opening. Probing the tract with a blunt metal probe may help with the dissection around the tract as it heads toward the tonsillar fossa. When the fistula is long, a second incision (stepladder) may be needed for complete excision of the tract. Care must be taken to avoid injury to vital structures, such as glossopharyngeal and hypoglossal nerves and carotid arteries, in the vicinity of the fistula (Fig. 3A–D). Dissection ends at the level of the tonsillar fossa where the fistula is ligated. The reported recurrence rate, usually a consequence of incomplete excision of the fistula, is less than 7% [10].

Lymphangioma: cystic hygroma

Clinical presentation and diagnosis

Lymphangiomas are congenital malformations of the lymphatic system and most commonly occur in the head and neck region. They might be present at birth or develop later during infancy or adulthood. Approximately 90% are detected before the age of 2 years [11]. Classically, lymphangiomas present as painless cystic masses. Diagnosis is based on clinical history,

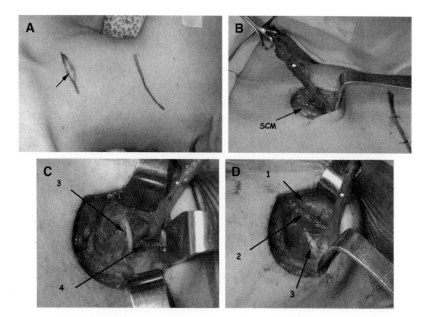

Fig. 3. Second branchial cleft fistula operation. (*A*) Stepladder incision. Notice secretion from the branchial fistula (*arrow*) at the center of the lower incision. (*B*) The lower incision allows extensive dissection of the inferior part of the fistula's tract (*), anterior to the sternocleidomastoid muscle (SCM). (*C, D*) The upper incision allows meticulous dissection of vital structures of the neck. 1, Submandibular gland; 2, Digastric muscle; 3, Hypoglossal nerve; 4, Glossopharyngeal nerve.

examination, and imaging. Ultrasound and CT are helpful, although MRI remains the imaging method of choice.

Two methods of classification are useful for determining treatment. Classification based on size would divide the malformation into microcystic or capillary lymphangiomas, in which the lesions are less than 1 cm in diameter, and macrocystic cystic hygromas, in which the cysts are larger than 1 cm. The other classification is based on location and extent of the involvement. As an example, De Serres and colleagues [12] proposed a five-stage classification for lymphangiomas. Lesions were categorized as being unilateral or bilateral and suprahyoid or infrahyoid.

Stage I: unilateral infrahyoid
Stage II: unilateral suprahyoid
Stage III: unilateral supra- and infrahyoid
Stage IV: bilateral suprahyoid
Stage V: bilateral supra- and infrahyoid

Treatment

There are three major therapeutic options for cervical lymphangiomas: surgical resection, injection of sclerosing agents, and observation.

Surgical resection

Historically, and even currently for many pediatric surgeons, resection is the treatment of choice for lymphangiomas [12–17]. The goal of surgical treatment is complete excision of the lesions without causing damage to important neck structures, such as carotid arteries, cranial nerves, tongue, or facial musculature. The ability to achieve this goal depends mostly on the type of the lymphangioma (macro- or microcystic) and its location (infra- or suprahyoid). De Serres and colleagues [12] reviewed the outcome of 56 patients who underwent surgical treatment of cervical lymphangiomas. They reviewed preoperative respiratory distress, dysphagia, and infection. They also evaluated postoperative complications, including cranial nerve paralysis, infection, and seroma formation. The report was based on their proposed anatomic staging system for lymphangiomas. The percentage of complications ranged from 17% in stage I to 100% in stage V. Long-term morbidity, such as cosmetic deformity, speech problems, and malocclusion, was also more frequent in higher stages.

Orvidas and Kasperbauer [15] reviewed 65 pediatric patients treated for head and neck lymphangiomas. Forty-nine patients underwent surgical treatment. The number of surgical interventions ranged from one surgical excision in 31 patients to more than ten procedures in 4 patients. This number correlated with the size and location of the lesion. Most patients with involvement of three or more head and neck anatomic sites needed more than one surgical procedure. Patients who had lesions that involved upper aerodigestive tract (eg, tongue, pharynx, and larynx) suffered higher rates of recurrence or persistent disease. Twenty percent of patients suffered from permanent cranial nerve paralysis (VII, XI, XII) caused by the surgical resection.

Sclerotherapy

Sclerotherapy of lymphangiomas is a well-established treatment. Multiple agents have been used, such as sodium morrhuate, dextrose, tetracycline, doxycycline, bleomycin, and ethanol [18]. The main complication of this therapy is the possible diffusion of the sclerosing agent into the tissues surrounding the lymphangioma, which causes tissue fibrosis and complicates an eventual complementary surgery. After their first publication in 1987, Ogita and colleagues [19] reported a series of 64 patients treated with sclerotherapy using OK-432 [20]. OK-432 is composed of lyophilized, low-virulence Su strain of group A *Streptococcus pyogenes* treated with benzylpenicillin potassium. Its main advantage over other products is the absence of perilesional fibrosis after injection. Several authors have reported the absence of scar tissue in patients who needed surgical excision after failure of treatment with OK-432 [21–23]. Appropriate selection of patients is the key to successful treatment with OK-432. Most recent reports emphasized the good results in macrocystic type of lymphangiomas in contrast to poor or absent results in the microcystic type [22–27].

After injection of OK-432, a local inflammatory reaction occurs. Pain, redness of the skin over the lesions, and low-grade fever are usually seen for approximately 3 days [23]. This local reaction is expected as part of the treatment and does not necessitate further treatment except for an analgesic agent. In lymphangiomas that surround the trachea or are close to the upper aerodigestive tract, however, swelling may cause temporary airway impairment and may necessitate emergency intubation or tracheostomy [14].

Observation

Debate exists among authors about the likelihood and frequency of spontaneous regression of lymphangiomas. In a series of 74 patients who suffered from lymphangiomas, Kennedy and colleagues [28] reported 12 patients who were observed without other treatment. Among them, 8 were followed up for more than 2 years (range, 2–7 years). Seven of 8 (87.5%) patients who had lymphangioma had complete resolution, whereas the eighth patient demonstrated an incomplete involution. Giguere and colleagues [11] reported spontaneous regression to be as high as 15%, whereas Cohen and Thompson [29], on the basis of a review of 160 patients, stated that "spontaneous resolution rarely, if ever, occurs", and thus "postponement of surgery is inadvisable and injudicious."

Other modalities of treatment have been described. CO_2 laser is especially useful for vaporization of mucosal lesions of the tongue or the larynx. Interstitial radiofrequency treatment has been described occasionally as a treatment for invasive lymphangioma of the upper aerodigestive tract [11].

A rational selection of treatment depends on the type of lymphangioma. We believe that when dealing with the macrocystic type of lymphangiomas, especially in cases in which there is only one cystic cavity (Fig. 4A, B), sclerotherapy with OK-432 is the best option [23]. In microcystic and mixed types or in macrocystic with multiple cysts (Fig. 5), surgical resection is the first line of treatment. Observation may be considered in selected cases when there is no concern for airway impairment, especially if surgical resection may endanger cranial nerves. Unfortunately, in the most complex cases of lymphangiomas (eg, suprahyoid location and mucosal involvement), sclerotherapy is usually ineffective and complete surgical excision almost impossible. Management of the airway is a significant part of treatment in these difficult cases. Tracheostomy must be considered in extensive lesions of the tongue or the larynx (Fig. 6) [12,13,17,18]. Unfortunately, these patients typically have experienced multiple surgical procedures and complications, and long-term sequelae are more the rule than the exception.

Summary

Surgical excision is the primary treatment for the congenital cervical lesions reviewed. Complete excision of TDC and branchial cleft cyst and

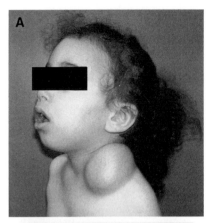

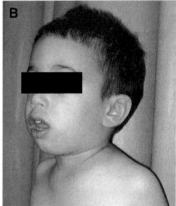

Fig. 4. Supraclavicular macrocystic lymphangioma in a 3-year-old boy. (*A*) Before injection of OK-432. (*B*) The same patient 6 months after sclerotherapy with OK-432.

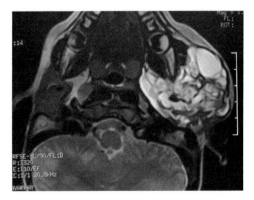

Fig. 5. T$_2$-weighted image (axial section) from an MRI study of a 5-year-old boy with lymphangioma (mixed macro- and microcystic type) of the left parotid area and parapharyngeal space. He was treated by surgical resection of the lesion.

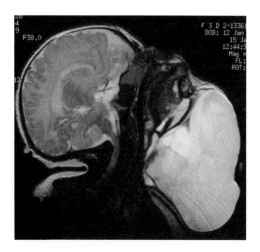

Fig. 6. T$_2$-weighted image (sagittal section) from an MRI of a 2-week-old girl with a large mixed macro- and microcystic lymphangioma of the anterior neck that invaded the base of tongue and the larynx and caused inspiratory stridor. After unsuccessful treatment with OK-432, she underwent a partial resection of the mass and tracheostomy.

fistula is imperative to avoid recurrences. A tailored treatment plan that includes conservative surgery, staged excisions, sclerotherapy, or observation alone is suggested for children who have cervical lymphangiomas.

References

[1] Sadler TW. Head and neck. In: Langman's medical embryology. 5th edition. Baltimore: Williams & Wilkins; 1985. p. 281–310.

[2] Koeller KK, Alamo L, Adair CF, et al. Congenital cystic masses of the neck: radiologic-pathologic correlation. Radiographics 1999;19:121–46.

[3] Telander RL, Deane SA. Thyroglossal and branchial cleft cysts and sinuses. Surg Clin North Am 1977;57:779–91.

[4] Lim-Dunham J, Feinstein K, Yousefzadeh D, et al. Sonographic demonstration of a normal thyroid gland excludes ectopic thyroid in patients with thyroglossal duct cyst. Am J Radiol 1993;161:183–6.

[5] Sistrunk WE. The surgical treatment of cysts of the thyroglossal tract. Ann Surg 1920;71: 121–2.

[6] Roback SA, Telander RL. Thyroglossal duct cyst and branchial cleft anomalies. Semin Pediatr Surg 1994;3:142–6.

[7] Ozturk O, Demirci L, Eglei E, et al. Papillary carcinoma of the thyroglossal duct cyst in childhood. Eur Arch Otorhinolaryngol 2003;260:541–3.

[8] Kaplan HJ, Tamkin JA. Invasive duct carcinoma in childhood. Ear Nose Throat J 1989;68: 460–2.

[9] Telander RL, Filston HC. Review of head and neck lesions in infancy and childhood. Surg Clin North Am 1992;72:1429–47.

[10] Rowe MI, et al. Neck lesions. In: Rowe MI, O'Neill JA, Grosfeld JL, et al, editors. Essentials of pediatric surgery. St. Louis: Mosby-Year Book; 1995. p. 325–34.

[11] Giguere CM, Bauman NM, Smith RJH. New treatment options for lymphangioma in infants and children. Ann Otol Rhinol Laryngol 2002;111:1066–75.

[12] De Serres LM, Sie KCY, Richardson MA. Lymphatic malformations of the head and neck: a proposal for staging. Arch Otolaryngol Head Neck Surg 1995;121:577–82.

[13] Pawda BL, Hayward PG, Ferraro NF, et al. Cervicofacial lymphatic malformation: clinical course, surgical intervention, and pathogenesis of skeletal hypertrophy. Plast Reconstr Surg 1995;95:951–60.

[14] Riechelmann H, Muehlfay G, Keck T, et al. Total, subtotal, and partial surgical removal of cervicofacial lymphangiomas. Arch Otolaryngol Head Neck Surg 1999;125:643–8.

[15] Orvidas LJ, Kasperbauer JL. Pediatric lymphangiomas of the head and neck. Ann Otol Rhinol Laryngol 2000;109:411–21.

[16] Fageeh N, Manoukian J, Tewfik T, et al. Management of head and neck lymphatic malformations in children. J Otolaryngol 1997;26:253–8.

[17] Ricciardelli EJ, Richardson MA. Cervicofacial cystic hygroma: patterns of recurrence and management of the difficult case. Arch Otolaryngol Head Neck Surg 1991;117:546–53.

[18] Molitch HI, Unger EC, Witte CL, et al. Percutaneous sclerotherapy of lymphangiomas. Radiology 1995;194:343–7.

[19] Ogita S, Tsuto T, Tokiwa K, et al. Intracystic injection of OK-432: a new sclerosing therapy for cystic hygroma in children. Br J Surg 1987;74:690–1.

[20] Ogita S, Tsuto T, Nakamura K, et al. OK-432 therapy in 64 patients with lymphangioma. J Pediatr Surg 1994;29:784–5.

[21] Greinwald JH, Burke DK, Sato Y, et al. Treatment of lymphangiomas in children: an update of Picibanil (OK-432) sclerotherapy. Otolaryngol Head Neck Surg 1999;121:381–7.

[22] Luzzatto C, Midrio P, Tchaprassian Z, et al. Sclerosing treatment of lymphangiomas with OK-432. Arch Dis Child 2000;82:316–8.

[23] Sichel JY, Udassin R, Gozal D, et al. OK-432 therapy for cervical lymphangioma. Laryngoscope 2004;114:1805–9.

[24] Giguere CM, Bauman NM, Sato Y, et al. Treatment of lymphangiomas with OK-432 (Picibanil) sclerotherapy: a prospective multi-institutional trial. Arch Otolaryngol Head Neck Surg 2002;128:1137–44.

[25] Banieghbal B, Davies MR. Guidelines for the successful treatment of lymphangioma with OK-432. Eur J Pediatr Surg 2003;13:103–7.

[26] Laranne J, Kieki-Nisula L, Rautio R, et al. OK-432 (Picibanil) therapy for lymphangiomas in children. Eur Arch Otorhinolaryngol 2002;259:274–8.

[27] Claesson G, Kuylenstierna R. OK-432 therapy for lymphatic malformation in 32 patients (28 children). Int J Pediatr Otorhinolaryngol 2002;65:1–6.

[28] Kennedy TL, Whitaker M, Pellitteri P, et al. Cystic hygroma/lymphangioma: a rational approach to management. Laryngoscope 2001;111:1929–37.

[29] Cohen SR, Thompson JW. Lymphangiomas of the larynx in infants and children: a survey of pediatric lymphangioma. Ann Otol Rhinol Laryngol 1986;127(Suppl):1–20.

SURGICAL
CLINICS OF
NORTH AMERICA

Surg Clin N Am 86 (2006) 393–425

Vascular Anomalies

Emily R. Christison-Lagay, MD, Steven J. Fishman, MD*

Department of Surgery, Children's Hospital, 300 Longwood Avenue, Fegan 3, Boston, MA 02115, USA

Most vascular anomalies involve the skin, the largest organ of the body, and, therefore, are notable at birth. For centuries, vascular birthmarks (nevi) were referred to by vernacular names derived from traditional beliefs that a mother's emotions or patterns of ingestion could indelibly imprint her unborn fetus. Old medicals texts are dotted with references to brightly colored edibles appropriated to describe the appearance of an unusual cutaneous lesion. Depending on culture and sensitivity, the mother was blamed for eating too much or too little red fruit during her pregnancy. The modern use of such terms as "cherry," "port wine stain," and "strawberry" can be referenced to this false doctrine of maternal impressions [1].

Virchow may be the first to have categorized vascular anomalies based on histologic features. He called them angioma simplex, angioma cavernosum, or angioma racemosum [2]. Angioma simplex became synonymous with capillary or strawberry hemangioma. Angioma cavernosum interchangeably described either a regressing subcutaneous infantile hemangioma or nonregressing venous abnormality. Angioma racemosum was modified to racemose (cirsoid) aneurysm or arteriovenous hemangioma, a slowly expanding lesion. Although these more formal terms attempted a more microanatomic-based classification of vascular lesions, the lack of specificity or identifying features perpetuated the confusion over vascular anomalies well into the late twentieth century.

* Corresponding author.
E-mail address: steven.fishman@childrens.harvard.edu (S.J. Fishman).

0039-6109/06/$ - see front matter © 2006 Elsevier Inc. All rights reserved.
doi:10.1016/j.suc.2005.12.017
surgical.theclinics.com

Vascular anomalies may be categorized into tumors and malformations. Although this distinction is clinically and heuristically useful, some anomalies seem to span both categories. It is hoped that our understanding of the biology and pathogenesis of these lesions eventually will permit a more comprehensive molecular classification. Genetic aberrations have been determined for several types of vascular lesions [3].

Hemangiomas and other vascular tumors

Incidence

Hemangioma is the most common tumor in infancy, with a perinatal incidence of 1% to 2.6% with a rising presence in the first year. They are speculated to affect 4% to 12% of white children [4]. The incidence seems to be lower in Asian infants and is low in children of African descent. Up to 30% of preterm infants with low birth weight (<1000 g) may have hemangioma [5]. A female-to-male ratio of 3:1 to 5:1 is reported and there is no clear genetic predisposition [6,7]. Approximately 10% of infants have a positive family history, but there is no difference in the frequency of coexpression in monozygotic and dizygotic twins [8].

History and physical examination

Hemangiomas typically appear around the first or second week of life. Approximately one third are nascent at birth and present as a premonitory pink macular stain, pale spot, telangectasia, or purplish ecchymotic patch (Fig. 1). The typical cutaneous hemangioma permeates the dermis

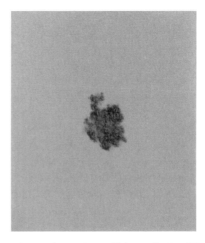

Fig. 1. Common cutaneous hemangioma. (*From* Fishman SJ, Fox VL. Visceral vascular anomalies. Gastrointest Endoscopy Clin 2001;11(4):816.)

so that the skin becomes raised, bosselated, and vivid crimson in color. Radial draining subcutaneous veins may be visible. This knobby, scarlet appearance of the superficial hemangioma gave rise to its common name of strawberry hemangioma.

Deeper hemangiomas located in the lower dermis, subcutis, or muscle may present as raised bluish lesions with indistinct borders that manifest at 2 to 3 months of life or later. Frequently, draining radial veins may be prominent. These tumors historically were referred to as cavernous hemangiomas [1,9], which is a misnomer and should be avoided to prevent confusion with venous or lymphatic malformations (LMs) that share the same historic appellation.

Congenital hemangiomas evolve in utero and present fully mature at birth [10]. They vary in appearance but most commonly present as raised gray to violaceous telangiectasias or ectatic veins, often surrounded by a pale halo. Occasionally, a congenital hemangioma exhibits an area of central necrosis.

Hemangiomas are most commonly located in the head and neck region (60%), followed by the trunk (25%) and extremities (15%) [11]. Approximately 20% of hemangiomas are in multiple locations. Infants with multiple lesions also are more likely to have hemangiomas of the gastrointestinal tract and liver. Infants with liver hemangioma(s) typically present at 1 to 16 weeks postnatally with hepatomegaly, congestive heart failure, anemia, or one or more asymptomatic masses, sometimes detected antenatally. When accompanied by cutaneous tumors, these are typically small (3–5 mm in diameter), red, and dome-shaped, although more banal hemangiomas also can occur. Multiple gastrointestinal hemangiomas can manifest as infantile anemia and bleeding.

Clinical course

The infantile hemangioma exhibits unique biologic behavior. In the first 6 to 12 months of life, it grows rapidly during what is termed the proliferative phase. In the second stage, it grows in proportion with the child, after which it enters a phase of slow regression known as the involuting phase, which lasts 1 to 7 years. During this time, the endothelial matrix of hemangiomas is replaced by loose fibrous or fibrofatty tissue (Fig. 2). Cellular studies have demonstrated that maximum apoptosis occurs at 2 years [12]. Regression is complete in half of the children by age 5, in 70% of children by age 7, and in the remainder by age 10 to 12. In the involuted phase, nearly normal skin is restored in approximately 50% of children [13]. Otherwise, the involved skin is damaged with telangiectasias, crepe-like laxity (secondary to destruction of elastic fibers), and yellowish discoloration or scarred patches (present if ulceration occurred during the proliferative phase). If the tumor was formerly large and protuberant, fibrofatty residuum and redundant skin may remain. Hemangioma of the scalp often destroys hair follicles. In rare

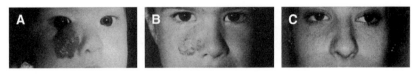

Fig. 2. Superficial hemangioma. (*A*) Proliferating phase (age 6 months). (*B*) Involuting phase (age 3 years). (*C*) Involuted phase (age 14 years). (*From* Mulliken JB, Fishman SJ, Burrows PE. Vascular anomalies. Curr Probl Surg 2000;37(8):533.)

cases, a large facial tumor can be associated with cartilaginous or bony overgrowth (presumably secondary to a local environment of increased blood flow) or produce a mass effect on the local facial skeleton.

Congenital hemangioma, defined as a tumor fully grown at birth, has a more rapid natural history than the common postnatal infantile hemangioma. Often, the tumor begins to regress during early infancy and is fully involuted by age 12 to 14 months (Fig. 3).

Pathogenesis

Despite its overwhelming incidence, little is known about the pathogenesis of infantile hemangioma. Evidence supports the development of hemangiomas from clonal expansion of endothelial cells subject to either abnormal local cellular signals or an initial somatic mutation favoring rapid expansion [6]. The tissue of origin of these endothelial progenitors remains elusive. Some studies suggest that a population of resident angioblasts, arrested in an early stage of vascular development, give rise to these endothelial cells [14]. A second theory suggests that these endothelial cells are derived from a distant population of endothelial precursors carried by existing vascular pathways to a receptive environment [5,15,16]. Potential sources include the bone marrow and the placenta. A small embolic nidus of placental endothelial cells could reach fetal tissues through the permissive right to left shunt of fetal circulation. This occurrence could, in part, explain the

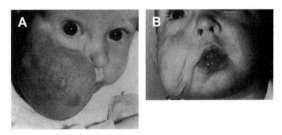

Fig. 3. Congenital hemangioma. (*A*) Appearance at birth. (*B*) Accelerated regression at 7 months of age. (*From* Mulliken JB, Fishman SJ, Burrows PE. Vascular anomalies. Curr Probl Surg 2000;37(8):535.)

threefold increased risk of hemangiomas observed in infants subjected in utero to chorionic villus sampling, because local placental injury might predispose the shedding of cells into the fetal circulation. At least five markers of hemangiomas are uniquely coexpressed in the placenta: GLUT1, merosin, Lewis Y antigen, Fcγ-RIIb, and type III iodothyronine deiodinase [15,17,18]. Recently, a comparison of the transcriptomes of human placenta and infantile hemangioma supported a placental origin of the tumor [19].

During the proliferative phase, hemangiomas overexpress such molecules as fibroblast growth factor-2, vascular endothelial growth factor-A (VEGF-A), and matrix metalloproteinases. With the exception of fibroblast growth factor-2, these molecules are downregulated during involution [20,21]. Involution is also marked by the appearance of mast cells and the induction of tissue inhibitors of metalloproteinases. Proapoptotic markers, such as mitochondrial cytochrome b and homer-2a, are also expressed [11,22]. Other key elements that may explain the behavior of hemangiomas, including the trigger toward involution, its female predominance, and its trophism, remain a mystery, however.

Associated malformative anomalies

Historical association of hemangiomas with a wide variety of syndromes is most likely secondary to misappellation of another vascular lesion. Certain true hemangiomas occasionally occur in association with other malformations, however. A large cervicofacial hemangioma can be accompanied by ocular abnormalities (eg, microphthalmia, congenital cataract, or optic nerve hypoplasia), sternal clefting, supraumbilical raphe, persistent intracranial and extracranial embryonic arteries, absence of ipsilateral carotid or vertebral vessels [23], coarctation of a right-sided aortic arch [24], and Dandy-Walker cystic malformation or other posterior fossa malformations (PHACES association) [25]. Lumbosacral hemangioma is one of several ectodermal lesions, such as hypertrichosis, capillary malformation (CM) (port-wine stain), achordoma, and sacral dimple, that are known to signal underlying occult spinal dysraphism (eg, lipomenigocele, tethered spinal cord) [26,27]. In patients who have sacral hemangioma, ultrasound can be used to screen infants younger than 4 months of age for occult spinal dysraphism, whereas MRI is usually necessary to identify spinal cord abnormalities in older children. There are rare reported incidences in which pelvic and perineal hemangioma is associated with urogenital and anorectal anomalies [24].

Differential diagnosis

Kasabach-Merritt phenomenon

In 1940, radiologist Kasabach and pediatrician Merritt reported a child with profound thrombocytopenia, petechiae, and bleeding in the presence of a giant hemangioma [28]. Only recently has it become known that persistent, profound thrombocytopenia is never associated with common hemangioma of infancy. Common infantile hemangioma markers Glut1 and Lewis Antigen Y are absent in the vascular tumors associated with Kasabach-Merritt phenomenon [29]. Instead, the so-called Kasabach-Merritt phenomenon occurs with a more invasive type of infantile vascular tumor called kaposiform hemangioendothelioma (KHE) or tufted angioma [30–32]. Both types of tumor are typically present at birth. Unlike infantile hemangioma, KHE and tufted angioma affect both sexes equally, are unifocal, and generally involve the trunk, shoulder, thigh, or retroperitoneum. The overlying skin is deep red-purple in color, tense, and shiny. Ecchymosis appears over and around the tumor in association with generalized petechiae and may raise concern for child abuse. Thrombocytopenia unresponsive to platelet transfusion can be profound ($<$10,000 mm^3), but coagulation values are normal to mildly elevated (Fig. 4). A child with Kasabach-Merritt thrombocytopenia is at risk for intracranial, pleural-pulmonic, intraperitoneal, or gastrointestinal hemorrhage, with an associated mortality of 20% to 30% [29]. Diagnosis can be aided by MRI, which demonstrates enhanced signal on T2-weighted images and a poorly defined tumor margin that extends across tissues and small vessels relative to tumor size. Histologically, KHE has an aggressive cellular pattern of infiltrating sheets or nodules of slender epithelial cells, slit-like vascular spaces filled with hemosiderin and fragments of red blood cells, and coexistent dilated lymphatic spaces. Tufted angioma, although macroscopically similar to KHE, is histologically composed of small tufts of capillaries (cannonballs) in the middle to lower dermis with lymphatics present at the periphery [18,32]. This heterogeneous pathogenesis of Kasabach-Merritt

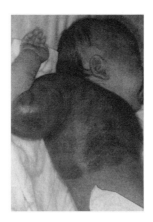

Fig. 4. KHE of the upper limb and trunk with Kasabach-Merritt coagulopathy (platelet count, $<$5000/mm^3). (*From* Mulliken JB, Fishman SJ, Burrows PE. Vascular anomalies. Curr Probl Surg 2000;37(8):540.)

coagulopathy makes it better designated as a phenomenon and not a syndrome.

Other conditions

Several dermatologic entities of early infancy are sometimes confused with an infantile hemangioma. The nevus flammeus neonatorum, known by lay terms as angel's kiss, stork bite, or salmon patch, is a nonevolving macular stain that typically vanishes by the first year of life. A deep hemangioma can be confused with either a localized lymphatic or venous malformation (VM) causing the overlying skin to assume a bluish tinge with a few telangiectasias or draining veins. Diagnosis may be aided by palpation of the lesion; just as with a superficial hemangioma, those of the deeper tissues are fibrofatty. VMs and LMs are usually soft and compressible unless intralesional bleeding or thrombosis has occurred. Hemangiomas also can imitate port-wine stains (CMs) and the blush of silent arteriovenous malformations (AVMs) [33].

Hemangiomas can be confused with a common, fruitlike cutaneous vascular tumor known as a pyogenic granuloma (Fig. 5). These small lesions rarely appear before 6 months of age (average age, 6.7 years) [34]. There is an association of pyogenic granulomas with port-wine stains. The lesions grow rapidly and erupt through the skin on a stalk or pedicle. Epidermal breakdown with crusting is the norm associated with recurrent, often copious, bleeding. The best treatment is curettage or excision [32].

Multifocal hemangiopericytoma is another uncommon congenital vascular tumor that can present with low-grade thrombocytopenia [35]. Other rare lesions that can masquerade as congenital hemangiomas include nasal glioma and infantile fibrosarcoma [36].

Treatment

Most hemangiomas are small and regress without need for cosmetic or therapeutic intervention. They should be allowed to undergo proliferation and involution under the careful observation of a pediatrician with gentle and sympathetic parental education and reassurance, recognizing the

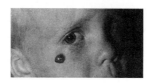

Fig. 5. Pyogenic granuloma in a 2-year-old child who experienced episodic bleeding for several months. (*From* Mulliken JB, Fishman SJ, Burrows PE. Vascular anomalies. Curr Probl Surg 2000;37(8):536.)

anguish caused by the appearance of a tumor on a previously unblemished infant. Referral to a specialty center should occur in the event of equivocal diagnosis, dangerous location, large size, rapidity of growth, or potential for other complications.

Ulceration

Spontaneous epithelial breakdown, crusting, ulceration, and necrosis occur in 5% of cutaneous hemangiomas and are most common in mucosal hemangiomas of the lips or anogenital region (Fig. 6) [37]. Initial treatment should include the application of a petroleum-based antibiotic salve along with viscous lidocaine to assist with pain control. If there is an eschar on the tumor, sharp débridement and wet-to-dry dressing changes are used to stimulate granulation tissue. Ulceration of more than several millimeters is an indication for referral. Superficial ulcerations usually heal within days to weeks, whereas a deep ulceration can take several weeks. Pharmacologic treatment with corticosteroid can accelerate healing and minimize recurrence. Flashlamp pulsed-dye laser is also reported to aid healing and alleviate pain [38]. Total resection of an ulcerated hemangioma is often the most expedient treatment and should be considered if the resultant scar would be the same as if the regressing tumor were removed later in childhood.

Punctate bleeding occasionally can complicate a bosselated, protuberant hemangioma. Parents should be instructed to apply a full 10 minutes of pressure to the area with a clean pad. In rare instances, a suture is required for control of a local bleeding site.

Endangering complications

The incidence of fatal or significantly morbid complications caused by hemangioma has been estimated at 10% [39]. Such complications are most commonly localized to the cervicofacial region and may cause destruction, distortion, or obstruction. Ulceration can destroy part of an eyelid, ear, nose, or lip. A large hemangioma can cause a mass effect and expansion of tissue. A periorbital hemangioma can block the visual axis and cause

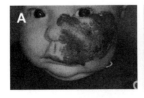 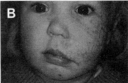

Fig. 6. A 2-month-old girl with ulcerated cheek hemangioma. (*A*) Before a 6-month course of systemic corticosteroid. (*B*) At 1.5 years of age. Note the hastened regression and residual scarring. (*From* Mulliken JB, Fishman SJ, Burrows PE. Vascular anomalies. Curr Probl Surg 2000;37(8):547.)

deprivation amblyopia or extend into the retrobulbar space and cause ocular proptosis. Similarly, a hemangioma of the upper eyelid can distort the growing cornea and produce astigmatic amblyopia. Such cases should be referred for immediate evaluation by a pediatric ophthalmologist.

Even a small hemangioma can obstruct the subglottis; any cervical hemangioma should be treated with a high index of suspicion. Symptoms include hoarseness and later—typically around 6 to 8 weeks of age—biphasic stridor, which may be confused with croup. Approximately one half of these infants have cutaneous cervical hemangioma, often in the beard distribution [40].

Other rare (approximately 1%) complications include high-output congestive heart failure in association with a hepatic hemangioma and gastrointestinal bleeding from mucosal hemangiomas of the bowel. Many gastrointestinal hemangiomas may be symptomatically controlled with pharmacologic treatment, endoscopy, or surgery. Large, diffusely infiltrating hemangiomas are often unamenable to surgical resection, however, and should be managed by transfusion, parenteral nutrition, and antiangiogenic drug therapy. Hepatic hemangiomas rarely may cause massive hepatomegaly and abdominal compartment syndrome (Fig. 7). These massive lesions also may cause profound hypothyroidism because of the expression of a deiodinase that inactivates thyroid hormones [18]. They should be treated with aggressive pharmacologic therapy and thyroid replacement. Care should be taken to distinguish intra-abdominal hemangiomas from more common vascular malformations.

Pharmacologic therapy

Small, well-localized cutaneous hemangiomas may be considered for intralesional injection of corticosteroid. Triamcinolone (25 mg/mL) is injected slowly at low pressure, with the periphery of the lesion compressed to minimize the chances of embolization through a draining vein. Three to 5 mg/kg are injected three to five times at a 6- to 8-week interval. Systemic therapy using oral prednisololone, 2 mg/kg/d, each morning for 2 to 3 weeks, is favored as a first line of treatment of large, problematic, or life-threatening hemangiomas. For an acute situation, such as an upper airway constriction, an equivalent dose of intravenous corticosteroid may result in a rapid involution of a sensitive tumor. Approximately 30% of hemangiomas demonstrate accelerated regression in response to corticosteroids, approximately 40% have stabilized growth, and the remaining 30% demonstrate no response [41]. Signs of responsiveness occur within several days to 1 week after initiation of the treatment and include a diminished rate of growth, fading color, and softening of the tumor. Typically, treatment is terminated at approximately 10 months of age and may be tapered toward the end of the treatment course to minimize steroid-associated complications.

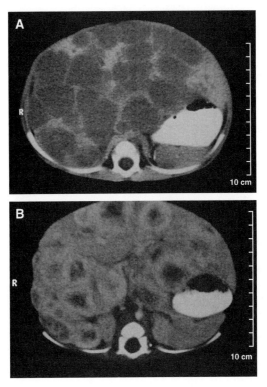

Fig. 7. Abdominal CT scan showing multiple hepatic hemangiomas in an infant. (*A*) Before intravenous contrast. (*B*) After intravenous contrast showing early-phase peripheral enhancement. (*From* Fishman SJ, Fox VL. Visceral vascular anomalies. Gastrointest Endoscopy Clin 2001;11(4):818.)

Until recently, recombinant interferon alpha 2a or 2b was considered a second-line agent for endangering or life-threatening hemangiomas after failure of or contraindication to corticosteroid treatment [42–44]. Toxicity has significantly curtailed its use, however. Complications and side effects include a low-grade fever, reversible elevation in hepatic transaminases, transient neutropenia, and anemia. The most concerning toxicity with the use of interferon is the idiopathic occurrence of spastic diplegia, with an incidence estimated at 5% [45]. Children who demonstrate evidence of neural impairment should be followed closely by a neurologist and interferon should be discontinued if the long-tract signs appear. Spastic diplegia generally improves after discontinuation of the drug.

Vincristine has been effective in some children unresponsive to interferon and is chosen by some practitioners as the second-line agent after corticosteroids for hemangioma and KHE [46,47]. In managing thrombocytopenia associated with KHE, platelet transfusion should be avoided unless there is active bleeding or a planned surgical procedure, and heparin should not be administered because it can stimulate tumor growth and aggravate platelet trapping.

Embolic therapy

Embolization may be indicated for hemangiomas that cause severe congestive heart failure and do not respond sufficiently to drug therapy. Hepatic hemangiomas are the most common lesions that necessitate embolization. Recognition and treatment of arteriovenous collaterals and portohepatic shunts are crucial for an effective embolization strategy. The shunts—and not the proximal hepatic artery branches—should be embolized. It is best to continue antiangiogenic therapy even after successful embolization. Rarely, embolization of the feeding arteries is indicated in infants who have complicated cutaneous or musculoskeletal vascular tumors.

Laser therapy

Although there is widespread interest in laser technology for the treatment of hemangiomas, useful indications are relatively few. Some investigators advocate prompt lasering of nascent hemangioma in the belief that it will prevent tumor growth and subsequent complication. Flashlamp pulsed-dye laser only penetrates 0.75 to 1.2 mm into the dermis, which typically affects only a superficial portion of a hemangioma. The laser reduces the surface color, but it does not affect subsequent proliferation. Small, flat lesions can be treated successfully, but these same lesions would regress naturally to leave little or no scar. Overzealous use of the laser can result in ulceration, partial-thickness skin loss, and consequent scarring. Two well-accepted indications for laser use are the obliteration of telangiectasias that persist into the involuting/involuted phase of hemangioma growth and excision of a unilateral subglottic hemangioma with a continuous-wave carbon dioxide laser [48].

Surgical therapy

Surgical excision of a hemangioma may be indicated in any stage of its life cycle. Indications include ulceration or recurrent bleeding. Similarly, problematic hemangiomas of the upper eyelid that do not respond to corticosteroid therapy should be considered for surgical excision to prevent the attendant changes in vision. Focal or multifocal gastrointestinal hemangiomas that persist in bleeding despite pharmacotherapy may be considered for removal, although one cannot always assume that an endoscopically visualized lesion is the only source of bleeding.

As children progress through their preschool years and develop a sense of physical awareness, consideration should be given to staged or total excision of a large or protuberant involuting phase hemangioma if the

lesion significantly compromises a child's body image. Excision of a hemangioma in early childhood can be considered if (1) it is obvious that resection is inevitable, (2) the scar would be the same if the excision were
postponed until the involuted phase, and (3) the scar is easily hidden
(Fig. 8). More commonly, waiting until late childhood is preferable for removal of the hemangiomas that persist. Protrusive hemangiomas frequently
leave unsightly expanded skin and fibrofatty tissue. Staged resection is
often indicated to minimize distortion and recreate a cosmetically acceptable outcome.

There is almost no role for surgical intervention in the treatment of
hepatic hemangiomas. Asymptomatic lesions without shunt can be
observed. Lesions with shunts can be treated with steroids or, if necessary,
shunt embolization. Hepatic artery ligation should be chosen only if a skilled
interventional radiologist is unavailable in such situations. In rare instances,
massive hepatomegaly that causes compartment syndrome refractory to
pharmacotherapy should stimulate evaluation for liver transplantation.

Vascular malformations

Vascular malformations are localized or diffuse errors of embryonic
development that may affect any segment of the vascular tree, including arterial, venous, capillary, and lymphatic vessels. They can be subcategorized
based on the predominant type of channel abnormality and flow characteristics. Using these criteria, two major categories exist: (1) slow-flow anomalies
(CMs, LMs, and VMs) and (2) fast-flow anomalies (arterial malformations,
such as aneurysm, coarctation, ectasia, and stenosis, AVMs, and arteriovenous fistulas [AVFs]). Complex, combined vascular malformations also exist,
including slow-flow (capillary-lymphatic, capillary-lymphaticovenous, and
lymphaticovenous) malformations and fast-slow (capillary-lymphatic
AVMs and capillary-lymphatic AVFs). The prevalence of congenital vascular
malformations is 1.2% to 1.5%, which makes them a common defect in
embryogenesis. Most vascular malformations are sporadic (ie, nonfamilial),
but some exhibit classic mendelian inheritance. Although much of the pathogenesis of vascular malformations remains unelucidated, recent progress in

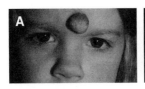 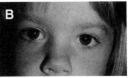

Fig. 8. (*A*) Residual involuting hemangioma in a 6-year-old girl. (*B*) Same girl after vertical len-
ticular excision. (*From* Mulliken JB, Fishman SJ, Burrows PE. Vascular anomalies. Curr Probl
Surg 2000;37(8):552.)

clarifying the development of the vascular and lymphatic systems has provided more insight into observed aberrancies.

Embryology and development of the vascular and lymphatic systems

During embryogenesis, the development of the vascular system occurs by two separate—but related—processes: vasculogenesis and angiogenesis [18]. Vasculogenesis describes the de novo differentiation of endothelial cells from mesoderm-derived precursor cells (hemangioblasts). Hemangioblasts congregate to form primary blood islands out of which two cell types develop. The inner cells of the blood islands become hematopoietic stem cells, whereas the cells of the outer layer differentiate into endothelial cell precursors called angioblasts. Proliferating angioblasts form a capillary-like network of tubes that constitute the primary vascular plexus. Reorganization of this plexus into a functional vascular system along with the sprouting of new capillaries is termed angiogenesis.

The recruitment of periendothelial cells to the vessel wall results in stabilization by inhibiting endothelial proliferation and migration and stimulating the production of extracellular matrix and the deposition of a basement membrane. Angiopoietin/Tie, the platelet derived growth factor-B (PDGF-B) and the transforming growth factor receptor systems appear to regulate this periendothelial cell-endothelial cell interaction [49].

Development of the lymphatic system begins in the sixth to seventh week of gestation, approximately 4 weeks after the onset of vasculogenesis. Existing veins give rise to lymph sacs which then bud lymphatic capillaries in a centrifugal manner [50]. Data suggest that there is in situ differentiation of lymphangioblasts from mesenchymal cells into lymphatic endothelial cells with subsequent recruitment of these cells into developing lymphatic vessels [51].

Vasculogenesis, angiogenesis, and lymphangiogenesis are subject to precise regulation of growth factors, intercellular and extracellular matrix signaling molecules including vascular endothelial growth factor (VEGF) and the VEGF receptor families, angiopoietins and the Tie-2 receptor, transforming growth factor-β and its receptor, PDGF-B and its receptor, the Notch and Jagged families of membrane-associated molecules and the integrin family of cell surface receptors [18]. The VEGF-A knock-out mouse fails to develop blood islands, endothelial cells or organized vessels, which suggests its role in the earliest stages of vasculogenesis [18]. Targeted disruption of the VEGFR-2 gene is similarly associated with failure of blood island development and vessel formation and is embryonic lethal [52]. Overexpression of the isoforms VEGF-C and VEGF-D in transgenic mice induces the formation of hyperplastic lymphatic vessels [53]. The VEGFR-3 knockout mouse dies at midgestation before lymphatic development as a consequence of defective vascular remodeling [54]. The

Tie receptor tyrosine kinase family seems to be involved in vascular remodeling. Tie-2–deficient mouse embryos demonstrate normal initial vasculogenesis but have a disorganized vascular network that lacks appropriate hierarchical organization [55]. Tie-1–deficient models demonstrate decreased endothelial cell integration leading to embryonic edema, hemorrhage, and death [50,56]. Ang1-4, members of the angiopoietin family, likely have roles in vessel stabilization and lymphatic development [57,58]. The TGR and PDGF family of signaling pathways seems to play a role in pericyte recruitment, vessel stabilization, and endothelial wall integrity. Targeted inactivations are embryonic lethal [59]. Notch signaling is activated by the binding of its ligands, Delta or Jagged. Jagged1 and Jagged2 are expressed exclusively by developing arterial endothelial cells, and Notch seems to be integral in vascular stabilization and arteriovenous differentiation [60]. Not surprisingly, the integrins, which mediate interactions within the extracellular matrix as cellular adhesion molecules and as signal tranducers, seem to be important in the formation of the vascular and lymphatic systems. Some integrins coprecipitate with the receptor isoforms for VEGF, and mutations or deletions in specific integrin subtypes can lead to abnormal lymphatic development [61].

Capillary malformation

Still commonly referred to as port-wine or claret stains, capillary malformations (CMs) are dermal vascular anomalies that are reported to occur in 0.3% of newborns, with an even gender distribution. CM must be differentiated from the fading macular stain nevus flammeus neonatorum, the most common vascular birthmark. These latter nevus represent a minor transient dilation of dermal vessels and must be relabeled if they persist into childhood. CMs are composed of dilated, ectatic capillary-to-venule–sized vessels in the superficial dermis. Immunohistochemical studies demonstrate normal endothelial and smooth muscle cell morphology and mitotic index but a paucity of surrounding normal nerve fibers [62]. With age, the vessels gradually dilate, probably accounting for the darkening color and tendency to nodular ectasias. Although CMs are usually sporadic, a familial pattern of autosomal dominant inheritance with incomplete penetration has been reported. Linkage analysis identified a locus on chromosome 5q13-15 termed CMC1, with the causative gene a negative regulator of ras termed RASA1 [63,64].

CMs can be localized or extensive and are rarely multiple; they can occur anywhere on the body. Facial CMs typically become deep in hue with age and are prone to nodular fibrovascular overgrowth in adulthood. Cutaneous CM is often associated with hypertrophy of the soft tissue and underlying skeleton. In the face, there can be enlargement of the affected lip and gingiva, usually with maxillary or mandibular overgrowth. Extensive CM of a limb is associated with hypertrophy of length and girth.

A CM can be a signal of underlying structural abnormality. A midline occipital CM can overlie an encephalocele or ectopic meninges. A CM over the cervical or lumbosacral spine can be a clue to occult spinal dysraphism. A child with a CM of the first or first-second trigeminal nerve distribution should be evaluated for Sturge-Weber syndrome, an associated vascular anomaly of the ipsilateral choroid and leptomeninges with clinical manifestations of seizures, contralateral hemiplegia, and variable developmental motor and cognitive delay. Choroid involvement leads to increased risk for retinal detachment, glaucoma, and blindness. Fundoscopic examination and tonometry are essential and should be performed twice annually for 2 years and yearly thereafter for life. Early diagnosis can be suggested by MRI that demonstrates pial vascular enhancement. Angiographic findings include parenchymal blush and apparent cortical venous occlusions and collaterals. Other syndromes associated with CM include Klippel-Trenaunay syndrome, a combined slow-flow capillary-lymphaticovenous malformation with axial elongation and overgrowth in girth involving one or more extremities, and Parkes Weber syndrome, a fast-flow vascular anomaly comprised of a capillary stain with AVM or AVFs of a limb.

Flashlamp pulsed-dye laser is currently the treatment of choice for selective photothermolysis of CM. The optimal timing is controversial [65,66]. In general, significant lightening is observed in approximately 70% of patients, with better outcomes observed on the face than on the trunk and limbs (Fig. 9). Soft tissue and skeletal hypertrophy require surgical strategies. Contour resection for labial ptosis and macrochelia is effective but often requires repeated procedures because growth does not end in adulthood. Children who have Sturge-Weber syndrome and seizures refractory to pharmacologic treatment may require neurosurgical resection of the involved brain.

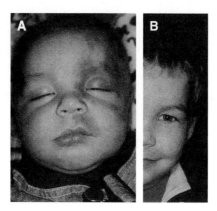

Fig. 9. (*A*) An infant with V1-V2 CM but no other signs of Sturge-Weber syndrome. (*B*) After laser photocoagulation at age 5 years. (*From* Mulliken JB, Fishman SJ, Burrows PE. Vascular anomalies. Curr Probl Surg 2000;37(8):556.)

Telangiectasias

Tiny acquired capillary vascular marks, commonly known as spider nevus or spider telangiectasis, typically appear on children in the preschool and school-aged years. Epidemiologic studies suggest that they may be present in nearly half of all children with an equal gender distribution. Spontaneous disappearance is possible, but pulsed-dye laser successfully removes the lesion.

Cutaneous marbling of the skin of white infants placed at a low temperature, so-called "cutis marmorata" or "livido reticularis," is an accentuated pattern of normal cutaneous vascularity that improves with age as the skin thickens. In one rare congenital pathologic disorder, the newborn has a distinctive deep purple, serpiginous, reticulated vascular staining pattern called cutis marmorata telangiectatica congenital. This vascular birthmark occurs in a localized, segmental distribution and usually involves the trunk and extremities. Neonatal ulceration of the depressed purple areas can occur; sometimes there is hypoplasia of the affected limb and subcutaneous tissues. Almost all infants with cutis marmorata telangiectatica congenital demonstrate steady improvement during the first year of life. In time, venous dilation becomes more prominent and persists into adulthood, together with residual cutaneous atrophy and staining [1].

Hereditary hemorrhagic telangiectasia (Rendu-Osler-Weber syndrome) is an autosomal dominant disorder with high penetrance and an age-dependent phenotype estimated to occur at a frequency among whites of 1 to 2 per 100,000. Patients who have hereditary hemorrhagic telangiectasia have mucocutaneous telangiectasias, cerebral and pulmonary AVMs, and hepatic vascular anomalies. Two causative genes have been identified, both of which are associated with loss of function of transforming growth factor-β. Hereditary hemorrhagic telangiectasia 1, located on chromosome 9q, is caused by a mutation in endoglin, a gene that encodes an endothelial glycoprotein and is involved in vascular remodeling [67]. A second mutation is associated with a mutation in activin receptor-like kinase 1 and maps to chromosome 12q [68]. Activin receptor-like kinase 1 seems to regulate the resolution phase of angiogenesis, which is characterized by cessation of proliferation and smooth muscle cell recruitment. Mice heterozygous for activin receptor-like kinase 1 mutation develop a phenotype similar to hereditary hemorrhagic telangiectasia, and the gene is embryonic lethal in its homozygous form [69].

Ataxia telangiectasia (Louis-Bar syndrome) is an autosomal recessive neurovascular disorder that appears at age 3 to 6 years. Bright red telangiectasias are first noted on the nasal and temporal area of the bulbar conjunctiva and subsequently manifest on the face, neck, upper chest, and flexor surfaces of the forearms. Cerebellar ataxia begins nearly synchronously followed by progressive motor neuron dysfunction. Endocrine and immunologic deficiencies become manifest, and death usually occurs in the second decade from recurrent sinopulmonary infections or lymphoreticular malignancy. The defective gene (ATM) is believed to cause abnormalities in DNA repair, because its primary function is to detect double-stranded breaks [70].

Lymphatic malformation

Historically termed lymphangioma or cystic hygroma, slow-flow vascular anomalies of the lymphatic system consist of localized or diffuse malformations of lymphatic channels best characterized as microcystic, macrocystic, or both. LMs most commonly appear as ballottable masses with normal overlying skin, although a blue hue may result if large underlying cysts are present. Less common dermal involvement manifests as puckering or deep cutaneous dimpling. LMs in the subcutis or submucosa manifest as tiny vesicles. Intravesicular bleeding is evidenced by tiny, dark red, dome-shaped nodules.

Prenatal ultrasound can detect macrocystic LM in the late first trimester. LMs not diagnosed prenatally are generally evident at birth or before age 2; occasionally, however, they can manifest suddenly in older children and adults. Radiologic documentation is best performed by MRI, although ultrasound is a useful auxiliary agent to confirm the presence of macrocystic LMs. LMs, like hemangiomas and VMs, demonstrate hyperintense signal intensity in T2-weighted and turbo-STIR images [71]. LMs demonstrate rim enhancement after contrast application. Microcystic lesions have an intermediate signal in T1 sequences and an intermediate to high signal on T2 sequences. Macrocystic lesions show low intensity in T1 and high intensity in T2 (Fig. 10). Although conventional contrast lymphangiography is rarely performed, it may be useful for determining the precise location of lymphatic or chylous leaks in a patient who has a diffuse thoracic lymphatic anomaly [72].

LMs are most commonly located in the axilla/chest, cervicofacial region (70%–80%) [66], mediastinum, retroperitoneum, buttock, and anogenital areas. LMs in the forehead and orbit cause proptosis and localized overgrowth. Facial LM is the most common basis for macrocheilia, macroglossia, macrotia, and macromala. Cervicofacial LM is associated with the overgrowth of the mandibular body, which causes an open bite and underbite (Fig. 11) [73] LMs in the floor of the mouth and tongue are characterized by vesicles, intermittent swelling, bleeding, and the possibility of oropharyngeal obstruction. Cervical LMs involving the supraglottic airway may necessitate early tracheostomy. Mediastinal LMs often accompany cervical LMs or axillary LMs. Diffuse thoracic lymphatic anomalies or rare abnormalities of the thoracic duct or cisterna chili can manifest as recurrent pleural and pericardial chylous effusion or chylous ascites. Anomalous lymphatics in the gastrointestinal tract can cause hypoalbuminemia as the result of chronic protein-losing enteropathy. LMs in an extremity cause diffuse or localized

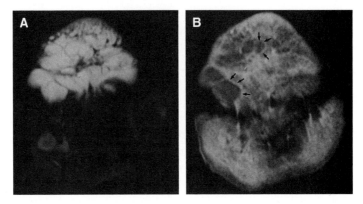

Fig. 10. MRI evaluation of cervicofacial LM. (*A*) Fat-suppressed axial T2-weighted image through submental area shows a hyperintense lesion composed of multiple macrocysts (posteriorly) and diffuse microcystic component (anteriorly). (*B*) T1-weighted axial image at same level as *A* with fat suppression and gadolinium shows contrast-enhancement of septations and rims of cysts (*arrows*) but not cyst contents. (*From* Mulliken JB, Fishman SJ, Burrows PE. Vascular anomalies. Curr Probl Surg 2000;37(8):558.)

swelling or gigantism with soft tissue and skeletal overgrowth. Pelvic LMs are accompanied by bladder outlet obstruction, constipation, or recurrent infection. Progressive osteolysis, caused by diffuse soft tissue and skeletal LM, is called Gorham-Stout syndrome and is known also as disappearing bone disease or phantom bone disease [74]. Lymphedema also should be included as a type of LM. Type I hereditary lymphedema (Milroy disease) is an autosomal dominant disorder that presents early in life with localized areas of edema. The initial superficial lymphatics of these areas are thought to be hypoplastic or absent, although superficial lymphatics are observed in nonedematous areas. Linkage analysis demonstrated the locus of mutation on chromosome 5q35.3 with the gene subsequently identified as VEGFR-3 [75,76]. Type II hereditary lymphedema (Meige disease) is a late-onset autosomal dominant

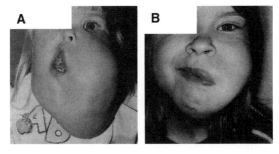

Fig. 11. (*A*) An infant with a large left hemifacial LM. (*B*) The same patient (age 10 years) after staged surgical resection and mandibular osteotomies. (*From* Mulliken JB, Fishman SJ, Burrows PE. Vascular anomalies. Curr Probl Surg 2000;37(8):557.)

disorder with variable penetrance and phenotype. Associated features include distichiasis (a double row of eyelashes), ptosis, cleft palate, yellow nails, and congenital heart disease. The disorder is thought to arise from an impairment of lymphatic drainage, and lymphoscintigraphy demonstrates numerous dilated lymphatic vessels. The putative gene is FOXC2, which is a member of the forkhead/winged helix family of transcription factors and is thought to play a role in somite development [77].

Treatment

The two main complications of LMs are intralesional bleeding and infection. Bleeding, whether spontaneous or the result of local trauma, causes rapid, painful enlargement of an LM. The LM becomes firm and ecchymotic. Analgesia, rest, and time are generally sufficient. Prophylactic antibiotics should be prescribed if there is a large collection of intraluminal blood. Hemorrhage and infection can transform a macrocystic lesion into a microcystic and scarred lesion.

LMs often swell in the event of a viral or bacterial infection. Most often this is a harmless event likely related to change in flow or alterations in lymphocytic component in the walls of the anomalous channels. Bacterial cellulitis, however, is a more dangerous condition. An infection in a cervicofacial LM can cause obstruction of the upper airway and dysphagia. Prolonged intravenous antibiotic therapy is frequently indicated, with choice of antibiotic agents based on the presumption of oral pathogens in the head and neck or enteric organisms in the trunk or perineum.

The two strategies for treating lymphatic anomalies are sclerotherapy and surgical resection. Sclerotherapy works through obliteration of the lymphatic lumen by endothelial destruction with subsequent sclerosis/fibrosis. Success depends on the sclerotic agent selected and the damage inflicted on the endothelial and deeper muscular and connective tissue layers. Macrocystic LM is more likely than microcystic tissue to shrink after an injection of sclerosant. Ethanol is widely considered to be the most effective sclerosing agent for low-flow malformations, although it has experienced greater success with VMs than LMs. Injection is painful and often requires general anesthesia and subsequent pharmacologic pain relief. Edema after sclerosant injection is associated with prolonged recovery and increased therapeutic effect. Side effects include local necrosis, blistering, and local neuropathy. Systemic absorption of ethanol may lead to cardiac arrest, pulmonary vasoconstriction, or systemic hypotension. Ethibloc, a solution of ethanol, amino acids, and contrast agent available in Europe, also has been used in treatment of venous and LMs with a success rate of 20% to 65% [66]. OK-432 is a lyophilized preparation derived from a strain of *Streptococcus pyogenes*, which induces a significant local inflammatory response with fibrosis and has demonstrated excellent success with shrinkage of lymphatic tissue (60%–100%) [66,78]. The mechanism of action of OK-432 has yet to be elucidated fully, but it is known to activate multiple components of the immunologic system, including neutrophils, macrophages, natural killer cells, and T cells. No significant toxicity has been recorded, but OK-436 has not yet been approved for use by the US Food and Drug Administration.

Resection is the only way to potentially cure LM. Often staged excision is necessary and total excision is often possible. In each resection a surgeon should focus on a defined anatomic region, attempt to limit blood loss, perform as thorough a dissection as possible, and be prepared to operate as long as necessary. Even with such an intensive approach to resection, the recurrence rate is reported to be 40% after an incomplete excision and 17% after a macroscopically complete excision [79].

Venous malformation

VMs are the most common of all vascular anomalies and are frequently misdiagnosed as hemangiomas or mislabeled as cavernous hemangiomas. Although present at birth, they are not always immediately evident. The typical description of a VM is of being blue, soft, and compressible. VMs can vary greatly in size, shape, and degree of associated deformation (Fig. 12). VMs demonstrate proportional growth with the growth of the child. Histologically, VMs are composed of thin-walled, dilated, spongelike abnormal channels. The normal architecture of vascular smooth muscle is distorted into clumps. This mural muscular abnormality is likely responsible for the tendency of VMs toward gradual expansion. Microscopy often reveals evidence of clot formation, fibrovascular ingrowth, and phleboliths. Phlebothrombosis is common and can be painful.

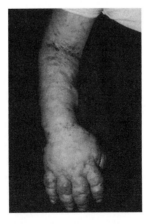

Fig. 12. Extensive VMs of the skin and muscle of the upper limb. VMs with glomus cells in the lower limb. Note the cobblestone appearance. (*From* Mulliken JB, Fishman SJ, Burrows PE. Vascular anomalies. Curr Probl Surg 2000;37(8):561.)

Most VMs are solitary, but multiple cutaneous or visceral lesions can occur. There are well-documented pedigrees of familial, usually multifocal, VMs. Familial multiple glomovenosus malformation is an autosomal-dominant disorder with high penetrance (70% by age 20) that manifests multiple tender, blue, nodular dermal lesions in the skin. Histologically, the lesions consist of ectatic, dilated blood vessels surrounded by cuboidal epithelioid-like glomus cells that express smooth muscle actin and vimentin [18]. The affected gene has been termed glomulin. Although widely expressed, little is known about its function [80]. Familial cutaneous mucosal VM is another autosomal-dominant condition that exhibits millimeter- to centimeter-sized dome-shaped lesions in the skin and mucosa of the gastrointestinal tract [81]. The malformations are progressive, and the degree of venous irregularity increases with age. A rapid expansion may be seen after trauma or with hormonal modulation (during pregnancy). On histopathologic examination the vessels are thin walled and lack an internal elastic membrane. The disease gene has been identified as Tie-2, and it is postulated that the abnormal vessel development associated with the syndrome is secondary to local uncoupling of endothelial smooth muscle cell signaling [82].

Cerebral cavernous VMs are also familial; a subset of these patients has hyperkeratotic capillary venous cutaneous lesions. Cerebral cavernous VMs are small, well-localized, bosselated vascular lesions that histologically appear as dilated sinusoidal vascular spaces lined by a single layer of endothelium. Mutations have been linked to the KRIT1 gene, which encodes a protein speculated to modulate integrin-microtubule signaling and is important in integrin-dependent angiogenesis [83,84]. Blue-rubber bleb nevus syndrome is a rare, sporadic disorder composed of cutaneous and gastrointestinal VMs. It is the most common vascular anomaly causing chronic gastrointestinal bleeding. Cutaneous lesions can occur anywhere on the body, but there is a predilection for the trunk, palms, and soles of the feet (Fig. 13) [85]. The lesions increase in size and become more apparent with age. Gastrointestinal lesions are located throughout the gastrointestinal tract but are most frequently located in the small bowel. In addition to bleeding, these lesions can provide a lead point for intussusception or volvulus.

Complications of VMs depend on their location. VMs of the head and neck can cause progressive distortion of facial features, exophthalmia, dental malalignment, and obstructive sleep apnea. VMs of the extremities can cause limb length discrepancies, painful hemarthrosis, and degenerative arthritis. Intraosseous VMs can cause structural weakening of the bone shaft and pathologic fracture. VMs of the gastrointestinal tract can manifest with chronic bleeding and anemia [86]. Although VMs may be localized throughout the length of the bowel, they are most commonly found encompassing the entire left colon and rectum and surrounding pelvic and retroperitoneal structures. Lesions that involve the foregut can be associated with central mesenteric and portal venous anomalies.

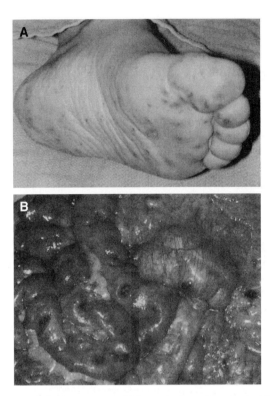

Fig. 13. (*A*) Numerous dark blue cutaneous VMs on the foot of a patient with blue rubber bleb nevus syndrome. (*B*) Extensive involvement of small and large bowel with VMs in a patient with blue rubber bleb nevus syndrome. (*From* Fishman SJ, Fox VL. Visceral vascular anomalies. Gastrointest Endoscopy Clin 2001;11(4):824, 826.)

Like other vascular malformations, VMs are best imaged by MRI, which demonstrates T2 enhancement and differs from lymphatic slow-flow lesions by the presence of contrast enhancement of the vascular spaces. Phleboliths can manifest as flow voids. Flow-sensitive sequences should show no evidence of arterial flow. MR venography is useful for the evaluation of an extensive VM of the extremities; direct phlebography is sometimes helpful as a presurgical planning tool (Fig. 14).

Treatment

As with LMs, the mainstay of therapy for VM is sclerotherapy and surgical resection. For small cutaneous or oromucosal VMs, injection with 1% sodium tetradecylsulfate is often successful. Ethanol, Ethibloc (outside of the United States), and OK-432 have been used as described for LMs [66]. Venous anomalies have a propensity for recanalization and recurrence. A recently described treatment using an injectable fibroblast-based

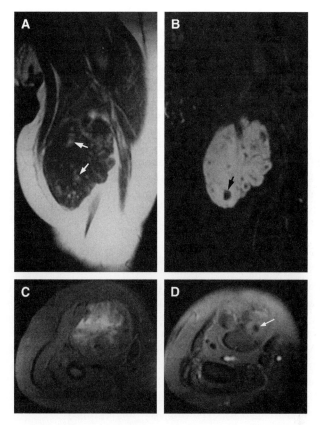

Fig. 14. Intramuscular VMs of the quadriceps. (*A*) Coronal T1-aweighted sequence shows a lesion isointense to the muscle with areas of focal hyperintensity that represent the thrombi (*arrows*). (*B*) Coronal T2-weighted image with fat suppression at same level as *A* shows a hyperintense, discrete soft tissue mass with linear septations and hypointense areas consistent with thrombi or phlebitis (*arrow*). (*C*) Axial T1-weighted image with fat suppression and after intravenous gadolinium shows inhomogeneous contrast enhancement within lesion that involves the vastus medialis. (*D*) Axial gradient recalled echo sequence through the VM shows flow enhancement (*white areas*) in the femoral and saphenous vessels but no rapid flow in the VM. Note the black signal void, which indicates a phlebolith (*arrow*). (*From* Mulliken JB, Fishman SJ, Burrows PE. Vascular anomalies. Curr Probl Surg 2000;37(8):564.)

tissue construct as an adjunct to sclerotherapy reduced the rates of venous recanalization in a leporine model, but this modality has not yet been extended into a population of human subjects [87].

Excision of a VM is usually successful for small, well-localized lesions. In some locations, staged subtotal surgical removal can be accomplished without preoperative sclerotherapy. Generally, however, sclerotherapy is used as a first-line approach to shrink the VM before surgical resection. Complete resection of large, focal gastrointestinal VMs is often necessary because of chronic bleeding, anemia, and transfusion dependence. Multifocal gastrointestinal lesions are best treated by multiple excisions (which sometimes number in the hundreds) [86,88]. Bowel resections should be minimized and used only in segments in which there is a high density of VMs.

Diffuse VMs of the colorectum and surrounding pelvic structures can be left alone if bleeding does not necessitate blood transfusions. When bleeding is more severe, control should be attempted with sclerotherapy. The definitive surgical alternatives are to divert the fecal stream by colostomy or, preferably, to perform a colectomy with endorectal mucosectomy and coloanal endorectal pull-through [89]. This procedure entails a risk of pulmonary embolism because of the manipulation of abnormal pelvic veins.

Elastic support stockings are indispensable in the treatment of VM of the extremities. Low-dose aspirin (81 mg/d or every other day) helps to minimize phlebothromboses.

Arteriovenous malformations

AVMs generally are latent during infancy and childhood and expand during adolescence as a warm, pink patch in the skin with an underlying thrill or bruit. Later, cutaneous consequences may include ischemic changes, ulceration, pain, and intermittent bleeding. The hormonal changes of puberty or local trauma seem to trigger expansion. There are rare examples of an AVM or AVF presenting at birth with life-threatening high output heart failure (eg, an AVF into the vein of Galen or a hepatic AVM). The natural history of AVMs can be documented by a clinical staging system introduced by Schobinger (Table 1) [90]. Like other vascular malformations, AVMs are best imaged by MRI and MR angiography.

Treatment

Prompt embolization may be necessary in the uncommon occurrence of postnatal congestive heart failure caused by an AVF or AVM. Treatment is rarely indicated during infancy or early childhood for a quiescent (stage I) AVM; however, children should be re-examined annually for signs of expansion. Conventional dogma dictates that intervention should be delayed until

Table 1
Schobinger clinical staging system for arteriovenous malformations

Stage	Description
I (Quiescence)	Pink-bluish stain, warmth, and arteriovascular shunting by continuous Doppler scanning or 20 MHz color Doppler scanning
II (Expansion)	Same as stage I plus enlargement, pulsations, thrill, and bruit and tortuous/tense veins
III (Destruction)	Same as stage II plus dystrophic skin changes, ulceration, bleeding, persistent pain, or tissue necrosis
IV (Decompensation)	Same as stage III plus cardiac failure

there are symptoms or endangering signs (eg, recurrent ulceration refractory to treatment, pain, bleeding, increased cardiac output [Branham's sign] or Schobinger stage III-IV). Ligation or proximal embolization of feeding vessels should not be attempted because it causes the rapid recruitment of flow from nearby arteries to supply the malformation. Rather, the usual strategy is arterial embolization for the temporary occlusion of the nidus 24 to 72 hours before surgical resection. If the arteries are tortuous or if the feeding arteries have been ligated, sclerotherapy may play a role in conjunction with local arterial and venous occlusion. Whenever possible, the lesion should be resected completely. Extensive preoperative planning is often necessary to determine the exact extent of resection necessary. Intraoperative frozen sectioning of the resection margins can be helpful, but the most accurate way to determine whether resection is complete is to observe the pattern of bleeding from the wound edges. Unfortunately, many AVMs are not localized and may permeate throughout the deep craniofacial structures or the soft and skeletal tissues of an extremity. In these instances, embolization is usually palliative and surgical resection is rarely indicated (Fig. 15).

Combined (eponymous) vascular malformations

Combined (or complex) vascular malformations are associated with the overgrowth of soft tissue and the skeleton. Many are named after the physicians who are credited with the most memorable description of the condition.

Slow-flow anomalies

Klippel-Trenaunay syndrome is a well-described combined capillary-lymphaticovenous anomaly associated with soft tissue and skeletal hypertrophy

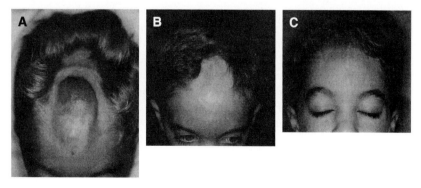

Fig. 15. (*A*) An AVM of the forehead in a 7-year-old boy. (*B*) The same boy after embolization, resection, and temporary closure of defect with split-thickness skin graft. (*C*) Appearance after tissue expansion , excision of graft, and linear closure 1 year after the resection. (*From* Mulliken JB, Fishman SJ, Burrows PE. Vascular anomalies. Curr Probl Surg 2000;37(8):568.)

of a limb or trunk. The CMs are multiple and typically arranged in a geographic pattern over the lateral side of the extremity, buttock, or thorax (Fig. 16). The CM component is macular in the newborn but becomes studded with lymphatic vesicles as a child ages. Anomalous lateral veins become prominent because of incompetent valves and deep venous abnormalities. Lymphatic hypoplasia is present in more than 50% of patients, with associated lymphedema or isolated lymphatic microcysts [1]. Pelvic involvement is frequently asymptomatic but can be associated with constipation, bladder outlet obstruction, and recurrent infection. Thrombophlebitis occurs in 20% to 45% of patients, and pulmonary embolism can occur [91,92]. Management is fundamentally conservative. Children should be seen annually and limb length followed by serial radiographs. If a limb length discrepancy of more than 1.5 cm develops, a shoe lift is prescribed to prevent limping and secondary scoliosis. Elastic compression stockings are recommended. Grotesque enlargement of the foot requires selective ablative procedures (ie, ray, midfoot, or Syme amputation) to allow the child to wear proper footwear. In selected patients, sclerotherapy can be used to obliterate incompetent superficial veins and shrink focal VMs or lymphatic cysts. Debulking procedures can be effective in selected patients. Laser photocoagulation or injection with 1% sodium tetradecyl sulfate can provide control over intermittent lymphatic oozing or bleeding from the lymphatic vesicles.

Proteus syndrome is a sporadic vascular, skeletal, and soft tissue disorder of asymmetric overgrowth and gigantism. Its salient clinical features include verrucous nevus, lipomas and lipomatosis, macrocephaly, asymmetric limbs with partial gigantism of the hands and feet or both, and cerebriform plantar thickening (moccasin feet). It has been suggested that Joseph Merrick, the unfortunately entitled "Elephant Man," suffered from Proteus syndrome.

Maffucci syndrome, a variant of Ollier's disease, is a low-flow malformation of exophytic vascular anomalies associated with multiple enchondromas and bony exostoses. Children who have this syndrome appear normal at birth, with osseous lesions manifesting as small nodules on a finger or toe during childhood and the vascular lesions appearing later. The vascular anomalies are predominantly venous and occur in the subcutaneous tissue and bones of the extremities. Early recognition is important because more than half of these patients develop spindle cell tumors with potential for malignant transformation into chondrosarcoma [93,94].

Fast-flow anomalies

Parkes Weber syndrome shares many similarities with Klippel-Trenaunay syndrome but should be distinguished by a component of an additional capillary-AVM/fistula (Fig. 17). The lesions are obvious at birth and the involved, asymmetrically enlarged limb is covered by a geographic pink, warm, macular stain with an underlying bruit or thrill. There may be

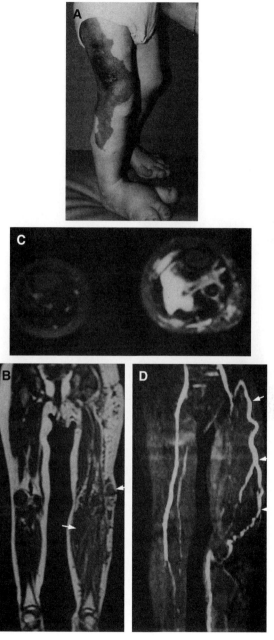

Fig. 16. (*A–D*) Capillary-lymphaticovenous (Klippel-trenaunay syndrome) of the pelvis and lower limb. Note the hypertrophy of the opposite foot. (*From* Mulliken JB, Fishman SJ, Burrows PE. Vascular anomalies. Curr Probl Surg 2000;37(8):570.)

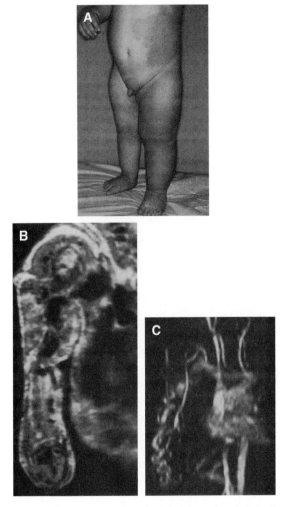

Fig. 17. (*A–C*) CAVM (Parkes Weber syndrome) of the left trunk, pelvis, and lower limb. (*From* Mulliken JB, Fishman SJ, Burrows PE. Vascular anomalies. Curr Probl Surg 2000;37(8):573.)

associated lymphatic abnormalities, and large lesions may be associated with high output cardiac failure. MRI complemented by MR angiography is important for diagnosis and anatomic delineation.

Summary

The last two decades have witnessed remarkable improvement in delineating the pathogenesis of vascular anomalies. Improved definitions based on this genetic-anatomic-histologic classification have allowed the development of multidisciplinary approaches toward disease treatment and management. As our appreciation of the embryonic and developmental contributions to disease increases, so does our ability to develop novel strategies for management of previously insurmountably complex lesions. Molecular and pharmacologic manipulation of vascular anomalies holds great promise.

References

[1] Mulliken JB, Young AE. Vascular birthmarks: hemangiomas and malformations. Philadelphia: WB Saunders; 1988.

[2] Virchow R. Angioma in die krankhaften geschwülste. Berlin: Hirshwald; 1863. p. 306–425.

[3] Vikkula M, et al. Molecular basis of vascular anomalies. Trends Cardiovasc Med 1998;8(7): 281–92.

[4] Holmdahl K. Cutaneous hemangiomas in premature and mature infants. Acta Paediatr Scand 1955;44:370–9.

[5] Amir J, Metzker A, Krikler R, et al. Strawberry hemangioma in preterm infants. Pediatr Dermatol 1986;3:331–2.

[6] Marchuk DA. Pathogenesis of hemangioma. J Clin Invest 2001;107(6):665–6.

[7] Boye E, Yu Y, Paranya G, et al. Clonality and altered behavior of endothelial cells from hemangiomas. J Clin Invest 2001;107(6):745–52.

[8] Cheung DS, Warmen ML, Mulliken JB. Hemangioma in twins. Ann Plast Surg 1997;38: 269–74.

[9] Mulliken JB, Glowacki J. Hemangiomas and vascular malformations in infants and children: a classification based on endothelial characteristics. Plast Reconstr Surg 1982;69: 412–20.

[10] Boon LM, Enjolras O, Mulliken JB. Congenital hemangioma: evidence of accelerated involution. J Pediatr 1996;128:329–35.

[11] Finn MC, Glowacki J, Mulliken JB. Congenital vascular lesions: clinical application of a new classification. J Pediatr Surg 1983;18:894–900.

[12] Razon MJ, Kraling BM, Mulliken JB, et al. Increased apoptosis coincides with onset of involution in infantile hemangioma. Microcirculation 1998;5(2–3):188–95.

[13] Bowers RE, Graham EA, Tomlinson KM. The natural history of the strawberry birthmark. Arch Dermatol 1960;82:667–80.

[14] Dadras SS, North PE, et al. Infantile hemangiomas are arrested in an early developmental vascular differentiation state. Mod Pathol 2004;17:1068–79.

[15] Bree AF, Siegfried E, et al. Infantile hemangiomas: speculation on placental trophoblastic origin. Arch Dermatol 2001;137(5):573–7.

[16] North PE, Waner M, Miterzaki A, et al. A unique microvascular phenotype shared by juvenile hemangiomas and human placenta. Arch Dermatol 2001;137(5):559–70.

[17] Leon-Villapalos J, Wolfe K, Kangesu L. GLUT-1: an extra diagnostic tool to differentiate between haemangiomas and vascular malformations. Br J Plast Surg 2005;58(3): 348–52.

[18] Huang SA, et al. Severe hypothyroidism caused by type 3 iodothyronine deiodinase in infantile hemangiomas. N Engl J Med 2000;343(3):185–9.

[19] Barnes CM, Huang S, Kaipainen A, et al. Evidence by molecular profiling for a placental origin of infantile hemangioma. PNAS, in press.

[20] Tille JC, Pepper MS. Hereditary vascular anomalies: new insights into their pathogenesis. Arterioscler Thromb Vasc Biol 2004;24:1578–90.

[21] Chang J, Most D, Bresnick S, et al. Proliferative hemangiomas: analysis of cytokine gene expression and angiogenesis. Plast Reconstr Surg 1999;103:1–10.

[22] Takahashi K, Mulliken JB, et al. Cellular markers that distinguish the phases of hemangioma during infancy and childhood. J Clin Invest 1994;93:2357–64.

[23] Pasqual-Castroviejo I, Viano J, Moreno F, et al. Hemangiomas of the head, neck and chest with associated vascular brain anomalies: a complex neurocutaneous syndrome. AJNR Am J Neuroradiol 1996;17:461–71.

[24] Burrows PE, Robertson RL, Mulliken JB, et al. Cerebral vasculopathy and neurologic sequelae in infants with cervicofacial hemangioma: report of eight patients. Radiology 1998; 207:601–7.

[25] Frieden IJ, Reese V, Cohen D. PHACE syndrome: the association of posterior fossa brain malformations, hemangiomas, arterial anomalies, coarcation of the aorta and cardiac defects and eye abnormalities. Arch Dermatol 1996;132:307–11.

[26] Goldberg NS, Hebert AA, Esterly NB. Sacral hemangiomas and multiple congenital abnormalities. Arch Dermatol 1986;122:684–7.

[27] Albright AL, Gartner JC, Wiener ES. Lumbar cutaneous hemangiomas as indicators of tethered spinal cords. Pediatrics 1989;83:977–80.

[28] Kasabach HH, Merritt KK. Capillary hemangioma with extensive purpura: report of a case. Am J Dis Child 1940;59:1063–70.

[29] Lyons LL, North PE, Mac-Moune LF, et al. Kaposiform hemangioendothelioma: a study of 33 cases emphasizing its pathologic, immunophenotypic, and biologic uniqueness from juvenile hemangioma. Am J Surg Pathol 2004;28(5):559–68.

[30] Enjolras O, Wassef M, Mazoyer E, et al. Infants with Kasabach-Merritt syndrome do not have "true" hemangiomas. J Pediatr 1997;130:631–40.

[31] Sarkar M, Mulliken JB, Kozakewich HP, et al. Thrombocytopenic coagulopathy (Kasabach-Merritt phenomenon) is associated with kaposiform hemangioendothelioma and not with common infantile hemangioma. Plast Reconstr Surg 1997;100:1377–86.

[32] Jones EW, Orkin M. Tufted angioma (angioblastoma): a benign progressive angioma, not to be confused with Kaposi's sarcoma or low grade angiosarcoma. J Am Acad Dermatol 1989; 20:214–25.

[33] Martinez-Perez D, Fine NA, Boon LM, et al. Not all hemangiomas look like strawberries: uncommon presentations of the most common tumor of infancy. Pediatr Dermatol 1995; 12:1–6.

[34] Patrice SJ, Wiss K, Mulliken JB. Pyogenic granuloma (lobular capillary hemangioma): a clinicopathologic of 178 cases. Pediatr Dermatol 1991;8:267–76.

[35] Chung KC, Weiss SW, Kuzon WM Jr. Multifocal congenital hemangiopericytomas associated with Kasabach-Merritt syndrome. Br J Plast Surg 1995;48:240–2.

[36] Boon LM, Fishman SJ, Lund DP, et al. Congenital fibrosarcoma masquerading as congenital hemangioma: report of two cases. J Pediatr Surg 1995;30:1378–81.

[37] Margileth AM, Museles M. Cutaneous hemangiomas in children: diagnosis and conservative management. JAMA 1965;194:523–6.

[38] Morelli JG, Tan OT, Yohn JJ, et al. Treatment of ulcerated hemangiomas in infancy. Arch Pediatr Adolesc Med 1994;148:1104–5.

[39] Enjolras O, Gelbert F. Superficial hemangiomas: associations and management. Pediatr Dermatol 1997;14:174–9.

[40] Orlow SJ, Isakoff MS, Blei F. Increased risk of symptomatic hemangiomas of the airway in association with cutaneous hemangiomas in a "beard" distribution. J Pediatr 1997;131: 643–6.

[41] Enjolras O, Riche MC, Merland JJ, et al. Management of alarming hemangiomas in infancy: a review of 25 cases. Pediatrics 1990;85:491–8.

[42] White CW, Wolf SJ, Korones DN, et al. Treatment of childhood angiomatous diseases with recombinant interferon alfa-2a. J Pediatr 1991;118:59–66.

[43] Ezekowitz RAB, Mulliken JB, Folkman J. Interferon alpha-2a therapy for life-threatening hemangiomas of infancy and childhood. N Engl J Med 1992;326:1456–63.

[44] Grienwald JH, Burke DK, Bonthius DJ, et al. An update on the treatment of hemangiomas in children with interferon alpha-2a. Arch Otolaryngol Head Neck Surg 1999;125:21–7.

[45] Barlow CF, Preibe CJ, Mulliken JB, et al. Spastic diplegia as a complication of interferon alpha-2a treatment of hemangiomas of infancy. J Pediatr 1998;132(3 Pt 1):527–30.

[46] Perez J, Pardo J, Gomez C. Vincristine: an effective treatment of corticoid-resistant life-threatening infantile hemangiomas. Acta Oncol 2002;41(2):197–9.

[47] Haisley-Royster C, Enjolras O, Frieden IJ, et al. Kasabach-Merritt phenomenon: a retrospective study of treatment with vincristine. J Pediatr Hematol Oncol 2002;24(6): 459–62.

[48] Sie KC, McGill T, Healy GB. Subglottic hemangioma: ten years' experience with carbon dioxide laser. Ann Otol Rhinol Laryngol 1994;103:167–72.

[49] Ramsauer M, D'Amore PA. Getting Tie(2)d up in angiogenesis. J Clin Invest 2002;110: 1615–7.

[50] Rodriguez-Niedenfuhr M, Papoutsi M, Christ B, et al. Prox1 is a marker of ectodermal placodes, endodermal compartments, lymphatic endothelium and lymphangioblasts. Anat Embryol (Berl) 2001;204:399–406.

[51] Oliver G. Lymphatic vasculature development. Nat Rev Immunol 2004;4:35–45.

[52] Bellomo D, Headrick JP, Silins GU, et al. Mice lacking the vascular endothelial growth factor-B gene (VEGF-b) have smaller hearts, dysfunctional coronary vasculature, and impaired recovery from cardiac ischemia. Circ Res 2000;86:E29–36.

[53] Jussila L, Alitalo K. Vascular growth factors and lymphangiogenesis. Physiol Rev 2002;82: 673–700.

[54] Dumont DJ, Jussila L, Taipale J, et al. Cardiovascular failure in mouse embryos deficient in VEGF receptor 3. Science 1998;282:946–9.

[55] Sato RN, Tozawa Y, Deutsch U, et al. Distinct roles of the receptor tyrosine kinases Tie-1 and Tie-2 in blood vessel formation. Nature 1995;376:70–4.

[56] Puri MC, Rossant J, Alitalo K, et al. The receptor tyrosine kinase TIE is required for integrity and survival of vascular endothelial cells. EMBO J 1995;14:5884–91.

[57] Suri C, Jones PF, Patan S, et al. Requisite role of angiopoietin-1, a ligand for the TIE2 receptor, during embryonic angiogenesis. Cell 1996;87:1171–80.

[58] Maisonpierre PC, Suri C, Jones PF, et al. Angiopoietin-2, a natural antagonist for Tie2 that disrupts in vivo angiogenesis. Science 1997;277:55–60.

[59] Dickson MC, Martin JS, Cousins FM, et al. Defective haematopoiesis and vasculogenesis in transforming growth factor-β 1 knock out mice. Development 1995;121:1845–54.

[60] Shawber CJ, Kitajewski J. Notch function in the vasculature: insights from zebrafish, mouse and man. Bioessays 2004;26:225–34.

[61] Soldi R, Mitola S, et al. Role of αvβ3 integrin in the activation of vascular endothelial growth factor receptor-2. EMBO J 1999;18:882–92.

[62] Smoller BR, Rosen S. Port-wine stains: a disease of altered neural modulation of blood vessels? Arch Dermatol 1986;122:177–9.

[63] Breugem CC, Alders M, Salieb-Beugelaar GB, et al. A locus for hereditary capillary malformations mapped on chromosome 5q. Hum Genet 2002;110:343–7.

[64] Eerola I, Boon LM, Mulliken JB, et al. Capillary malformation-arteriovenous malformation: a new clinical and genetic disorder caused by RASA1 mutations. Am J Hum Genet 2003;73:1240–9.

[65] Tan OT, Sherwood K, Gilchrest BA. Treatment of children with port wine stains using the flashlamp pumped tunable dye laser. N Engl J Med 1989;320:416–21.

[66] van der Horst CM, Koster PH, deBorgie CA, et al. Effect of the timing of treatment of port-wine stains with the flash lamp pulsed dye laser. N Engl J Med 1998;338:1028–33.

[67] McAllister KA, Grogg KM, Johnson DW, et al. Endoglin, a TGF-β binding protein of endothelial cells, is the gene for hereditary haemorrhagic telangiectasia type I. Nat Genet 1994;8:345–51.

[68] Johnson DW, Berg JN, et al. Mutations in the activin receptor-like kinase 1 gene in hereditary haemorrhagic telangiectasia type 2. Nat Genet 1996;13:189–95.

[69] Johnson DW, Berg JN, Baldwin MA, et al. A mouse model for hereditary hemorrhagic telangiectasia (HHT) type 2. Hum Mol Genet 2003;12:473–82.

[70] Lee JH, Paull TT. ATM activation by DNA double-strand breaks through the Mre11-Rad50-Nbs1 complex. Science 2005;308(5721):551–4.

[71] Puig S, Casati B, Staudenherz A, et al. Vascular low-flow malformations in children: current concepts for classification, diagnosis and therapy. Eur J Radiol 2005;53:35–45.

[72] Fishman SJ, Burrows PE, Upton J, et al. Life-threatening anomalies of the thoracic duct: anatomic delineation dictates management. J Pediatr Surg 2001;36(8):1269–72.

[73] Padwa BL, Hayward PG, Ferraro NF, et al. Cervicofacial lymphatic malformation, clinical course, surgical intervention, and pathogenesis of skeletal hypertrophy. Plast Reconstr Surg 1995;95:951–60.

[74] Gorham LW, Stout AP. Massive osteolysis (acute spontaneous absorption of bone, phantom bone, disappearing bone): its relations to hemangiomatosis. J Bone Joint Surg Am 1955;37:986–1004.

[75] Karkkainen MJ, Ferrell RE, Lawrence EC, et al. Missense mutations interfere with VEGFR-3 signaling in primary lymphoedema. Nat Genet 2000;25:153–9.

[76] Irrthum A, Karkkainen MJ, Devriendt K, et al. Congenital hereditary lymphedema caused by a mutations that inactivates VEGFR3. Am J Hum Genet 2000;67:295–301.

[77] Fang J, Dagenais SL, Erickson RP, et al. Mutations in FOXC2 (MFH-1), a forkhead family transcription factor, are responsible for the hereditary lymphedema-distichiasis syndrome. Am J Hum Genet 2000;67:1382–8.

[78] Ogita S, Tsuto T, Nakamura K, et al. OK-432 therapy in 64 patients with lymphangioma. J Pediatr Surg 1994;29:784–5.

[79] Algahtani A, Nguyen LT, Flageole H, et al. 25 years' experience with lymphangiomas in children. J Pediatr Surg 1999;34:1164–8.

[80] Brouillard P, Boon LM, Mulliken JB, et al. Mutations in a novel factor, glomulin, are responsible for glomuvenous malformations ("glomangiomas"). Am J Hum Genet 2002;70:866–74.

[81] Boon LM, Mulliken JB, Vikkula M, et al. Assignment of a locus for dominantly inherited venous malformations to chromosome 9. Hum Mol Genet 1994;3:1583–7.

[82] Vikkula M, Boon LM, Carraway KL, et al. Vascular dysmorphogenesis caused by an activating mutation in the receptor tyrosine kinase TIE2. Cell 1996;87:1181–90.

[83] Laberge-le CS, Jung HH, Houtteville JP, et al. Truncating mutations in CCM1, encoding KRIT1, cause hereditary cavernous angiomas. Nat Genet 1999;23:189–93.

[84] Zhang J, Clatterbuck RE, Rigamonti D, et al. Interaction between krit1 and icap1α infers perturbation of integrin β1-mediated angiogenesis in the pathogenesis of cerebral cavernous malformation. Hum Mol Genet 2001;10:2953–60.

[85] Oranje AP. Blue rubber bleb nevus syndrome. Pediatr Dermatol 1986;3:304–10.

[86] Fishman SJ, Burrows PE, Leichtner AM, et al. Gastrointestinal manifestations of vascular anomalies in childhood. J Pediatr Surg 1998;33:1163–7.

[87] Smithers CJ, Vogel AM, Kozakewich HP, et al. An injectable tissue-engineered embolus prevents luminal recanalization after vascular sclerotherapy. J Pediatr Surg 2005;40:920–5.

[88] Fishman SJ, Smithers CJ, Folkman J, et al. Blue rubber bleb nevus syndrome: surgical eradication of gastrointestinal bleeding. Ann Surg 2005;241(3):523–8.

[89] Fishman SJ, Shamberger RC, Fox VL, et al. Endorectal pull-through abates gastrointestinal hemorrhage for colorectal venous malformations. J Pediatr Surg 2000;35:982–4.

[90] Kohout MP, Hansen M, Pribaz JJ, et al. Arteriovenous malformations of the head and neck: natural history and management. Plast Reconstr Surg 1998;102:643–54.

[91] Gloviczki P, Stanson AW, Stickler GB, et al. Klippel-Trenaunay syndrome: the risks and benefits of vascular interventions. Surgery 1991;110:469–79.

[92] Baskerville PA, Akroyd JS, Thomas ML, et al. The Klippel-Trenaunay syndrome: clinical,
      radiological, and hemodynamic features and management. Br J Surg 1985;82:757–61.
[93] Yanez S, Val-Bernal JF, Mira C, et al. Spindle cell hemangioendotheliomas associated with
      multiple skeletal enchondromas: a variant of Maffucci's syndrome. Gen Diagn Pathol 1998;
      143:331–5.
[94] Sun T-C, Swee RG, Shives TC, et al. Chondrosarcoma in Maffucci's syndrome. J Bone Joint
      Surg Am 1985;67:1214–9.

ELSEVIER
SAUNDERS

SURGICAL
CLINICS OF
NORTH AMERICA

Surg Clin N Am 86 (2006) 427–439

Surgical Management of Pediatric Hematologic Disorders

Ai-Xuan L. Holterman, MD[a,*],
Kumari N. Adams, BS[b], Ruth A. Seeler, MD[c]

[a]Department of Surgery, Division of Pediatric Surgery, University of Illinois at Chicago,
840 South Wood Street, M/C 958 Chicago, IL 60612, USA
[b]University of Illinois College of Medicine at Chicago, 1853 West Polk Street,
M/C 785, Chicago, IL 60612, USA
[c]Department of Pediatrics, University of Illinois at Chicago, 840 South Wood Street,
M/C 856 Chicago, IL 60612, USA

Hemolytic uremic syndrome

The hemolytic uremic syndrome (HUS) is an acquired systemic disease arising from toxic injury to the endothelial lining of the small blood vessels, which results in microangiopathic hemolytic anemia and thrombocytopenia. The kidney is the major target organ, making HUS the most common cause of acute renal failure requiring dialysis in infants and children.

Etiology and pathophysiology

In children, 90% of the cases of HUS follow an episode of acute hemorrhagic enteritis caused by the Shiga toxin–producing *Escherichia coli* 0157:H7 or *E coli* 011. The Shiga toxin is absorbed from the intestines and inhibits protein synthesis in target cells in the kidney, gut, or other vital organs. Endothelial damage within the small vessels activates the coagulation system, resulting in platelet thrombi that trap erythrocytes in the microvascular circulation and cause hemolytic anemia and thrombocytopenia. Less often, HUS is associated with non–*E coli* infections involving streptococcus pneumonia or with other conditions including transplantation and medications. An atypical recurrent form of HUS from factor H deficiency or von Willebrand's factor cleaving protease enzyme (ADAMTS 13) deficiency is characterized by excessive accumulation of large von Willebrand's

---

* Corresponding author.
E-mail address: aithanh@uic.edu (A-X.L. Holterman).

0039-6109/06/$ - see front matter © 2006 Elsevier Inc. All rights reserved.
doi:10.1016/j.suc.2005.12.004
surgical.theclinics.com

factor multimers, leading to complement deposition within renal endothelial cells and secondary glomerular thrombotic microangiopathy [1].

Clinical course and treatment

Supportive care with attention to fluid and electrolytes, aggressive nutrition, management of hypertension, and early institution of dialysis have reduced the mortality rate from 80% to less than 10% over the past 30 years. Because antibiotics may accelerate the acute release of large amounts of preformed toxin from the bacteria and increase the risk of developing overt HUS in children who have E coli 0157:H7 enteritis [2], caution should be exercised in antibiotics use unless the enteritis is known to be Shiga toxin negative. No specific therapy against the microangiopathic process has yet been proved to affect the course of the disease in children. Although the efficacy of plasmapheresis in treating the diarrheal form of HUS is unclear, randomized controlled clinical trials have shown survival benefits for plasma exchange in the treatment of HUS associated with factor H or ADAMTS-13 deficiency [3]. Recent treatments include the use of monoclonal antibodies or Shiga toxin receptor analogs to neutralize E coli 0157:H7 Shiga toxins in the early colitis stage [4,5]. Angiotensin-converting enzyme inhibitors have also been shown to be beneficial in slowing the progression of renal injury [6,7]. Patients who have the atypical form of HUS (eg, factor H deficiency) have a high risk of recurrence [8] and are managed with repeated plasma and cryoprecipitate infusions. Despite aggressive management of acute renal failure, approximately 50% of the patients who have the diarrheal form of HUS still require dialysis and have long-term renal damage or hypertension [9]. Kidney transplantation remains the only alternative to life-long dialysis in 5% to 10% of the patients who have E coli 0157:H7–mediated end-stage renal disease.

The surgeons' role in HUS is to help evaluate patients who have abdominal pain or bloody diarrhea, provide dialysis access, and manage the rare complications of HUS pancreatitis.

Henoch-Schönlein purpura

Henoch-Schönlein purpura (HSP) is the most common form of vasculitis in children. It is of presumed autoimmune etiology and has a self-limited course, although life-threatening organ specific complications can occur [10,11].

Etiology and pathophysiology

The etiology of HSP remains unknown, but in 30% to 50% of the cases, HSP follows upper respiratory tract infections caused by group A Steptococcus. The underlying pathology is believed to be an autoimmune IgA-mediated small vessel panvasculitis that predominantly affects the skin, gastrointestinal tract, joints, and kidneys [10,11]. Immunofluorescence microscopy often reveals IgA and C3 deposition in the involved small vessels but the pathophysiologic role of complement activation remains controversial. A predisposition toward HSP has also been described for patients who have specific HLA haplotypes or who have familial Mediterranean fever [10,11].

Clinical manifestations

Children typically develop abdominal pain, polyarthritis, rash, and nephritis. Skin manifestations begin as an erythematous maculopapular rash and progress to purpura primarily in the posterior legs, buttocks, eyelids, or scrotum. Arthritis/arthralgia occurs in more than 50% and nephritis in 40% of the children [11]. Other complications include ophthalmitis, cardiomyositis, mononeuropathies, pulmonary or intramuscular hemorrhage, and central nervous system involvement with seizures, paresis, or coma. Gastrointestinal tract vasculitis is seen in up to 60% of the patients and presents as hemorrhagic pancreatitis, hydrops of the gall bladder, mesenteric lymphadenopathy, pseudomembranous colitis, or more commonly, intestinal edema, hemorrhage, or hematoma with cramping abdominal pain and bloody stools. An important differential diagnosis for these intestinal symptoms is intussusception, which occurs in 5% of the patients [12,13].

Prognosis and treatment

Supportive treatment includes adequate hydration and pain control. Although steroids have been advocated for the treatment of nephritis, central nervous system complications, or intestinal obstruction, randomized controlled studies have not shown a benefit for the early use of steroids in preventing HSP-related complications or in improving outcomes [14]. The mortality rate from renal, intestinal, or central nervous system complications is low. Residual renal damage persists in up to 50% of the patients, with relapses occurring as late as several years after the onset of HSP with 4% progressing to end-stage kidney disease [15]. HSP is fortunately a self-limited disease that has little significant sequelae in most children.

The pediatric surgeon is involved in the evaluation and management of gastrointestinal complications, mainly intussusception. In contrast to the usual ileocolic intussusception in pediatric patients, 60% of HSP intussusception are ileoileal or jejunoileal [13] and unamenable to hydrostatic retrograde enema diagnosis or reduction. Although upper gastrointestinal barium studies or abdominal CT scans are well-established diagnostic tools, ultrasonography is becoming a reliable imaging technique for defining the anatomic location, assessing the extent of the intestinal edema, assessing the progression of intussusception, and guiding surgical decisions [16,17]. Immediate surgical reduction with open or laparoscopic techniques has been espoused for the treatment of upper intestinal tract intussusception. Spontaneous resolution of symptoms can however occur [18]. In the absence of absolute surgical indications such as perforation, complete obstruction, or recalcitrant hemorrhage, patients can be carefully followed with serial sonograms, frequent re-examinations, and supportive care. Prompt surgical intervention is recommended if sonographic findings and clinical symptoms do not improve within 24 hours.

An important differential diagnosis of HSP-related vasculitis such as epidydimitis or orchitis is testicular torsion. Because true testicular torsion during the course of HSP is rare [19], surgical exploration is rarely justified unless the diagnosis is less obvious when scrotal manifestations are the sole symptoms. High-resolution color Doppler assessment of testicular blood flow can help resolve this diagnostic dilemma [20].

Idiopathic thrombocytopenic purpura

The most common cause of acute-onset thrombocytopenia in an otherwise healthy child is idiopathic (immune) thrombocytopenic purpura (ITP). ITP is an autoimmune disease with a benign self-limited course in children. Splenectomy is often required for the management of hemorrhagic complications from chronic ITP.

Etiology and pathophysiology

ITP is characterized by antiplatelet autoantibodies and complement-mediated platelet destruction [21]. The etiology of ITP remains unclear, although 50% to 65% of cases of childhood ITP are associated with a recent history of a viral illness. The severity of the disease is likely modulated by genetic polymorphism in the host inflammatory response [22]. A number of viruses have been implicated, including Epstein-Barr virus and HIV.

Clinical manifestations

A previously healthy child typically develops sudden-onset generalized petechiae and purpura or epitaxis without any other symptoms. Less commonly, the patient develops oral mucosal or gingival bleeding, hematuria, hematochezia, or rarely intracranial hemorrhage [23].

Prognosis and treatment

Spontaneous complete remission occurs within 6 months in 80% to 90% of children. Patients who have ITP lasting beyond 6 months of duration are considered to have chronic ITP [24]. Because medical therapy has not been shown to affect the long-term prognosis of ITP [25,26], the current treatment approach is minimal intervention for mildly symptomatic patients. Platelet transfusions are generally ineffective because of the presence of pre-existing antiplatelet antibodies but may be given as a last resort to transiently elevate the platelet count and control life-threatening hemorrhage. According to the American Society of Hematology, corticosteroids, intravenous immunoglobulin, or intravenous anti-D immunoglobulin therapy is restricted to patients at high risk of hemorrhagic complications, such as symptomatic patients who have platelet counts less than 20,000/μL [27].

Splenectomy in idiopathic thrombocytopenic purpura

Emergency splenectomy is performed in 60% of the rare 0.1% to 1% of ITP patients who develop life-threatening cerebral hemorrhage [28] and in 7% to 15% of the chronic ITP patients [29]. It currently offers the best chance for curative treatment, with an immediate remission rate of 70% to 90% and a long-term efficacy rate of 60% [27,30]. Although the contribution of residual accessory spleen in postsplenectomy ITP relapse remains controversial [31], accessory spleens are found in 10% to 30% of the patients and should be meticulously searched for in the splenic hilum, greater omentum, and gastrocolic and splenocolic ligament [32].

The benefits of splenectomy need to be weighed against postsplenectomy complications such as (1) postsplenectomy sepsis requiring life-long antibiotic prophylaxis with potential development of penicillin-resistant organisms; (2) ITP relapse (20%–40% incidence); and (3) other adverse events such as the long-term risks for venous thrombosis and pulmonary hypertension. Because of these concerns, splenectomy is not a first-line therapy for ITP. In the absence of short- and long-term risk/benefit analyses, the indications for splenectomy are currently restricted to patients who have symptomatic chronic ITP, to those who have complications of steroid use, or to those who relapse after medical therapy [24]. Polyvalent pneumococcal, meningococcal, and *Haemophilus influenzae* type B vaccination is administered at the time of diagnosis or before splenectomy. Penicillin prophylaxis has been recommended in all children younger than 5 years and in older children for the first 2 years after splenectomy [25,32] because this patient population is highly susceptible to post-splenectomy–related sepsis. The need for lifelong penicillin prophylaxis in the non immunocompromised host remains unresolved [33,34], but these controversies reflect risk assessment based on studies that preceded the 7- and 23-valent pneumococcal vaccines era.

Compared with open splenectomy, laparoscopic splenectomy is associated with similar remission outcome but lower surgical mortality and morbidity [35,36]. It is the procedure of choice in patients who have a normal-sized spleen, whereas the hand-assisted laparoscopic approach is a well-described alternative to open splenectomy in patients who have massive splenomegaly [37,38].

Most of the postsplenectomy ITP relapses occur during the first 2 years after surgery [39]. The management of postsplenectomy ITP failure or relapse remains challenging. Combination pharmacotherapy has been used with short-term success, but the sustained response rate is only approximately 30% [31]. Surgical exploration should be considered if residual splenic tissue is radiographically demonstrated in relapsing patients.

Hereditary spherocytosis

Hereditary spherocytosis (HS) is the most common congenital abnormality of the erythrocyte membrane, causing nonimmune chronic hemolytic anemia. It is characterized by a highly heterogenous mode of inheritance, underlying genetic defects, and clinical expression. Splenectomy and cholecystectomy are often needed to manage the complications of chronic hemolysis.

Etiology and pathophysiology

The underlying molecular pathologies are defects in genes encoding the membrane components of erythrocyte lipid bilayers. The red cells become more permeable to water, acquire a spherocyte shape, and lose their deformability. Spherocytes are prematurely trapped in the splenic microvasculature where they hemolyze, leading to chronic hemolysis. The autosomal dominant genetic defect is found principally in patients of Northern European descent, although 25% the cases are thought to arise from spontaneous mutations. Hereditary elliptocytosis, ovalocytosis, and pyropoikilocytosis are hemolytic diseases involving different red cell membrane abnormalities with similar molecular pathology [40,41].

Clinical manifestations

The clinical expression ranges from no symptoms or neonatal hyperbilirubinemia to severe transfusion-dependent hemolytic anemia. The most common features of HS include mild anemia, jaundice, and mild splenomegaly. Hematologic analysis shows increased red cell indices and reticulocyte count. Peripheral blood smears reveal diverse red cell morphologies such as spherocytes, acanthocytes, and poikilocytes. Cholelithiasis occurs in up to 40% of patients older than 10 years [42]. It can present as the first manifestation of HUS and should be suspected in patients who have a strong family history of gallstone disease. Other patients may present with hemolytic, megaloblastic, or aplastic crises (following human parvovirus B19 infection) and growth failure [41].

Prognosis and treatment

Severe neonatal hyperbilirubinemia is managed with phototherapy and occasionally with exchange red cell transfusions. Erythropoietin may be useful in reducing the transfusion needs in infants who have severe HS [43], and folate supplements are given to patients who have chronic hemolysis to help maintain erythropoiesis. In general, hemoglobin level alone is not an indication for transfusion unless patients are symptomatic.

There is no evidence that splenectomy is beneficial in mild or well-compensated HS, although hemoglobin levels of 6 to 8 g/dL, bilirubin of greater than 34 μmol/L, reticulocyte count of greater than 6%, and erythrocyte spectrin content of less than 60% are indicative of moderate or severe disease and have been used as guidelines for recommending splenectomy [44]. Because spherocytes are destroyed almost exclusively in the spleen, osmotic fragility and anemia often improves following splenectomy, along with a decreased incidence of gallstones [41]. Subtotal splenectomy [45] and near total splenectomy [46] have recently been advocated in children younger than 5 years. The potential benefit of splenic preservation in immunologically immature young children should be carefully weighed against the risks of residual hemolysis, secondary cholelithiasis, and aplastic crisis [47], which may necessitate reoperative completion splenectomy.

Computer-modeled decision analysis has shown that combined cholecystectomy and splenectomy can be of benefit in children who have concurrent cholelithiasis and mild HS [48]. Patients who qualify for splenectomy should therefore be screened for the presence of silent stones. Because the risks of developing gallstones after splenectomy are low [49], cholecystectomy is not indicated in HS patients who do not have biliary diseases.

Sickle cell disease

Sickle cell disease (SCD) is one of the most common inherited diseases worldwide that involves a heterogenous group of related hemoglobinopathies associated with complications of ischemic multiorgan systemic damage and chronic hemolytic anemia. Recent advances in neonatal screening and comprehensive follow-up care have reduced historical mortality rates of as high as 20% to less than 2% by age 10 years.

Etiology and pathophysiology

The underlying molecular defect is a single point mutation in the β-globin gene that results in abnormal sickle hemoglobin (hemoglobin S). In the deoxygenated state, hemoglobin S polymerizes and erythrocytes become rigid and adhere to the endothelium, leading to microvascular occlusion and end-organ damage. SCD includes the more severe form of homozygous hemoglobin S disease, also known as sickle cell anemia, and various forms of hemoglobin S heterozygosity, β-thalassemias, and hemoglobin C hemoglobinopathies [50]. The differential diagnosis is resolved by hemoglobin electrophoresis.

Clinical manifestations

Newborns are frequently asymptomatic because of the protective effect of fetal hemoglobin (hemoglobin F) which interferes with hemoglobin S polymerization and attenuates disease severity [51]. The cardinal feature of SCD is vasocclusion leading to end-organ acute or chronic ischemic damage and chronic hemolytic anemia. Patients present with painful episodes or "crises" of bone marrow microvascular occlusion, acute splenic sequestration, dactylitis (hand-foot syndrome) from epiphyseal infarction of the digits, sepsis, and acute chest syndrome from pulmonary infarction, which is the leading cause of death in children who have SCD. Aplastic anemia precipitated by human parvovirus B19 can present as life-threatening acute anemia and thrombocytopenia from hypersplenism. Chronic complications of silent ischemia lead to stroke, cardiomyopathy, pulmonary and hepatic fibrosis, glomerular sclerosis, retinal disease, avascular femoral head necrosis, chronic osteomyelitis, and cholelithiasis [52]. The spleen is the first organ affected by chronic vaso-occlusion, and autoinfarction leads to functional hyposplenism early in life.

Prognosis and treatment

In patients who have no symptoms or mild disease, treatment is expectant with folate supplementation and prevention of bacterial infection by immunizations and prophylactic penicillin. Symptomatic patients are treated with analgesics, hydration, and sometimes red cell transfusions. Preventive treatment consists of chronic red cell transfusion therapies; pharmacologic induction of fetal hemoglobin with hydroxyurea; or experimental stem cell transplantation to reduce transfusion needs, attenuate the ischemic complications (especially cerebral infarcts), and improve survival [53–56]. Red cell transfusions are also indicated for aplastic crisis and splenic sequestration. The benefits of red cell transfusion should be balanced against the complications of transmittable diseases, chronic iron overload, and alloimmunization. Partial phenotype matching for minor red cell antigens should be done for chronic transfusion patients to reduce the risks of alloimmunization.

Perioperative management

The underlying management principles are to maximize erythrocyte oxygen-carrying capacity and to prevent hypoxia. The preoperative work-up includes careful screening for pre-existing SCD comorbidities. Perioperative management involves judicious hydration; avoidance of hypoxia, hypothermia, or acidosis; optimal pain control; intensive pulmonary toilet; and early mobilization [57]. Advances in modern anesthetic care leading to improved SCD-related perioperative morbidities have significantly simplified the perioperative transfusion management of SCD patients. Current data show that the minimal SCD complication rates associated with low-risk elective surgical procedures such as pediatric inguinal hernia repair in stable SCD patients do not justify the need for preoperative transfusion [58]. The Preoperative Transfusion in Sickle Cell Disease Study Group compared simple preoperative blood transfusion to bring the hemoglobin level to 10 g/dL (a "top-off" transfusion approach) with aggressive transfusion to lower hemoglobin S levels to less than 30% (with exchange transfusion). No difference was demonstrated in the incidence (10%) of postoperative acute chest syndrome between the two groups, but higher transfusion-related complications were found in the aggressive transfusion group [59]. For medically stable patients undergoing intermediate-risk surgery such as elective laparoscopic surgery, a top-off transfusion approach is an accepted procedure. In patients undergoing elective major abdominal surgery such as open cholecystectomy or thoracotomy, optimal hemoglobin A levels can be achieved with a 3- to 4-week schedule of weekly transfusions as an alternative to preoperative exchange transfusion. Evidence-based studies are still needed to address controversial issues such as the impact of hemoglobin S levels on perioperative morbidities, the preoperative indications for exchange transfusion, and the optimal transfusion preparation. The current transfusion management is therefore highly individualized and must be balanced against the risks of transfusion-related complications.

Cholelithiasis

The prevalence of cholelithiasis is at least 20% in pediatric SCD. In agreement with findings from several pediatric retrospective studies [60,61], the National Preoperative Transfusion Study randomized trial found no difference in SCD-related complication rates between elective laparoscopic and open cholecystectomy [62], making laparoscopic cholecystectomy the most common surgical procedure performed in SCD patients [63]. Because of the high morbidity and mortality of emergency cholecystectomy in SCD, prophylactic elective cholecystectomy is recommended in SCD patients who have asymptomatic cholelithiasis. Choledocholithiasis (reported to be ≥10% in SCD patients [64]) should be evaluated by intraoperative cholangiography at the time of cholecystectomy. Combining open or laparoscopic cholecystectomy with elective splenectomy without aggressive preoperative transfusion in patients who have concomitant cholelithiasis can be achieved with minimal SCD-related complications so long as adequate hemoglobin levels are maintained [65].

Splenectomy

The most common indications for splenectomy are symptomatic hypersplenism and life-threatening acute splenic sequestration. The Cooperative Study of Sickle Cell Disease reported a 3% incidence of emergency splenectomy for acute splenic sequestration in pediatric SCD [66]. Acute splenic sequestration more commonly occurs in patients younger than 5 years, but older pediatric patients who have persistent splenomegaly are also at risk. Accelerated destruction of sickled red cells and hypersplenism lead to acute anemia, thrombocytopenia, and reticulocytosis. The long-term management options include preventive transfusion or splenectomy to reduce the risks of lethal recurrent acute splenic sequestration, although there is insufficient evidence in support of either treatment in preventing acute splenic sequestration recurrence and in improving the survival [67]. The size of the residual spleen, the patient age, and the degree of severity of the initial attack as risk factors for acute splenic sequestration recurrence and mortality are important considerations in deliberating further treatment approaches. Parental education in regular assessment of the child's splenic size and in early recognition of the signs of acute splenic sequestration is essential.

Summary

The optimal care of patients who have hematologic disorders requires a good understanding of the underlying pathophysiology and the disease course to integrate the surgical and the medical management of these complex multiorgan system diseases. Advanced anesthetic care and minimally invasive surgery can be credited for recent changes in the operative indications for these diseases and for a less aggressive transfusion approach in the perioperative care of SCD patients. The authors' recommendations are for the most part based on their assessment of the risk/benefit ratio of the various interventions, on data from case control series, and on their practical experience. Advances in molecular pathophysiology to enhance the understanding of disease mechanism and in outcome-related research to provide best practice data are essential to provide clinicians with scientifically based management of these challenging patients.

References

[1] Zimmerhackl LB. E. coli, antibiotics, and the hemolytic-uremic syndrome. N Engl J Med 2000;342(26):1990–1.
[2] Siegler R, Oakes R. Hemolytic uremic syndrome; pathogenesis, treatment, and outcome. Curr Opin Pediatr 2005;17(2):200–4.
[3] Rock GA. Management of thrombotic thrombocytopenic purpura. Br J Haematol 2000; 109(3):496–507.
[4] Karmali MA. Prospects for preventing serious systemic toxemic complications of Shiga toxin-producing Escherichia coli infections using Shiga toxin receptor analogues. J Infect Dis 2004;189(3):355–9.
[5] Tazzari PL, Ricci F, Carnicelli D, et al. Flow cytometry detection of Shiga toxins in the blood from children with hemolytic uremic syndrome. Cytometry B Clin Cytom 2004;61(1):40–4.
[6] Caletti MG, Lejarraga H, Kelmansky D, et al. Two different therapeutic regimes in patients with sequelae of hemolytic-uremic syndrome. Pediatr Nephrol 2004;19(10):1148–52.
[7] Van Dyck M, Proesmans W. Renoprotection by ACE inhibitors after severe hemolytic uremic syndrome. Pediatr Nephrol 2004;19(6):688–90.
[8] Loirat C, Niaudet P. The risk of recurrence of hemolytic uremic syndrome after renal transplantation in children. Pediatr Nephrol 2003;18(11):1095–101.
[9] De Petris L, Gianviti A, Giordano U, et al. Blood pressure in the long-term follow-up of children with hemolytic uremic syndrome. Pediatr Nephrol 2004;19(11):1241–4.

[10] Szer IS. Henoch-Schonlein purpura. Curr Opin Rheumatol 1994;6(1):25–31.

[11] Saulsbury FT. Henoch-Schonlein purpura in children. Report of 100 patients and review of the literature. Medicine (Baltimore) 1999;78(6):395–409.

[12] Chang WL, Yang YH, Lin YT, et al. Gastrointestinal manifestations in Henoch-Schonlein purpura: a review of 261 patients. Acta Paediatr 2004;93(11):1427–31.

[13] Choong CK, Beasley SW. Intra-abdominal manifestations of Henoch-Schonlein purpura. J Paediatr Child Health 1998;34(5):405–9.

[14] Huber AM, King J, McLaine P, et al. A randomized, placebo-controlled trial of prednisone in early Henoch Schonlein purpura [ISRCTN85109383]. BMC Med 2004;2(1):7.

[15] Kawasaki Y, Suzuki J, Sakai N, et al. Clinical and pathological features of children with Henoch-Schoenlein purpura nephritis: risk factors associated with poor prognosis. Clin Nephrol 2003;60(3):153–60.

[16] Couture A, Veyrac C, Baud C, et al. Evaluation of abdominal pain in Henoch-Schonlein syndrome by high frequency ultrasound. Pediatr Radiol 1992;22(1):12–7.

[17] Connolly B, O'Halpin D. Sonographic evaluation of the abdomen in Henoch-Schonlein purpura. Clin Radiol 1994;49(5):320–3.

[18] Sonmez K, Turkyilmaz Z, Demirogullari B, et al. Conservative treatment for small intestinal intussusception associated with Henoch-Schonlein's purpura. Surg Today 2002;32(12): 1031–4.

[19] Ioannides AS, Turnock R. An audit of the management of the acute scrotum in children with Henoch-Schonlein purpura. J R Coll Surg Edinb 2001;46(2):98–9.

[20] Ben-Sira L, Laor T. Severe scrotal pain in boys with Henoch-Schonlein purpura: incidence and sonography. Pediatr Radiol 2000;30(2):125–8.

[21] McMillan R. Autoantibodies and autoantigens in chronic immune thrombocytopenic purpura. Semin Hematol 2000;37(3):239–48.

[22] Chanock S. The etiology of childhood immune thrombocytopenic purpura: how complex is it? J Pediatr Hematol Oncol 2003;25(Suppl 1):S7–10.

[23] Kaplan RN, Bussel JB. Differential diagnosis and management of thrombocytopenia in childhood. Pediatr Clin North Am 2004;51(4):1109–40 [xi].

[24] Bolton-Maggs PH. Idiopathic thrombocytopenic purpura. Arch Dis Child 2000;83(3):220–2.

[25] Blanchette VS, Price V. Childhood chronic immune thrombocytopenic purpura: unresolved issues. J Pediatr Hematol Oncol 2003;25(Suppl 1):S28–33.

[26] Yetman RJ. Evaluation and management of childhood idiopathic (immune) thrombocyto-penia. J Pediatr Health Care 2003;17(5):261–3.

[27] George JN, Woolf SH, Raskob GE, et al. Idiopathic thrombocytopenic purpura: a practice guideline developed by explicit methods for the American Society of Hematology. Blood 1996;88(1):3–40.

[28] Butros LJ, Bussel JB. Intracranial hemorrhage in immune thrombocytopenic purpura: a ret-rospective analysis. J Pediatr Hematol Oncol 2003;25(8):660–4.

[29] Aronis S, Platokouki H, Avgeri M, et al. Retrospective evaluation of long-term efficacy and safety of splenectomy in chronic idiopathic thrombocytopenic purpura in children. Acta Paediatr 2004;93(5):638–42.

[30] Gadenstatter M, Lamprecht B, Klingler A, et al. Splenectomy versus medical treatment for idiopathic thrombocytopenic purpura. Am J Surg 2002;184(6):606–9 [discussion: 609–10].

[31] Kumar S, Diehn FE, Gertz MA, et al. Splenectomy for immune thrombocytopenic purpura: long-term results and treatment of postsplenectomy relapses. Ann Hematol 2002;81(6): 312–9.

[32] Eraklis AJ, Filler RM. Splenectomy in childhood: a review of 1413 cases. J Pediatr Surg 1972; 7(4):382–8.

[33] Read RC, Finch RG. Prophylaxis after splenectomy. J Antimicrob Chemother 1994;33(1): 4–6.

[34] Waghorn DJ. Overwhelming infection in asplenic patients: current best practice preventive measures are not being followed. J Clin Pathol 2001;54(3):214–8.

[35] Rescorla FJ, Engum SA, West KW, et al. Laparoscopic splenectomy has become the gold standard in children. Am Surg 2002;68(3):297–301 [discussion: 301–2].

[36] Pace DE, Chiasson PM, Schlachta CM, et al. Laparoscopic splenectomy for idiopathic thrombocytopenic purpura (ITP). Surg Endosc 2003;17(1):95–8.

[37] Kercher KW, Matthews BD, Walsh RM, et al. Laparoscopic splenectomy for massive splenomegaly. Am J Surg 2002;183(2):192–6.

[38] Tarr PI. Basic fibroblast growth factor and Shiga toxin-O157:H7-associated hemolytic uremic syndrome. J Am Soc Nephrol 2002;13(3):817–20.

[39] El-Alfy MS, El-Tawil MM, Shahein N. 5- to 16-year follow-up following splenectomy in chronic immune thrombocytopenic purpura in children. Acta Haematol 2003;110(1):20–4.

[40] Shah S, Vega R. Hereditary spherocytosis. Pediatr Rev 2004;25(5):168–72.

[41] Bolton-Maggs PH, Stevens RF, Dodd NJ, et al. Guidelines for the diagnosis and management of hereditary spherocytosis. Br J Haematol 2004;126(4):455–74.

[42] Rutkow IM. Twenty years of splenectomy for hereditary spherocytosis. Arch Surg 1981;116(3):306–8.

[43] Eber SW, Armbrust R, Schroter W. Variable clinical severity of hereditary spherocytosis: relation to erythrocytic spectrin concentration, osmotic fragility, and autohemolysis. J Pediatr 1990;117(3):409–16.

[44] Tchernia G, Delhommeau F, Perrotta S, et al. Recombinant erythropoietin therapy as an alternative to blood transfusions in infants with hereditary spherocytosis. Hematol J 2000;1(3):146–52.

[45] Bader-Meunier B, Gauthier F, Archambaud F, et al. Long-term evaluation of the beneficial effect of subtotal splenectomy for management of hereditary spherocytosis. Blood 2001;97(2):399–403.

[46] Stoehr GA, Stauffer UG, Eber SW. Near-total splenectomy: a new technique for the management of hereditary spherocytosis. Ann Surg 2005;241(1):40–7.

[47] de Buys Roessingh AS, de Lagausie P, Rohrlich P, et al. Follow-up of partial splenectomy in children with hereditary spherocytosis. J Pediatr Surg 2002;37(10):1459–63.

[48] Marchetti M, Quaglini S, Barosi G. Prophylactic splenectomy and cholecystectomy in mild hereditary spherocytosis: analyzing the decision in different clinical scenarios. J Intern Med 1998;244(3):217–26.

[49] Sandler A, Winkel G, Kimura K, et al. The role of prophylactic cholecystectomy during splenectomy in children with hereditary spherocytosis. J Pediatr Surg 1999;34(7):1077–8.

[50] Chui DH, Dover GJ. Sickle cell disease: no longer a single gene disorder. Curr Opin Pediatr 2001;13(1):22–7.

[51] Quinn CT, Miller ST. Risk factors and prediction of outcomes in children and adolescents who have sickle cell anemia. Hematol Oncol Clin North Am 2004;18(6):1339–54 [ix].

[52] Schnog JB, Duits AJ, Muskiet FA, et al. Sickle cell disease; a general overview. Neth J Med 2004;62(10):364–74.

[53] Atweh GF, DeSimone J, Saunthararajah Y, et al. Hemoglobinopathies. Hematology (Am Soc Hematol Educ Program) 2003;1:14–39.

[54] Hankins J, Jeng M, Harris S, et al. Chronic transfusion therapy for children with sickle cell disease and recurrent acute chest syndrome. J Pediatr Hematol Oncol 2005;27(3):158–61.

[55] Gaziev J, Lucarelli G. Stem cell transplantation for hemoglobinopathies. Curr Opin Pediatr 2003;15(1):24–31.

[56] Reed W, Vichinsky EP. Transfusion therapy: a coming-of-age treatment for patients with sickle cell disease. J Pediatr Hematol Oncol 2001;23(4):197–202.

[57] Firth PG, Head CA. Sickle cell disease and anesthesia. Anesthesiology 2004;101(3):766–85.

[58] Griffin TC, Buchanan GR. Elective surgery in children with sickle cell disease without preoperative blood transfusion. J Pediatr Surg 1993;28(5):681–5.

[59] Vichinsky EP, Haberkern CM, Neumayr L, et al. A comparison of conservative and aggressive transfusion regimens in the perioperative management of sickle cell disease. The Preoperative Transfusion in Sickle Cell Disease Study Group. N Engl J Med 1995;333(4):206–13.

[60] Wales PW, Carver E, Crawford MW, et al. Acute chest syndrome after abdominal surgery in children with sickle cell disease: is a laparoscopic approach better? J Pediatr Surg 2001;36(5): 718–21.

[61] Delatte SJ, Hebra A, Tagge EP, et al. Acute chest syndrome in the postoperative sickle cell patient. J Pediatr Surg 1999;34(1):188–91 [discussion: 191–2].

[62] Haberkern CM, Neumayr LD, Orringer EP, et al. Cholecystectomy in sickle cell anemia patients: perioperative outcome of 364 cases from the National Preoperative Transfusion Study. Preoperative Transfusion in Sickle Cell Disease Study Group. Blood 1997;89(5): 1533–42.

[63] Al-Salem AH, Qaisruddin S. The significance of biliary sludge in children with sickle cell disease. Pediatr Surg Int 1998;13(1):14–6.

[64] Al-Salem AH, Nourallah H. Sequential endoscopic/laparoscopic management of cholelithiasis and choledocholithiasis in children who have sickle cell disease. J Pediatr Surg 1997; 32(10):1432–5.

[65] Al-Salem AH. Should cholecystectomy be performed concomitantly with splenectomy in children with sickle-cell disease? Pediatr Surg Int 2003;19(1–2):71–4.

[66] Gill FM, Sleeper LA, Weiner SJ, et al. Clinical events in the first decade in a cohort of infants with sickle cell disease. Cooperative Study of Sickle Cell Disease. Blood 1995;86(2):776–83.

[67] Owusu-Ofori S, Riddington C. Splenectomy versus conservative management for acute sequestration crises in people with sickle cell disease. Cochrane Database Syst Rev 2002;4: CD003425.

SURGICAL
CLINICS OF
NORTH AMERICA

Surg Clin N Am 86 (2006) 441–454

Adolescent Obesity and Bariatric Surgery

Michael A. Helmrath, MD[a],*, Mary L. Brandt, MD[a], Thomas H. Inge, MD, PhD[b]

[a]Michael E. DeBakey Department of Surgery, Baylor College of Medicine,
Texas Children's Hospital Clinical Care Center, Suite 650, 6621 Fannin,
Houston TX 77030, USA
[b]Comprehensive Weight Management Center,
Division of Pediatric General and Thoracic Surgery,
Cincinnati Children's Hospital Medical Center, 3333 Burnet Avenue,
MLC 2023, Cincinnati, OH 45229-3039, USA

Obesity has become the most common nutritional disorder of children and adolescents in the United States. Along with this epidemic, there has been an increase in associated potentially life-threatening diseases. The World Health Organization classification in adults defines overweight as a body mass index (BMI) of 25 to 30 kg/m^2 and obesity as a BMI of 30 kg/m^2 or more. The BMI, which takes into account the relationship of weight and height, correlates with the amount of body fat in children and adults [1]. In children, the ratio of weight to height changes with growth. For that reason BMI growth charts have been developed for children by the US Centers for Disease Control and Prevention. The definition of obesity for children is ninety-fifth percentile or more of BMI for age. Children with a BMI between the eighty-fifth and ninety-fifth percentile are considered overweight [2]. Using these criteria, the prevalence of being obese doubled among children aged 6 to 11 years and tripled among children aged 12 and 17 years in the United States between 1980 and 2000. Currently more than 1 million adolescents and young adults in the United States are considered severely obese (BMI ≥ 40 kg/m^2). Groups that are at particularly high risk for morbid obesity include African Americans, Hispanics, Pima Indians, and other Native Americans.

The epidemic of obesity has multiple causes. Human beings are genetically predisposed to store fat, a survival mechanism that served well during lean times for our prehistoric ancestors. Currently our lifestyles, unlike those of our ancestors, are much more sedentary. Food in modern

---

* Corresponding author.
E-mail address: helmrath@bcm.tmc.edu (M.A. Helmrath).

society also is plentiful, processed, and energy dense. In general, it is thought that genetic predisposition plays a permissive role, interacting with environmental factors to promote obesity. It is estimated that 30% to 50% of the tendency toward excess adiposity can be explained by genetic variations [3]. Although numerous genetic markers are linked with obesity and its metabolic consequences, identifiable hormonal, syndromic, or molecular genetic abnormalities are present in less than 5% of obese individuals [4,5]. More than 430 genes, markers, and chromosomal regions have been associated or linked with human obesity phenotypes [6]. Every chromosome, except the Y chromosome, has a locus linked with the phenotype of obesity. The most frequent mutations that result in the obesity phenotype have been found in the melanocortin receptor 4, occurring in up to 4% of early-onset and severe childhood obesity [7]. Given recent genetic findings, it is highly probable that severe childhood obesity is polygenic, with susceptibility conferred via complex interactions among genetic factors, behavioral factors, and the environment.

Comorbidities of obesity

Obesity in many children is not a problem of "willpower" or "discipline" but is a potentially life-threatening disease. A dose-response relationship between BMI during young adulthood and the risk of death has been demonstrated, with extreme obesity resulting in a reduction of 20, 13, 5 and 8 years of life expectancy for black men, white men, white women, and black women, respectively [8]. Importantly, the loss of 5% to 10% of body weight results in a significant improvement of risk and comorbidities [9].

Metabolic abnormalities

Over the past decade, an alarming increase in the appearance of type 2 diabetes in children has occurred. Type 2 diabetes is responsible for approximately one fifth of the new diagnoses of diabetes in pubertal children. By some estimates, up to one third of all children and half of Hispanic and black children develop type 2 diabetes in their lifetime [10]. Diabetes can be diagnosed by a fasting plasma glucose >125 mg/dL in the presence of diabetes symptoms or two fasting plasma glucose values >125 mg/dL in the absence of symptoms or by measuring a serum glucose concentration >200 mg/dL 2 hours after an oral load of 75 g of glucose (oral glucose tolerance test).

In adults, the metabolic syndrome is defined by the US National Cholesterol Education Program's Adult Treatment Panel III as requiring three of five characteristics:

1. Abdominal obesity with a waist circumference more than 102 cm in men and 88 cm in women
2. Triglyceride concentration >150 mg/dL or 1.7 μmol/L

3. Abnormal cholesterol profile with high-density lipoprotein cholesterol <40 mg/dL or 1 μmol/L in men and <50 mg/dL or 1.3 μmol/L in women
4. Blood pressure >130/85 mm Hg
5. Impaired fasting glucose ≥100 mg/dL or 5.5 μmol/L [11]

The metabolic syndrome is a clustering of risk factors for later cardiac disease and diabetes. Approximately 47 million adults meet criteria for this syndrome, which elevates one's risk of later heart diseases twofold and the risk of diabetes fivefold. There is as yet no definition of metabolic syndrome for the pediatric age group, but using the adult criteria, the overall prevalence of metabolic syndrome among 12- to 19-year-old individuals in the United States was found to be 4.2% [12]. Using modified criteria, Weiss and colleagues [13] found that nearly 50% of severely obese adolescents met criteria for the metabolic syndrome and that the risk increased as BMI increased. Currently, there is a lack of certainty about the pathogenesis of the syndrome, and considerable controversy exists about whether the metabolic syndrome poses a greater health risk than the sum of its parts, especially for pediatric patients.

Acanthosis nigricans, another frequent manifestation of insulin resistance, is characterized by hyperpigmented, hyperkeratotic, velvety plaques on the dorsal surface of the neck and hands. Insulin resistance also stimulates ovarian and adrenal androgen and estrogen production. These hormonal perturbations place obese adolescent girls at high risk of menstrual disorders and early onset of polycystic ovary syndrome. Polycystic ovary syndrome, previously called Stein-Leventhal syndrome, is a complex metabolic disease that may present in adolescents and is associated with obesity. This syndrome is manifested by oligomenorrhea or amenorrhea associated with obesity, insulin resistance, hirsutism, acne, and acanthosis nigrans [14]. It is reasoned that weight loss, which results in decreases in insulin resistance, can be an important adjunct to treatment of polycystic ovary syndrome and menstrual abnormalities in obese patients [15].

Cardiac risk factors

Cardiac risk factors are common in obese children and include atherogenic dyslipidemia (low high-density lipoprotein cholesterol and elevated triglycerides or low-density lipoprotein cholesterol), hypertension, sleep apnea, and left ventricular hypertrophy. Fifty percent of overweight adolescents have one risk factor for developing cardiovascular disease and 20% have two factors [15]. Childhood obesity is the leading cause of pediatric hypertension. Systolic blood pressure correlates positively with BMI, skinfold thickness, and waist-to-hip ratio in children and adolescents [16]. Clinical hypertension is ten times more common in obese children than lean children, with up to 30% of obese children having elevated systolic or diastolic blood pressure [17,18]. Significant, irreversible consequences of hypertension, such as hypertensive cardiac disease, can present in childhood. In one study, 38% of children who had hypertension had left ventricular hypertrophy by echocardiography [18]. Others have noted that the prevalence of left ventricular hypertrophy increases as a function of overweight, with 3% of normal weight, 25% of overweight, 52% of obese, and 86% of morbidly obese youth fulfilling echocardiographic criteria for left ventricular hypertrophy (Thomas Kimball, MD, personal communication, 2005). Hyperlipidemia in obese children is most often manifested by elevated low-density lipoprotein cholesterol, elevated triglycerides, and decreased high-density lipoprotein cholesterol [19].

Obstructive sleep apnea syndrome

There is a strong association between obesity and obstructive sleep apnea syndrome (OSAS), because obese children are four to six times more likely to have OSAS when compared with lean subjects [20]. Symptoms of OSAS may include snoring, poor school performance because of daytime sleepiness, enuresis, and hyperactivity [21]. OSAS is diagnosed by an overnight sleep study to measure the apnea-hypopnea index. Twenty-six percent to 37% of obese children have an abnormal sleep study, although not all have significant obstruction [22]. We have found that OSAS correlates directly with BMI: 40%, 50%, and 70% of adolescents with BMI of 40 to 49, 50 to 59, and >60, respectively, meet polysomnographic criteria for OSAS [23]. For obese children, weight reduction improves obstructive sleep apnea, although it is important to rule out other anatomic causes of sleep apnea, such as tonsillar hypertrophy [24]. Obese children with sleep disorders may benefit from an evaluation by an otorhinolaryngologist.

Nonalcoholic fatty liver disease

Obesity is related to a spectrum of liver abnormalities, referred to as nonalcoholic fatty liver disease. This disease may present as isolated fatty infiltration of the liver to steatohepatitis (termed "NASH" for nonalcoholic steatosis/hepatitis) or may involve fibrosis and cirrhosis. Up to 40% of obese children have ultrasound findings that suggest infiltration of the liver, and up to 40% of these children also have abnormal liver function test results [17]. Because characteristic biochemical findings do not always correlate with histology, diagnosis requires a liver biopsy [25]. Nonalcoholic fatty liver disease has been diagnosed histologically in up to 50% of obese children and in 83% of morbidly obese teenagers [25a]. Nonalcoholic fatty liver disease in childhood may be characterized by a benign clinical course without progression. With escalating rates of pediatric obesity, however, there is concern that the prevalence and severity of NASH also may increase because of earlier and prolonged exposure to obesity and associated inflammation [26]. The long-term outcome of untreated NASH acquired in childhood is unknown, but the literature notes that 25% of adult patients who have NASH develop cirrhosis [27]. Currently, antioxidants are being used for the treatment of NASH, but weight loss may prove to be the only effective treatment for nonalcoholic fatty liver disease [28].

Orthopedic disorders

Overweight children are susceptible to developing orthopedic problems. Excess weight may cause injury to the growth plate and result in slipped capital femoral epiphysis, genu valga, tibia vara (Blount's disease), flat kneecap pressure/pain, spondylolisthesis, scoliosis, and osteoarthritis [29]. Blount's disease (tibia vara) is overgrowth of the medial aspect of the proximal tibial metaphysis, which occurs in response to and then accentuates bowing of the legs under the pressure of excess weight [19].

Pseudotumor cerebri

Pseudotumor cerebri is a rare disorder characterized by a gradual increase in intracranial pressure, which, if untreated, may result in visual impairment or even blindness. The usual presentation is headaches, but patients also may experience dizziness, unsteadiness, or diploplia [21]. Approximately 50% of children who have pseudotumor cerebri are obese [19]. There is no effective long-term therapy other than weight loss [19].

Psychology

Although not a life-threatening comorbidity, morbid obesity has a profound impact on normal adolescent development. In a recent study, Schwimmer and Varni demonstrated that the health-related quality of life experienced by obese children and adolescents was the same as that of children undergoing chemotherapy for cancer [30]. The challenge of adolescence is to make the transition to an emotionally and physically mature adult who is able to work and have meaningful relationships [31]. Obese children are more at risk for poor self-esteem, withdrawal from social interaction, depression, and anxiety [32]. The impact of peer teasing and changed body image can be profound in adolescents [33]. Among severely obese adolescents, 48% have moderate to severe depressive symptoms and 35% report a high level of anxiety. Extreme obesity is associated with an increased risk of suicide and suicidal ideation among adolescents [33,34]. This is particularly true for obese adolescent girls [35]. Obese adolescents are more likely to remain unmarried, have lower incomes, and live in poverty than their matched normal weight controls [17]. They are less likely to be accepted into college than normal weight adolescents with comparable scholastic achievement [36].

Treatment of morbid obesity in adolescence

Without question, obesity results from an imbalance in energy intake and expenditure. The ideal treatment for obesity involves decreasing caloric intake while increasing caloric expenditure through exercise or nonexercise thermogenesis. Successful weight loss and maintenance require great effort and commitment but are occasionally possible. In general, patients who are successful in keeping weight off long-term exercise consistently, eat breakfast regularly, control portions and fat in their diet, monitor their weight, and eat consistently during weekdays and weekends [37]. Although weight loss success is possible, most studies have shown that behavior modification and dieting are associated with poor weight loss, high attrition rates, and a high probability of weight regain [38]. For morbidly obese teenagers with comorbidities, failure in one of these programs leaves little chance to achieve and maintain a healthy weight into adulthood.

Behavioral and dietary measures have formed the cornerstone of treatment of obesity [39]. The abundance of diet books and programs available in our society reflects how ineffective most of these strategies are for adults, however. It is not surprising that 90% to 95% of adult patients who lose weight with dietary changes alone regain the weight. The lack of effective weight loss programs has intensified the ongoing search for effective and safe medications to aid in weight loss [39,40]. Currently, the only anorectic agent currently approved for use in obese adolescents (older than age 16) is sibutramine, a nonselective inhibitor of serotonin, norepinephrine, and dopamine. When combined with caloric restriction, exercise, and a comprehensive family-based behavioral program, sibutramine has been shown to be effective in the treatment of adolescent obesity. In a prospective, randomized trial of 60 adolescents, the group treated with sibutramine had an average weight loss of 10.3 kg compared with 2.4 kg in a placebo group [41]. Although previous trials had reported hypertension as a significant side effect, this was not a problem in this trial [41,42].

Orlistat also has been studied in the treatment of morbid obesity. Orlistat inhibits pancreatic lipase and increases fecal losses of triglyceride. In the United States, the Food and Drug Administration has approved orlistat in children older than age 12. In a 1-year, prospective, randomized trial of 539 adolescents, orlistat resulted in an improvement in weight control compared with a control group. BMI in patients on orlistat decreased by 0.55 compared with an increase of 0.31 in the control group, a statistically significant change but of no real clinical relevance [43]. Durable weight loss with orlistat requires maintenance of therapy; unfortunately, high study dropout rates occur because of unacceptable flatulence and diarrhea [44]. Metformin is a bisubstituted, short-chain hydrophilic guanidine derivative that activates AMP protein kinase and reduces fasting and postprandial insulin concentrations. It has been used primarily in obese adolescents who have polycystic ovarian syndrome to decrease weight and insulin resistance [45]. In preliminary studies, it also has improved obesity-related NASH [46]. Metformin is fairly well tolerated and is approved by the US Food and Drug Administration for the treatment of type 2 diabetes. It is not approved for the treatment of childhood obesity.

Bariatric surgery in adolescents

Resorting to surgery to change the metabolism of a growing child is a profound new concept, but adolescents with morbid obesity who have life-threatening comorbidities probably warrant such a radical therapy. Ethically, it is important that all adolescents first be treated with aggressive nonoperative approaches and, once surgery is considered, that the indications for surgery are considered carefully. The indications for bariatric surgery in adults were derived by an National Institutes of Health consensus panel in 1991 based on known risks factors of obesity and its associated comorbidities [47]. In general, adults with a BMI >40 with or without comorbidities and BMI >35 with comorbidities who have failed multiple attempts at medical management of their obesity are considered candidates for bariatric surgery. This panel specifically avoided making a recommendation for the treatment of patients younger than 18 years of age. Objective data to demonstrate the medical risk of being severely obese as an adolescent and carrying that obesity into adulthood would provide important insight required for developing objective criteria for this unique set of patients. In the absence of these data, the question remains: Will any adolescent patients benefit from bariatric surgery? A task force convened by the American Pediatric Surgical Association addressed this issue, taking into account the noncompliant nature of this population of patients, nutritional and developmental requirements, the ethical issue of assent versus consent in children younger than age 18, and the overall lack of medical data supporting the role for bariatric surgery in severely obese adolescents. The indications for surgery described by this task force are much more conservative than those for adults and include the necessity of studying these patients for long-term outcome [48].

Adolescents being considered for bariatric surgery require careful preoperative testing and preparation. Preoperative testing should focus on identifying comorbidities associated with severe obesity. Routine screening laboratories often performed on patients being evaluated for bariatric surgery include a complete blood count, liver profile, lipid profile, fasting insulin and glucose, oral glucose tolerance test at baseline, and vitamin B_1, B_{12}, and folate levels. All patients undergo a sleep study and ultrasound evaluation of the abdomen to look for steatohepatitis, gallstones, and, in girls, ovarian pathology. In addition to a structured clinical interview with an adolescent psychologist, objective tests are performed to assess personality traits, cognitive maturity, depression, eating behaviors, and weight-related quality of life, which may have a bearing on candidacy for bariatric surgery or postoperative adherence to medical and nutritional regimens. Screening evaluation of all patients by a pediatric dietitian and exercise physiologist who have experience with adolescent obesity has been helpful preoperatively and postoperatively. Participation in a monthly adolescent support group is also required as part of the preoperative preparation.

A multidisciplinary adolescent bariatric review board should deliberate indications and contraindications before scheduling an adolescent for bariatric surgery. Such a board should consist minimally of a medical director (pediatrician), surgical director (bariatric surgeon), pediatric psychologist, anesthesiologist, gynecologist, dietician, and ethicist. Such a board has been developed at Cincinnati Children's and Texas Children's Hospital. It has facilitated the development of the adolescent bariatric program throughout the hospital and community and been instrumental in resolving potential controversial patient selection and management decisions.

All patients are told that the long-term consequences of bariatric surgery in adolescents are not known and that a long-term study of outcomes is an integral part of this surgery. All patients who undergo surgery are asked to participate in a 10-year outcome study. Operative consent for surgery includes requiring all patients to write a letter describing their indications for having a bariatric procedure, the short- and long-term risks of having the procedure, dietary restrictions and expectations, need to adhere to medical and exercise regimen, their understanding of the procedure, and the lifelong commitment that comes with the decision. The patient and parents/guardians are required to sign the letter and a formal operative consent.

Gastric bypass is considered the gold standard obesity surgery and is the most commonly performed operation worldwide for obesity. Gastric bypass can be performed by laparotomy or laparoscopy. Recent data suggested that the laparoscopic technique may have some advantages over the open technique, but only surgeons with advanced training and expertise in laparoscopic and bariatric surgery should perform it [49,50]. Laparoscopic gastric bypass surgery results in consistent initial weight loss in >90% of patients. Expected weight loss after laparoscopic gastric bypass surgery is 20 to 30 pounds in the first month and approximately 10 pounds/mo until the weight loss plateaus after 12 to 18 months. Preliminary data from adolescents demonstrated a decrease of BMI from 59 kg/m^2 to 38 kg/m^2 by 1 year [51,52]. If a patient complies with the postoperative diet and exercise program, a weight loss of 80% of excess body weight can be expected at 1 year. Recidivism in the form of weight gain occurs in 20% to 30% of adults. Durable weight loss occurs in most adolescents, yet up to 15% of these patients may have late weight regain [53]. More important than the specific weight loss, laparoscopic gastric bypass surgery results in reversal of nearly all studied comorbidities, with marked improvement in patient health and long-term prognosis [53–55]. Treatment of morbid obesity with surgery results in improved educational and occupational status [56].

The ultimate success of all bariatric procedures depends on a patient's ability to adhere to a markedly changed and reduced diet. Given the propensity of adolescents to rebel against strict regimens, continued support must be available to all of these patients. Postoperative vitamin and mineral supplementation is critical and commonly consists of two pediatric chewable multivitamins, a calcium supplement (1500 mg calcium citrate/d), and supplementation of B-complex vitamins based on postoperative serum levels. All nonsteroidal anti-inflammatory medications should be avoided. Long-term nutritional complications can be avoided by the patient's adherence to the five basic rules: (1) Eat protein first. (2) Drink at least 64 ounces of liquids daily. (3) No snacking between meals. (4) Walk or exercise at least 30 minutes per day. (5) Always remember vitamins and minerals.

Early complications occur in 1% to 5% of patients who undergo a laparoscopic gastric bypass surgery and include death, acute gastric distention, pulmonary embolism (1%–2%), anastomotic leak (1%–2%), and wound infection (1%–5%) [57]. The mortality rate associated with gastric bypass is 0.5% to 1% in most reports. Population-based data from Washington suggest a mortality rate of up to 6% during a surgeon's first 20 bariatric procedures, decreasing to less than 0.4% beyond 100 procedures performed [58]. Acute gastric distention usually presents with hiccups, bloating, and left shoulder pain and is diagnosed by abdominal radiograph and ultrasound or CT scan demonstrating a dilated stomach. Differentiating this condition from a jejunojejunostomy anastomotic obstruction is important and often requires an experienced radiologist or bariatric surgeon to interpret the radiologic findings. Acute gastric distention may be treated by image-guided needle decompression, usually performed by an interventional radiologist. If distention recurs, an image-guided percutaneous gastrostomy tube can be placed. The diagnosis of an anastomotic leak in the early-postoperative period is difficult in obese patients who may not manifest peritoneal signs. To further complicate matters, an upper gastrointestinal series may not demonstrate the leak. The procedure of choice to evaluate a postoperative bariatric patient who has unexplained tachycardia, particularly in the presence of fever, shoulder, or pelvic pain, should be surgical re-exploration.

Late complications of laparoscopic gastric bypass surgery include anastomotic strictures, marginal ulcers, bowel obstructions from internal and incisional hernias, cholelithiasis, and dietary complications. Patients who have internal hernias often present with recurrent periumbilical abdominal pain or biliary colic in the absence of gallstones as their only symptom. Plain films and upper gastrointestinal scans are often normal, whereas a CT may demonstrate dilation of the biliary limb but also may be normal. The presence of persistent periumbilical pain, even in the face of normal imaging studies, mandates exploration [57]. Patients who have postprandial vomiting after bariatric surgery are at risk of developing dry beriberi, which most often presents with numbness in the extremities and ataxia. If left untreated, the patient may develop irreversible encephalopathy [59,60]. Previously, as many as 38% of adult obese patients who underwent bariatric surgery developed postoperative cholelithiasis. This number can be reduced substantially by prophylaxis with ursodeoxycholic acid therapy [61,62]. Although previously a concern, the weight loss associated with bariatric surgery does not affect the outcome of subsequent pregnancies, as long as the mother has achieved a stable weight. For that reason, pregnancy is contraindicated in the first 1 or 2 years after surgery [63].

Other surgical options exist for the treatment of morbid obesity in adults. One of the more popular approaches is the laparoscopic gastric band, which was approved in the United States for use in adults in 2001 but has been performed around the world since the early 1990s. The adjustable gastric band offers an enticing alternative to the gastric bypass because it is potentially reversible and carries a lower morbidity and mortality rate (0.1%) [64]. The adjustable gastric band or "lap band" is a prosthetic band with an adjustable inner diameter that is placed around the proximal stomach, which restricts food intake. An adjustable gastric band is connected to a subcutaneous port, which is accessed via a needle through which saline solution is injected to alter the inner diameter. The laparoscopic gastric band has been reported to be successful in European and Australian trials [65,66]. These trials have yet to be reproduced in the United States, most likely because of the difference in abilities to provide week-to-week postoperative adjustments and follow-up. Weight loss with an adjustable gastric band occurs more slowly than with other procedures, with maximal loss occurring 2 to 3 years postoperatively, compared with 12 to 18 months in gastric bypass. Complications of gastric banding include exacerbation of gastroesophageal reflux, esophageal dilation and dysmotility, and mechanical failure of port or device. Complications leading to reoperation have been reported in up to 41% of patients [67].

Summary

Morbid obesity in the United States has reached epidemic proportions. Families, physicians, and the government are finally hearing the message that obesity is an issue of health and not of appearance. Treating this epidemic requires a multidisciplinary approach and a commitment on the part of legislators, health care executives, and medical professionals. Prevention is critical, and all efforts should be made to support increasing safe physical activity for children and adolescents. Children and families also should be educated about appropriate food choices and portion sizes in schools and by their physicians. Decisions about foods in the schools and at home should be driven by education and not by advertising or other outside forces.

The treatment of morbid obesity in adolescence first and foremost should be based on aggressive behavioral and dietary modification. With only a small daily increase in caloric expenditure and a relatively small decrease in caloric intake, many adolescents can achieve and maintain weight loss. This goal requires constant encouragement and surveillance on the part of a "coach," whether that be family, a commercial weight loss program, or a physician. For adolescents with severe morbid obesity who have failed attempts at weight loss, the options are medical therapy or bariatric surgery. Medical therapy is occasionally effective in some patients and should be considered. Bariatric surgery is currently the most effective method of weight loss for morbid obesity. Current indications for bariatric surgery in adolescence are more conservative than for adults, because the long-term consequences of this surgery in growing children are not known. The unique psychological and physical issues of adolescence add another layer of complexity to the management of these patients. For that reason, morbidly obese teenagers are best treated in centers with special expertise in the care of adolescents. Because the long-term outcomes of bariatric surgery in adolescents are not known, it is ethically and clinically important that these patients be enrolled, whenever possible, in long-term prospective outcome studies.

References

[1] Freedman DS, Serdula MK, Dietz WH, et al. Inter-relationship among childhood BMI, childhood height, and adult obesity: the Bogalusa Heart Study. Int J Obes Relat Metab Disord 2004;28:10–6.

[2] Morrison JA, Barton BA, Waslawiw MA, et al. Overweight, fat patterning, and cardiovascular disease risk factors in black and white girls: the National Heart, Lung, and Blood Institute Growth and Health Study. J Pediatr 1999;135:458–64.

[3] Bouchard C. Genetic determinants of regional fat distribution. Hum Reprod 1997;12 (Suppl 1):1–5.

[4] O'Rahilly S, Yeo GS, Challis BG. Minireview: human obesity. Lessons from monogenic disorders. Endocrinology 2003;144:3757–64.

[5] Clement KFP. Genetics and the pathophysiology of obesity. Pediatr Res 2003;53:721–5.

[6] Grace C, Summerbell C, Jebb SA, et al. Energy metabolism in Bardet-Biedel syndrome. Int J Obes Relat Metab Disord 2003;27:1319–24.

[7] Vaisse C, Durand E, Hercberg S, et al. Melanocortin-4 receptor mutations are a frequent and heterogenous cause of morbid obesity. J Clin Invest 2000;106:253–62.

[8] Fontaine KR, Redden DT, Wang C, et al. Years of life lost due to obesity. JAMA 2003;289: 187–93.

[9] Finer N. Obesity. Clin Med 2003;3:23–7.

[10] Narayan KM, Boyle JP, Thompson TJ, et al. Lifetime risk for diabetes mellitus in the United States. JAMA 2003;290:1884–90.

[11] Genuth S, Bennett P, Buse J, et al. Follow-up report on the diagnosis of diabetes mellitus. Diabetes Care 2003;26:3160–7.

[12] Cook S, Auinger P, Nguyen M, et al. Prevalence of a metabolic syndrome phenotype in adolescents: findings from the third National Health and Nutrition Examination Survey, 1988–1994. Arch Pediatr Adolesc Med 2003;157:821–7.

[13] Weiss R, Burgert TS, Tamborlane WV, et al. Obesity and the metabolic syndrome in children and adolescents. N Engl J Med 2004;350:2362–74.

[14] Silfen ME, Denburg MR, Manibo AM, et al. Early endocrine, metabolic, and sonographic characteristics of polycystic ovary syndrome (PCOS): comparison between nonobese and obese adolescents. J Clin Endocrinol Metab 2003;88:4682–8.

[15] Freedman DS, Khan LK, Dietz WH, et al. Relationship of childhood obesity to coronary heart disease risk factors in adulthood: the Bogalusa Heart Study. Pediatrics 2001;108:712–8.

[16] Lurbe E, Redon J. Obesity, body fat distribution, and ambulatory blood pressure in children and adolescents. J Clin Hypertens (Greenwich) 2001;3:362–7.

[17] Must A. Risk and consequences of childhood and adolescent obesity. Int J Obes Relat Metab Disord 1999;23(Suppl 2):S2–11.

[18] Sorof J. Obesity hypertension in children: a problem of epidemic proportions. Hypertension 2002;40:441–7.

[19] Dietz W. Health consequences of obesity in youth: childhood predictors of adult disease. Pediatrics 1998;101:518–25.

[20] Young TPP, Gottlib DJ. Epidemiology of obstructive sleep apnea: a population health perspective. Am J Respir Crit Care Med 2002;165:1217–39.

[21] Styne D. Childhood and adolescent obesity: prevalence and predictors of adult disease. Pediatr Clin North Am 2001;48:823–54.

[22] Wing YK, Pak WM, Ho CK, et al. A controlled study of sleep related disordered breathing in obese children. Arch Dis Child 2003;88:1043–7.

[23] Karla M, Inge TH, Garcia VF, et al. Obstructive sleep apnea in morbidly obese adolescents: effect of bariatric surgical intervention. Obes Res 2005;13:175–9.

[24] Spector A, Scheid S, Hassink S, et al. Adenotonsillectomy in the morbidly obese child. Int J Pediatr Otorhinolaryngol 2003;67:359–64.

[25] Bray G. Risks of obesity. Endocrinol Metab Clin North Am 2003;32:787–804.

[25a] Xanthakos S, Miles L, Bucuvalas J, et al. Histologic spectrum of nonalcoholic fatty liver disease in morbidly obese adolescents. Clin Gastroenterol Hepatol 2006;4(2):226–32.

[26] Charlton M. Nonalcoholic fatty liver disease: a review of current understanding and future impact. Clin Gastroenterol Hepatol 2004;2(12):1048–58.

[27] Matteoni CA, Younossi ZM, Gramlich T, et al. Nonalcoholic fatty liver disease: a spectrum of clinical and pathological severity. Gastroenterology 1999;116(6):1413–9.

[28] Roberts E. Nonalcoholic steatohepatitis in children. Curr Gastroenterol Rep 2003;5:253–9.

[29] Yanovski J. Pediatric obesity. Rev Endocr Metab Disord 2001;2:371–83.

[30] Schwimmer JB, Varni W. Health-related quality of life of severely obese children and adolescents. JAMA 2003;239:1813–9.

[31] Culbertson JL, Newman JE, Willis DJ. Childhood and adolescent psychologic development. Pediatr Clin North Am 2003;50(4):741–64.

[32] Deckelbaum RJ. Childhood obesity: the health issue. Obes Res 2001;9(Suppl 4):239S–43S.

[33] Eisenberg ME, Neumark-Sztainer D, Story M. Associations of weight-based teasing and emotional well-being among adolescents. Arch Pediatr Adolesc Med 2003;157(8):733–8.

[34] Dong C, Li WD, Li D, et al. Extreme obesity is associated with attempted suicides: results from a family study. Int J Obes (Lond) 2006;30(2):388–90.

[35] Falkner NH, Story M, Jeffery RW, et al. Social, educational, and psychological correlates of weight status in adolescents. Obes Res 2001;9:32–42.

[36] Gortmaker SL, Perrin JM, Sobol AM, et al. Social and economic consequences of overweight in adolescence and young adulthood. N Engl J Med 1993;329:1008–12.

[37] Wing RR, Phelan S. Long-term weight loss maintenance. Am J Clin Nutr 2005;82(1 Suppl): 222S–5S.

[38] Tsai AG, Wadden TA. Systematic review: an evaluation of major commercial weight loss programs in the United States. Ann Intern Med 2005;142(1):56–66.

[39] Durant N, Cox J. Current treatment approaches to overweight in adolescents. Curr Opin Pediatr 2005;17(4):454–9.

[40] Ioannides-Demos LL, Proietto J, McNeil JJ. Pharmacotherapy for obesity. Drugs 2005; 65(10):1391–418.

[41] Godoy-Matos A, Carraro L, Vieira A, et al. Treatment of obese adolescents with sibutramine: a randomized, double-blind, controlled study. J Clin Endocrinol Metab 2005; 90(3):1460–5.

[42] Poston WS, Foreyt JP. Sibutramine and the management of obesity. Expert Opin Pharmacother 2004;5(3):633–42.

[43] Chanoine JP, Hampl S, Jensen C, et al. Effect of orlistat on weight and body composition in obese adolescents: a randomized controlled trial. JAMA 2005;293(23):2873–83.

[44] Ozkan B, Bereket A, Turan S, et al. Addition of orlistat to conventional treatment in adolescents with severe obesity. Eur J Pediatr 2004;163(12):738–41.

[45] Allen HF, Mazzoni C, Heptulla RA, et al. Randomized controlled trial evaluating response to metformin versus standard therapy in the treatment of adolescents with polycystic ovary syndrome. J Pediatr Endocrinol Metab 2005;18(8):761–8.

[46] Schwimmer JB, Middleton MS, Deutsch R, et al. A phase 2 clinical trial of metformin as a treatment for non-diabetic paediatric non-alcoholic steatohepatitis. Aliment Pharmacol Ther 2005;21(7):871–9.

[47] National Institutes for Health. Gastrointestinal surgery for severe obesity: Consensus Development Conference Panel. Ann Intern Med 1991;115:956–61.

[48] Inge TH, Krebs NF, Garcia VF, et al. Bariatric surgery for severely overweight adolescents: concerns and recommendations. Pediatrics 2004;114(1):217–23.

[49] Nguyen NT, Palmer LS, Wolfe BM. A comparison study of laparoscopic versus open gastric bypass for morbid obesity. J Am Coll Surg 2000;191:149–55.

[50] Schauer P, Hamad G, Gourash W. The learning curve for laparoscopic Roux-en-Y gastric bypass is 100 cases. Surg Endosc 2003;17:212–5.

[51] Inge TH, Garcia VK, Kirk S, et al. Body composition changes after gastric bypass in morbidly obese adolescents. Obes Res 2004;12:A53.

[52] Sugerman HJ, DeMaria EJ, Kellum JM, et al. Bariatric surgery for severely obese adolescents. J Gastrointest Surg 2003;7:102–8.

[53] Sugarman HJ, Sood RK, Engle K, et al. Long-term effects of gastric surgery for treating respiratory insufficiency of obesity. Am J Clin Nutr 1992;55:597S–601S.

[54] De Zwaan M, Mitchell JE, Howell LM, et al. Health-related quality of life in morbidly obese patients: effect of gastric bypass surgery. Obes Res 2002;12:773–80.

[55] Pories WJ, Morgan EJ, Sinha MK, et al. Surgical treatment of obesity and its effect on diabetes: 10-year follow-up. Am J Clin Nutr 1992;55:582S–5S.

[56] Kopec-Schrader EM, Ramsey-Stewart G, Beumont PJ. Psychosocial outcome and long-term weight loss after gastric restrictive surgery for morbid obesity. Obes Surg 1994;4: 336–9.

[57] Sugarman HJ. Gastric bypass surgery for severe obesity. Semin Laparosc Surg 2002;9(2): 79–85.

[58] Flum DR. Impact of gastric bypass operation on survival: a population-based analysis. J Am Coll Surg 2004;199:543–51.

[59] Gollobin C. Bariatric beriberi. Obes Surg 2002;12:309–11.

[60] Towbin A, Garcia VF, Roerig HR, et al. Beriberi after gastric bypass surgery in adolescents. J Pediatr 2004;45:263–7.

[61] Strauss RS, Brolin RE. Gastric bypass surgery in adolescents with morbid obesity. J Pediatr 2001;138:499–504.

[62] Fisher BL. Medical and surgical options in the treatment of severe obesity. Am J Surg 2002; 184:9S–16S.

[63] Sheiner E, Silverberg D, Menes TS, et al. Pregnancy after bariatric surgery is not associated with adverse perinatal outcome. Am J Obstet Gynecol 2004;190:1335–40.

[64] Fisher BL. Medical and surgical options in the treatment of morbid obesity. Am J Surg 2002; 184:9S–16S.

[65] O'Brien PE, Smith A, McMurrick PJ, et al. Prospective study of a laparoscopically placed, adjustable gastric band in the treatment of morbid obesity. Br J Surg 1999;86:113–8.

[66] Dolan K, Hopkins G, Fielding G. Laparoscopic gastric banding in morbidly obese adolescents. Obes Surg 2003;13:101–4.

[67] DeMaria E. Laparoscopic adjustable silicone gastric banding. Surg Clin North Am 2001;81: 1129–44.

ELSEVIER
SAUNDERS

SURGICAL
CLINICS OF
NORTH AMERICA

Surg Clin N Am 86 (2006) 455–467

Hepatobiliary Disorders

Max R. Langham, Jr, MD[a,b,c,*], Kristin L. Mekeel, MD[d]

[a]Division of Pediatric Surgery, University of Tennessee Health Science Center,
777 Washington Avenue, Suite P220, Memphis, TN 38105, USA
[b]Pediatric Surgery Residency Program, LeBonheur Children's Medical Center,
50 North Dunlap Street, Memphis, TN 38103, USA
[c]St. Jude Children's Research Hospital, 332 North Lauderdale Street, Memphis,
TN 38105, USA
[d]University of Florida College of Medicine, 1600 SW Archer Road, Gainesville,
FL 32608, USA

A variety of disorders involving the liver and biliary tract of infants and children may require surgical intervention. Clinical presentations of these children include jaundice, hepatic insufficiency, tumors, portal hypertension, and those effects caused by abdominal trauma. As in many areas of pediatric surgery, the age of the patient is relevant for formulating the differential diagnosis. Table 1 summarizes disorders and their associated clinical presentations that occur at different times during a child's growth and development. While not comprehensive, the table provides the surgeon a reasonable start on creating a differential diagnosis. The purpose of this chapter is to provide a focused review of updated information on three disorders commonly of interest to surgeons. These are biliary atresia, hepatoblastoma, and portal hypertension. Important new data have provided insight into the etiology of these disorders and resulted in changes in recommendations for their evaluation and surgical management.

Biliary atresia

In the past decade there has been considerable improvement in the scientific understanding of the disease process currently called biliary atresia. The clinical entity was recognized in the nineteenth century and Howard and

---

* Corresponding author. Division of Pediatric Surgery, University of Tennessee Health Science Center, 777 Washington Avenue, Suite P220, Memphis, TN 38105.
E-mail address: mlangham@utmem.edu (M.R. Langham,).

Table 1
Most common hepatobiliary diseases and injuries of childhood based on age and presentation

Age at presentation	Jaundice	Hepatic insufficiency	Portal hypertension	Tumors	Trauma
≤ 2 wk	Benign hyperbilirubinemia Congenital form of biliary atresia	Perinatal viral hepatitis Mitochondrial chain defects	Extremely rare	Hemangioma Hemangio-endothelioma	Birth trauma
2–8 wk	Biliary atresia Neonatal jaundice Alagille's syndrome Biliary hypoplasia Gallstones	Viral or bacterial infections	Extremely rare	Hepatoblastoma Mesenchymal hamartoma Hemangioma Hemangio-endothelioma	Child neglect or abuse
8 wk-1 y	Hemaglobinopathies Viral hepatitis	Viral hepatitis Biliary atresia	Biliary atresia	Hepatoblastoma Mesenchymal hamartoma Neuroblastoma	Child neglect or abuse
1–8 y	Viral hepatitis Stone disease Choledochal cysts	Viral hepatitis Biliary atresia	Biliary atresia Cavernous transformation of the portal vein Alpha 1-AT	Hepatoblastoma Hepatocellular carcinoma Metastatic disease	Child abuse Accidental trauma
8–18 y	Stone disease Viral hepatitis Drug overdose or toxicity	Viral disease Drug overdose or toxicity Autoimmune hepatitis Wilson's disease	Cystic fibrosis Congenital hepatic fibrosis Polycystic disease of liver	Adenomas Hepatocellular carcinoma Sarcomas Metastatic disease	Accidental trauma

Abbreviation: Alpha 1-AT, alpha 1-anti trypsin.

colleagues have outlined the historical aspects of the disorder [1]. Histologic examination of liver biopsies from affected children shows a mixed cellular inflammation composed of lymphocytes, macrophages, and eosinophils within expanded portal triads, along with proliferation of bile ductules and variable but progressive hepatic fibrosis [2]. Electron microscopy shows hepatocellular cholestasis, marked loss of bile canalicular microvilli, bile duct cell degeneration, and periductal inflammatory fibrosis [3]. There is a resultant and predictably progressive biliary cirrhosis that probably represents a common clinical phenotype caused by several pathogenic processes [4,5]. Two distinct forms of biliary atresia exist. One is a more common perinatal form that usually presents at several weeks of life. The other is a true congenital form associated with a variety of laterality abnormalities, including abdominal situs inversus, and absence or anomalies of the vena cava and portal vein. This form is also called embryonic or fetal biliary atresia. There are rare cases of a similar histologic pattern associated with choledochal cysts, which probably represent what was once termed "correctable biliary atresia" [6,7].

The natural history of the condition has been elegantly described by Potts [8]. Before Kasai's procedure was widely adopted, several series reported average survival of less than 2 years [9,10]. Death resulted from malnutrition, sepsis, or complications of portal hypertension. The inflammatory nature of the lesion has led to speculation about an infectious etiology. However, experts in this agree that it is unlikely that biliary atresia can be attributed to a specific infectious etiology. Building on observations by a number of investigators, Mack and Sokol have recently proposed a "unifying hypothesis" or mechanistic explanation for the common final clinical entity [11]. They postulate that an immune mediated attack on bile duct epithelium is fundamental to formation of the clinical phenotype of biliary atresia and that this may be triggered by a perinatal infection, a genetic mutation, or a combination of the two. This hypothesis is compatible with most clinical observations made to date and provides a framework within which specific nonsurgical therapy could be developed and tested. For now, the treatment options of proven benefit to babies with biliary atresia include the portoenterostomy, as described by Morio Kasai in 1959 [12], and liver transplantation, which was first successfully performed by Thomas Starzl [13].

Jaundice is the most common presenting symptom of biliary atresia. The most common cause of jaundice in newborns is benign hyperbilirubinemia occurring in the first days of life and associated with a limited ability to conjugate bilirubin via the glucuronyl transferase enzyme pathway. The importance of distinguishing this disorder from pathologic direct hyperbilirubinemia has been emphasized to generations of pediatricians. Early accurate diagnosis is critical in the management of babies with biliary atresia. The diagnosis is urgent because of the predictable and progressive destruction of the liver caused by the disease. While normal livers have an immense capability to regenerate, those damaged by biliary cirrhosis do not. Ohi has documented a decline in 10-year survival of patients with biliary atresia from 75%, if the operation is done before the 51st day of life, to 3%, if surgery is delayed more than 131 days. The drop appears linear between these time points [14]. Presumably, adequate drainage of bile limits the damage to the biliary epithelium caused by bile stasis. This decreases inflammation and thus slows the progressive hepatic fibrosis, bile duct proliferation, and obliteration of the major bile ducts, both intra- and extrahepatic, which is a hallmark of the disease. Unfortunately no group has documented any ability to sustain improvement in the timeliness of diagnosis.

The recommendations for evaluation of babies with direct hyperbilirubinemia remain unchanged. All jaundiced babies should have a direct bilirubin measured. An elevated level of conjugated (ie, direct) bilirubin should prompt a structured evaluation with the goal of rapidly making a definitive diagnosis [15]. While babies with biliary atresia frequently have stools with little pigment (ie, so-called "clay-colored stools"), stools are surprisingly variable and presence of some pigment in the stools should not delay a diagnostic workup, including an ultrasound examination and a hepatobiliary iminodiacetic acid (HIDA) scan. The ultrasound should focus on exclusion of choledochal cysts or intrahepatic biliary cysts, both of which may be present without jaundice. Biliary obstruction due to stones is rare but should be excluded. The absence of a gallbladder is suggestive of biliary atresia, while biliary hypoplasia should be suspected if the gallbladder and duct structures are visible but small. Biliary hypoplasia is especially likely in those infants with a heart murmur compatible with pulmonic stenosis, or in infants with other stigmata of Alagille's syndrome. HIDA scans in jaundiced babies with normal bile ducts frequently show absent flow of radionuclide into the intestine (ie, false positive), which may be less frequent if the baby is given phenobarbital before the study. If there is not unequivocal, rapid emptying of radionuclide into the bowel, imaging of the hepatobiliary system is mandatory. In the past, such imaging required an operative cholangiogram. The accuracy of magnetic resonance cholangiopancreatography has not been established, but holds promise as a less invasive alternative [16].

Liver biopsy is an integral part of the evaluation for biliary atresia. As noted above, the classic histologic findings include portal inflammation, with bile duct proliferation and architectural distortion [2]. The histopathology is somewhat variable, however, and caution should be exercised in interpreting a biopsy as definitively excluding biliary atresia [17]. The authors have had experience with several liver biopsies in the first months of life for infants whose histologic pattern was felt to exclude biliary atresia by pathologists with considerable experience and expertise in the disorder. These infants proved subsequently to have classic biliary atresia. These false negatives deprived the babies of the possible palliation afforded by a Kasai portoenterostomy and led to early liver transplantation. The authors therefore recommend a cholangiogram on any infant with direct hyperbilirubinemia who does not have a definitive diagnosis.

Kasai's portoenterostomy should be preceded by an attempt at operative cholangiography to confirm the diagnosis of "extrahepatic" biliary atresia, if a gallbladder exists. Findings of an obstructed gallbladder at surgery are very suggestive of biliary atresia. The cholangiogram should be done in a setting that permits proceeding to completion of the Kasai procedure under the same anesthetic. Technical considerations in performance of the cholangiogram were well described in the 1960s and 1970s and have changed little [18,19]. The authors perform this study with undiluted contrast (ie, iothalamate meglumine 60% or equivalent), slowly injected through a catheter placed in the fundus of the gallbladder, and secured with a purse string created with fine vascular suture. Imaging may be with fluoroscopy if the unit has a very high resolution. Small ducts are often better seen on plain radiographs although some digital radiograph systems also have inadequate resolution. The presence of bile ducts extending into the liver, even if very small, and the emptying of contrast into the duodenum are contraindications to portoenterostomy. The bypass has no utility in Alagille's syndrome or other forms of neonatal cholestasis.

After confirming the diagnosis, the surgeon's job is to obtain bile drainage from ductules present in the scar tissue within the portal triad. If the gallbladder and common bile duct are normal (true in fewer than 10% of cases), and the cystic artery is preserved, one may consider using the gallbladder as a conduit. In most cases, however, a Roux-en-Y intestinal bypass will be used and the operation begins with a cholecystectomy, followed by division of the scarred common-duct remnant. All scar tissue anterior to the portal vein is dissected from the vein and the hepatic artery and its branches to a point cephalad to the bifurcation of the portal vein. Different authors express different opinions about whether dissection should proceed into the liver substance [20,21]. The authors, in their personal practice, often proceed further out the left and right portal bundles, excising a small part of segment four to improve exposure for the portoenterostomy. This technique appears to improve the volume and quality of bile drainage visible during the procedure, and has not been associated with increased short-term problems. No clear long-term outcomes data has been published comparing the results of these technical nuances. A Kasai portoenterostomy done well in a young baby results in relief of jaundice in about one third of patients, significant improvement in about one third, and persistence of jaundice for the remaining one third [22,23].

Treatment after a Kasai portoenterostomy includes antibiotic prophylaxis against cholangitis [24]. The most common regimen is trimethoprim and sulfamethoxazole given daily for the first 6 months, 1 ml per day by mouth for infants under 1 year of age. All children should also receive fat-soluble vitamins (ie, A, D, E, and K), and careful follow-up of nutritional status, growth, and development. Perioperative steroids and choleretic drugs [25,26] are used by many surgeons, although the efficacy of these treatments has not been rigorously tested. Studies of Pediatric Liver

Transplant has clearly shown that mortality after Kasai portoenterostomy, but before liver transplantation, is significantly related to age, growth failure, serum albumin, total bilirubin levels, and prolongation of the international normalized ratio (INR) [27]. Thus, any baby after a Kasai who does not grow normally or who has hypoalbuminemia, a persistent elevation of the serum bilirubin, or a prolonged INR requiring supplemental vitamin K should be promptly referred for transplant evaluation.

Hepatoblastoma

Children with a mass in the liver are frequently asymptomatic or have only vague discomfort. As a result, the tumors are often enormous by the time of diagnosis. Vascular malformations or large hemangiomas may present with failure to thrive or congestive heart failure. In our experience, 65% of liver masses in children are malignant with hepatoblastoma (28.3%), hepatocellular carcinoma (23.3%), and sarcomas (13.3%) [28] representing the three distinct histologic types. However, if masses are found in the first year of life, they are slightly more likely to be benign. Other benign lesions seen in children include hemangioendotheliomas, mesenchymal hamartomas, inflammatory pseudotumors, and adenomas. Except for hepatoblastoma, surgical resection represents the only successful therapy in all of these lesions. Hepatoblastoma is the only primary hepatic malignancy in which chemotherapy has proven to be beneficial.

The incidence of hepatoblastoma appears to be increasing in the United States [29,30]. Hepatoblastoma is more common in premature infants than in full-term babies [31–33]. The malignancy is also more common in babies born to mothers who smoke than in babies born to nonsmokers [34]. These two risk factors may be related [35]. Hepatoblastoma is also more frequent in patients with anomalies in the familial adenomatosis polyposis gene [36]. Genetic analysis has documented gains on several chromosomes (1Q and 2Q are the most common). These chromosomal abnormalities may be related to prognosis and have importance for design of therapy [37].

Prognosis for children with hepatoblastoma is clearly related to pretreatment extent of disease, both local and metastatic [38]. Children with hepatoblastoma and an alpha fetoprotein of less than 100 tend to do worse than those who have higher levels, while those with pure fetal histology do better. Micro- or macroscopic invasion of blood vessels also indicates a poor prognosis [39].

Before any attempt at biopsy is performed, one must determine the extent of disease in the initial evaluation of a child with hepatoblastoma. Careful radiographic imaging is critical and both an MRI and a CT scan are recommended [40,41]. Angiography is rarely needed in children with liver masses. Our preferred study is a triple-phase CT of the abdomen with 2 mm slices through the liver and a CT scan of the chest. Three-dimensional reconstructions of the liver, and for very large resections, estimation of the residual volumes based on the reconstructions, are occasionally helpful. General anesthesia may be needed to obtain optimal imaging. Imaging should be adequate to determine the PRETEXT stage of the tumor. The importance of obtaining the best possible anatomic understanding of the tumor and its relationship to the segmental anatomy of the liver cannot be overstated. The surgeon should be directly involved in the radiographic workup to the extent necessary to obtain this level of understanding, which is vital for subsequent treatment planning. The accuracy of radiographic studies in determining resectability is unknown with one report citing a 20% error rate [41]. Scanners have improved so that errors should be less common but studies are frequently inadequate because of motion artifact, problems with timing of the contrast bolus, or slices that are too thick. Ultrasound is often helpful in determining specific relations of the tumor to hepatic veins and portal triad. If resectability is questionable, a repeat study should be done at an institution with special expertise in pediatric hepatobiliary problems.

The role of biopsy is somewhat controversial. Primary excision of the tumor provides optimal pathologic staging, but complications in adult patients and, by extension, probably in children are directly related to the extent of the resection [42]. Surgeons trained in the United States are in general agreement that a PRETEXT 1 lesion may be excised primarily. Biopsy should be performed for PRETEXT 2 or higher lesions when the results would alter disease management. The surgeon's goal should be to differentiate hepatoblastoma from a benign tumor, sarcoma, or hepatocellular carcinoma. A very high alpha fetoprotein (ie, > 10,000) in a child over a year of age with a typical lesion on CT scan may be adequate to make the diagnosis of hepatoblastoma without a biopsy, but a low alpha fetoprotein does not exclude hepatoblastoma, and treatment for other histologic subtypes of liver tumors vary from observation in some small, benign lesions to complete resection for hepatocellular carcinomas and sarcomas when feasible. Hepatoblastoma is chemosensitive and current data support the use of neoadjuvant chemotherapy for lesions that involve more than one sector of the liver, or have vascular involvement or metastatic disease [43]. In these situations, biopsy with pre-resection chemotherapy has resulted in excellent outcomes [44]. The authors recommend that all liver biopsies be planned in consultation with the surgeon responsible for the subsequent liver resection. Needle biopsy of hepatic lesions through an uninvolved portion of the liver, which for anatomic reasons will subsequently be included in the resection, diminishes the chance of tumor spillage and upstaging a malignant lesion. Transvenous biopsy should be avoided because of the possibility of vascular spread.

Effective chemotherapy currently available includes cisplatin, vincristine, and 5-flurouracil, or so-called "PLADO" chemotherapy with cisplatin and doxorubicin, although chemotherapy is probably not necessary for a stage 1 patient with pure fetal histology [45]. Four to six courses of effective chemotherapy are recommended for all other children with hepatoblastoma.

Current consensus recommendations are for surgical resection or transplantation after four cycles of chemotherapy with two cycles of postresection therapy for PRETEXT 2 or higher lesions.

Except in rare instances of very small lesions, liver resections should be done along intersectoral and segmental planes. This method should decrease both complications and the risk of a positive margin. Technical aspects of liver resection have been addressed elsewhere [46]. Close margins do not significantly increase mortality or tumor recurrence, but gross positive residual disease (ie, stage 3) does make treatment failures more likely. The surgeon's goal must be a complete resection [47].

In those patients with unresectable primary disease, total hepatectomy with liver transplantation has been performed with excellent short- and long-term outcomes [48]. While no direct comparisons with randomized data are available, the survival rates are twice as good as those published for children with incomplete resections. The role of extended hepatectomy, with or without reconstruction of the vena cava [49], hepatic veins [50], or portal vein, has not been defined in patients with hepatoblastoma. In select patients with multifocal disease, primary transplantation has achieved better disease-free survival than has conventional therapy [48].

Portal hypertension

The diagnosis and treatment of portal hypertension has changed dramatically in the past 10 to 15 years. More aggressive endoscopic therapy has allowed better planning for surgery and fewer emergent operations are needed. Long-term consequences of portosystemic shunts and improvement in the results of liver transplantation have also affected the choice of therapy. For children, portal hypertension is defined as a pressure over 11 mmHg in the portal vein or over 16 mmHg in the parenchyma of the spleen [51]. Esophageal varices as a consequence of portal hypertension remain the most common cause of spontaneous, massive gastrointestinal bleeding in children.

The most common etiology of portal hypertension in children is cirrhotic liver disease from biliary atresia or cystic fibrosis [52,53]. There are a variety of less common causes, which are summarized in Table 2 [54]. Children with these disorders should be monitored for development of portal hypertension by carefully following the abdominal exam for evidence of splenomegaly and serial determination of platelet counts looking for thrombocytopenia. Either of these findings should prompt referral for esophagoscopy. Other common manifestations of portal hypertension include the presence of hemorrhoids or rectal bleeding [55].

Treatment of portal hypertension in children, as in adults, should aim to reduce the portal pressure to normal while preserving normal hepatic blood flow and synthetic function with few long-term side effects. In many instances, current therapy falls far short of this ideal. Therapy may be focused on symptoms and palliation (eg, sclerotherapy or banding), or

Table 2
Causes of portal hypertension in children

Types of portal hypertension		Causes
"Cirrhotic"[a]		Cystic fibrosis
		Biliary atresia
		Alpha 1 antitrypsin deficiency
		Autoimmune hepatitis
		Hepatitis B
		Hepatitis C
Non cirrhotic	Prehepatic	Cavernous transformation of the portal vein
		Portal vein sclerosis
		Portal vein thrombosis
		Extrahepatic fistula between hepatic artery and portal vein
	Intrahepatic	Congenital hepatic fibrosis
		Nodular regenerative hyperplasia
		Veno-occlusive disease
		Intrahepatic arteriovenous fistula
	Suprahepatic	Budd-Chiari syndrome

[a] Disorders frequently present a picture of mixed portal hypertension and hepatic insufficiency. Best treated by liver transplantation.

may divert hepatic blood flow (eg, transjugular intrahepatic portosystemic shunt and most operative shunts), or result in long-term health issues and cost (eg, liver transplantation).

The authors have found few studies that address directly the central question of which patients benefit most from specific types of treatment. The answer to this vexing question would be a boon to these children and the surgeons and physicians caring for them. In the absence of such data, the authors believe that two factors are most likely to be the critical variables. These are the etiology of the portal hypertension and the degree of hepatic parenchymal disease. For children with biliary atresia after portoenterostomy, portal hypertension does not appear to be as important as cholestasis in predicting the outcome. In this population, treatment with sclerotherapy in patients with normal bilirubin levels can result in long-term survival [56], although caution must be exercised because of the demonstrated importance of other factors, such as age, growth, serum albumin, and international normalized ratio [27]. Data from a randomized study suggest that sclerotherapy decreases the number of bleeding episodes and the volume of blood lost but does not affect survival rate and may increase the incidence of portal hypertensive gastropathy [57]. Although portal hypertension alone is rarely an indication for transplantation in patients with biliary atresia, the authors believe that children with marginally compensated liver failure and symptomatic portal hypertension are best treated via liver transplantation.

The role of surgical shunting in this population and in children with cystic fibrosis as the etiology of their portal hypertension is a controversial subject. Portosystemic shunts are effective at stopping bleeding and can be done in children with little mortality [58]. In the short run, bleeding is relieved and many aspects of the child's overall health appear improved [59]. However, few long-term data are available. Complication rates for encephalopathy are not clearly delineated and other complications, such as portopulmonary hypertension, are underreported. This particular problem occurs in patients with long-standing portal hypertension or those who have had a surgical portosystemic shunt. Condino and colleagues found that symptoms occurred an average of 14 years after initial diagnosis [60]. The resulting hypoxemia can be devastating and is correctable by liver transplantation in some individuals.

An exciting new development in the treatment of portal hypertension has been the description of the Rex shunt. Originally devised as a technique for salvage treatment for portal vein thrombosis after liver transplant [61], the Rex shunt is now used in treating children with cavernous transformation of the portal vein [62]. In selected patients with a patent left portal vein, the shunt seems to be an ideal solution to this problem because it simultaneously relieves the portal hypertension and restores portal blood flow to an otherwise normal liver. While experience with the procedure is anecdotal in most instances, a few centers have reported a modest experience with excellent short-term outcomes [63]. Placing a Rex shunt is a technically demanding procedure, and should be done by those surgeons with expertise in both pediatric liver transplantation and hepatic resection.

Budd-Chiari syndrome is uncommon in children in the United States with the largest series reported from China [64]. The severity of the syndrome is variable but in the most severe cases, mortality is still high. Those children with a caval membrane may be cured by resection [65], but liver transplantation is the most commonly successful treatment for severely affected individuals [66]. Data are scarce in children but the careful reader is left with the impression that shunts rarely provide significant long-term palliation for children and are associated with a higher mortality than liver transplantation.

Summary

The treatment of hepatobiliary disorders in children is an evolving field with recent improvements that have dramatically affected children who previously had little hope of long-term survival. However, a large number of unsolved issues remain. They include the following:

1. The costs, availability, complications and long-term health effects of liver transplantation
2. The absence of alternative therapy for most children with biliary atresia
3. The absence of effective chemotherapy for children with hepatocellular carcinoma and hepatic sarcomas

4. Current limitations on the treatment of portal hypertension in children with both cirrhotic and posthepatic portal hypertension

References

[1] Howard ER. Biliary atresia: etiology, management and complications. In: Howard ER, Stringer MD, Colombani PM, editors. Surgery of the liver, bile ducts and pancreas in children. 2nd edition. London: Arnold; 2002. p. 103–4.

[2] Bill AH, Haas JE, Foster GL. Biliary atresia: histopathologic observations and reflections upon its natural history. J Pediatr Surg 1977;12:977–82.

[3] Park WH, Kim SP, Park KK, et al. Electron microscopic study of the liver with biliary atresia and neonatal hepatitis. J Pediatr Surg 1996;31(3):367–74.

[4] Sokol RJ, Mack C, Narkewicz MR, et al. Pathogenesis and outcome of biliary atresia: current concepts. J Pediatr Gastroenterol Nutr 2003;37:4–21.

[5] Perlmutter DH, Shepherd RW. Extrahepatic biliary atresia: a disease or a phenotype? Hepatology 2002;35(6):1297–304.

[6] Holmes JB. Congenital obliteration of the bile duct: diagnosis and suggestions for treatment. Am J Dis Child 1916;11:405–31.

[7] Ladd WE, Gross RE. Abdominal surgery of infancy and childhood. Philadelphia: WB Saunders; 1941.

[8] Potts WJ. The surgeon and the child. Philadelphia: WB Saunders; 1959.

[9] Hays DM, Snyder WH. Life-span in untreated biliary atresia. Surgery 1963;64:373–5.

[10] Bill AH. Biliary atresia—introduction. World J Surg 1978;2(5):557–9.

[11] Mack CL, Sokol RJ. Unraveling the pathogenesis and etiology of biliary atresia. Pediatr Res 2005;57(5 Pt 2):87R–94R.

[12] Kasai M, Suzuki S. A new operation for 'non-correctable' biliary atresia: hepatic portoenterostomy. Shujitsu 1959;13:733–9.

[13] Starzl TE, Groth CG, Brettschneider L, et al. Extended survival in 3 cases of orthotopic homotransplantations of the human liver. Surgery 1968;278(12):642–8.

[14] Ohi R. Biliary atresia: long-term outcomes. In: Howard RJ, Stringer MD, Colombani PM, editors. Surgery of the liver, bile ducts and pancreas in children. 2nd edition. London: Arnold; 2002. p. 133–47.

[15] Rosenthal P, Sinatra F. Jaundice in infancy. Pediatr Rev 1989;11(3):79–86.

[16] Miyazaki T, Yamashita Y, Tang Y, et al. Single-shot MR cholangiopancreatography of neonates, infants, and young children. AJR Am J Roentgenol 1998;170(1):33–7.

[17] Li MK, Crawford JM. The pathology of cholestasis. Semin Liver Dis 2004;24(1):21–42.

[18] Mason GR, Northway W, Cohn RB. Difficulties in the operative diagnosis of congenital atresia of the biliary ductal system. Am J Surg 1966;112:183–7.

[19] Lilly JR, Altman RP. The biliary tree. In: Ravitch MM, Welch KJ, Benson CD, editors. Pediatric surgery. 3rd edition. Chicago: Year Book Publishers; 1979. p. 827–38.

[20] Kimura K, Tsugawa C, Kubo M, et al. Technical aspects of hepatic portal dissection in biliary atresia. J Pediatr Surg 1979;14:27–32.

[21] Schweizer P, Kirschner H, Schittenhelm C. Anatomy of the porta hepatis as a basis for extended hepatoporto-enterostomy for extrahepatic biliary atresia—a new surgical technique. Eur J Pediatr Surg 2001;11(1):15–8.

[22] Howard ER, MacLean G, Nio M, et al. Survival patterns in biliary atresia and comparison of quality of life in long-term survivors in Japan and England. J Pediatr Surg 2001;36(6):892–7.

[23] Karrer FM, Lilly JR, Stewart BA, et al. Biliary atresia resgistry, 1976 to 1989. J Pediatr Surg 1990;25(10):1076–80.

[24] Bu LN, Chen HL, Chang CJ, et al. Prophylactic oral antibiotics in prevention of recurrent cholangitis after the Kasai portoenterostomy. J Pediatr Surg 2003;38(4):590–3.

[25] Muraji T, Nio M, Ohhama Y, et al. Postoperative corticosteroid therapy for bile drainage in biliary atresia—a nationwide survey. J Pediatr Surg 2004;39(12):1803–5.

[26] Meyers RL, Book LS, O'Gorman MA, et al. High-dose steroids, ursodeoxycholic acid, and chronic intravenous antibiotics improve bile flow after Kasai procedure in infants with biliary atresia. J Pediatr Surg 2003;38(3):406–11.
[27] Utterson EC, Shepherd RW, Sokol RJ, et al. Biliary atresia: clinical profiles, risk factors and outcomes of 755 patients listed for liver transplantation. J Pediatr 2005;147(2):142–3.
[28] Josephs MD, Langham MR Jr, Lauwers G, et al. Evidence based strategy for improving outcome of children with liver tumors. Presented at the International Society of Pediatric Surgical Oncology, Lake Buena Vista, Florida, May 2000.
[29] Ross JA, Gurney JG. Hepatoblastoma incidence in the United States from 1973 to 1992. Med Pediatr Oncol 1998;30(3):141–2.
[30] Darbari A, Sabin KM, Shapiro CN, et al. Epidemiology of primary hepatic malignancies in US children. Hepatology 2003;38(3):560–6.
[31] Tanimura M, Matsui I, Abe J, et al. Increased risk of hepatoblastoma among immature children with a lower birth weight. Cancer Res 1998;58(14):3032–5.
[32] Spector LG, Feusner JH, Ross JA. Hepatoblastoma and low birth weight. Pediatr Blood Cancer 2004;43(6):706.
[33] Reynolds P, Urayama KY, Von Behren J, et al. Birth characteristics and hepatoblastoma risk in young children. Cancer 2004;100(5):1070–6.
[34] Pang D, McNally R, Birch JM. Parental smoking and childhood cancer: results from the United Kingdom Childhood Cancer Study. Br J Cancer 2003;88(3):373–81.
[35] Spector LG, Ross JA. Smoking and hepatoblastoma: confounding by birth weight? Br J Cancer 2003;89(3):602.
[36] Kingston JE, Herbert A, Draper GJ, et al. Association between hepatoblastoma and polyposis coli. Arch Dis Child 1983;58(12):959–62.
[37] Weber RG, Pietsch T, von Schweinitz D, et al. Characterization of genomic alterations in hepatoblastoma. A role for gains on chromosomes 8q and 20 as predictors of poor outcome. Am J Pathol 2000;157(2):571–8.
[38] Brown J, Perilongo G, Shafford E, et al. Pretreatment prognostic factors for children with hepatoblastoma—results from the International Society of Paediatric Oncology (SIOP study SIOPEL 1). Eur J Cancer 2000;36(11):1418–25.
[39] Gregory JJ, Finlay JL. Alpha-fetoprotein and beta-human chorionic gonadotropin: their clinical significance as tumor markers. Drugs 1999;57(4):463–7.
[40] Rummeny E, Weissleder R, Stark DD, et al. Primary liver tumors: diagnosis by MR imaging. AJR Am J Roentgenol 1989;152(1):63–72.
[41] King SJ, Babyn PS, Greenberg ML, et al. Value of CT in determining the respectability of hepatoblastoma before and after chemotherapy. AJR Am J Roentgenol 1993;160(4): 793–8.
[42] Wei AC, Tung-Ping Poon R, Fan ST, et al. Risk factors for perioperative morbidity and mortality after extended hepatectomy for hepatocellular carcinoma. Br J Surg 2003;90(1): 33–41.
[43] Von Schweinitz D, Burger D, Mildenberger H. Is laparotomy the first step in treatment of childhood liver tumors? The experience from the German Cooperative Pediatric Liver Tumor Study HB-89. Eur J Pediatr Surg 1994;4(2):82–6.
[44] Schnater JM, Aronson DC, Plaschkes J, et al. Surgical view of the treatment of patients with hepatoblastoma: results from the first prospective trial of the International Society of Pediatric Oncology Liver Tumor Study Group. Cancer 2002;94(4):1111–20.
[45] Ortega JA, Douglass EC, Feusner JH, et al. Randomized comparison of cisplatin/vincristine/flurouracil and cisplatin/continuous-infusion doxorubicin for treatment of pediatric hepatoblastoma: a report from the Children's Cancer Group and the Pediatric Oncology Group. J Clin Oncol 2000;18:2665–75.
[46] Langham MR Jr, Hemming AW. Surgical liver disease. In: Oldham KT, Colombani PM, Foglia RP, et al, editors. Principles and practice of pediatric surgery. Philadelphia: Lippincott Williams & Wilkins; 2005. p. 1459–73.

[47] Dicken BJ, Bigam DL, Lees GM. Association between surgical margins and long-term outcome in advanced hepatoblastoma. J Pediatr Surg 2004;39(5):721–5.

[48] Otte JB, Pritchard J, Aronson DC, et al. Liver transplantation for hepatoblastoma: results of the International Society of Pediatric Oncology (SIOP) Study SIOPEL-1 and review of the world experience. Pediatr Blood Cancer 2004;42(1):74–83.

[49] Hemming AW, Langham MR, Reed AI, et al. Resection of the inferior vena cava for hepatic malignancy. Am Surg 2001;67(11):1081–8.

[50] Hemming AW, Reed AI, Langham MR, et al. Hepatic vein reconstruction for resection of hepatic tumors. Ann Surg 2002;235(6):850–8.

[51] Whitington PF. Portal hypertension in children. Pediatr Ann 1985;14(7):494–5, 498–9.

[52] Efrati O, Barak A, Modan-Moses D, et al. Liver cirrhosis and portal hypertension in cystic fibrosis. Eur J Gastroenterol Hepatol 2003;15(10):1073–8.

[53] Colombo C, Battezzati PM, Crosignani A, et al. Liver disease in cystic fibrosis: a prospective study on incidence, risk factors, and outcome. Hepatology 2002;36(6):1374–82.

[54] Howard ER. Etiology of portal hypertension and congenital anomalies of the portal venous system. In: Howard ER, Stringer MD, Colombani PM, editors. Surgery of the liver, bile ducts and pancreas in children. 2nd edition. London: Arnold; 2002. p. 287–95.

[55] Heaton ND, Davenport M, Howard ER. Incidence of haemorrhoids and anorectal varices in children with portal hypertension. Br J Surg 1993;80(5):616–8.

[56] Miga D, Sokol RJ, Mackenzie T, et al. Survival after first esophageal variceal hemorrhage in patients with biliary atresia. J Pediatr 2001;139(2):291–6.

[57] Goncalves ME, Cardoso SR, Maksoud JG. Prophylactic sclerotherapy in children with esophageal varices: long-term results of a controlled prospective randomized trial. J Pediatr Surg 2000;35(3):401–5.

[58] Botha JF, Campos BD, Grant WJ, et al. Portosystemic shunts in children: a 15-year experience. J Am Coll Surg 2004;199(2):179–85.

[59] Kato T, Romero R, Koutouby R, et al. Portosystemic shunting in children during the era of endoscopic therapy: improved postoperative growth parameters. J Pediatr Gastroenterol Nutr 2000;30(4):419–25.

[60] Condino AA, Ivy DD, O'Connor JA, et al. Portopulmonary hypertension in pediatric patients. J Pediatr 2005;147(1):20–6.

[61] De Ville de Goyet J, Gibbs P, Clapuyt P, et al. Original extrahilar approach for hepatic portal revascularization and relief of extrahepatic portal hypertension related to later portal vein thrombosis after pediatric liver transplantation. Long term results. Transplantation 1996. 15;62(1)71–5.

[62] Stenger AM, Malago M, Nolkemper D, et al. Mesentericoportal Rex-shunt as a treatment for extrahepatic portal vein thrombosis. Chirurg 1999;70(4):476–9.

[63] Bambini DA, Superina R, Almond PS, et al. Experience with the Rex shunt (mesenterico-left portal bypass) in children with extrahepatic portal hypertension. J Pediatr Surg 2000;35(1): 13–8.

[64] Wang ZG, Zhang FJ, Yi MQ, et al. Evolution and management for Budd-Chiari syndrome: a team's view from 2564 patients. ANZ J Surg 2005;75(1–2):55–63.

[65] Odell JA, Rode H, Millar AJ, et al. Surgical repair in children with the Budd-Chiari syndrome. J Thorac Cardiovasc Surg 1995;110(4 pt 1):916–23.

[66] Ringe B, Lang H, Oldhafer KJ, et al. Which is the best surgery for Budd-Chiari syndrome: venous decompression or liver transplantation? A single-center experience with 50 patients. Hepatology 1995;21(5):1337–44.

SURGICAL
CLINICS OF
NORTH AMERICA

ELSEVIER
SAUNDERS

Surg Clin N Am 86 (2006) 469–487

Pediatric Solid Malignancies: Neuroblastoma and Wilms' Tumor

Sunghoon Kim, MD[a], Dai H. Chung, MD[b],*

[a]Children's Hospital and Research Center Oakland, 747 Fifty-Second Street,
Oakland, CA 94609, USA
[b]The University of Texas Medical Branch, 301 University Blvd.,
Galveston, TX 77555, USA

Neuroblastoma is the most common extracranial solid tumor in infants and children, accounting for 6% to 10% of all childhood cancers and 15% of all pediatric cancer deaths in the United States. The overall incidence is estimated at about 1 case per 10,000 live births, representing just over 500 new cases in the United States annually [1]. The incidence is highest in the first year of life during which approximately 30% of all cases occur; nearly half of newly diagnosed neuroblastomas are encountered between ages 1 and 4 years. Despite extensive ongoing clinical and basic science research, neuroblastoma remains an enigmatic tumor with unknown etiology and unpredictable clinical course.

Pathology

Neuroblastomas arise from primordial neural crest cells, which migrate during embryogenesis to form the adrenal medulla and sympathetic ganglia. As a result, neuroblastomas occur in the adrenal medulla or anywhere along the sympathetic ganglia, most notably in the retroperitoneum and posterior mediastinum. The broad nomenclature of neuroblastomas is based on a spectrum of cellular differentiation. Neuroblastoma typically represents poorly differentiated tumor, whereas ganglioneuroma is its well-differentiated, benign counterpart [2]. Ganglioneuroblastoma represents both, having features of immature, poorly differentiated neuroblasts and matured ganglion cells [3].

* Corresponding author.
  E-mail address: dhchung@utmb.edu (D.H. Chung).

0039-6109/06/$ - see front matter © 2006 Elsevier Inc. All rights reserved.
doi:10.1016/j.suc.2005.12.008   *surgical.theclinics.com*

Histology

Neuroblastomas are made up of immature neuroblasts of small, uniform cells with dense, hyperchromatic nuclei and scant cytoplasm. Differentiated cells have a more mature ganglion cell appearance with well-defined nucleoli and eosinophilic cytoplasm. Abundance of neuropil is also a distinctive feature of differentiated tumors. Shimada classification has been widely used to characterize and predict tumor behavior, taking into consideration patient age along with histologic features such as degree of schwannian stroma, cellular differentiation, and the mitosis-karyorrhexis index [4,5]. The Shimada classification, modified in 1999 as the International Neuroblastoma Pathology Classification [6], strongly predicts the biologic behavior and prognosis of tumors. Nonmorphologic favorable prognostic indicators are age less than 1 year, clinical stages 1, 2, and 4S, and N-*myc* nonamplification. Other favorable prognostic factors identified are differentiation, low mitosis-karyorrhexis index (defined as fewer than 100 mitotic or karyorrhectic cells per 5000 cells), and stroma-rich tumors.

Cytogenetics

Several cytogenetic abnormalities have been identified in neuroblastoma. In particular, a loss of heterzygosity (LOH) on chromosome 1 (deletion of 1p36 region) occurs in greater than 70% of tumors [7,8]. This defect strongly correlates with N-*myc* amplification and unfavorable prognosis [9]. Deletions of chromosome 11q and 14q are also commonly found in neuroblastoma [10]. A recent report showed that 1p36 LOH and unbalanced 11q LOH are strongly associated with worse outcome in patients who have neuroblastoma, suggesting the addition of these cytogenetic markers to currently used prognostic variables [11]. Others have found allelic gain on chromosomes 17q to be of clinical significance [12]. Although these common chromosomal features of neuroblastoma suggest presence of a tumor suppressor gene (or genes) in these regions, none has been found to date. Moreover, DNA index of neuroblastomas correlates with their chemosensitivity and overall prognosis. The presence of hyperdiploid DNA content is associated with early tumor stage and improved prognosis [13]. Tumors with diploid DNA content are found in approximately two thirds of advanced-stage neuroblastomas and are often resistant to chemotherapeutic options.

Tumor biomarkers

Neuroblastomas are characterized by numerous biochemical and molecular markers. The clinical significance of these biomarkers remains the major focus of research to predict tumor behavior and overall patient outcome and as potential targets for novel therapeutic options. Traditional biochemical markers of importance include neuron-specific enolase (NSE), ferritin, and lactate dehydrogenase. N-*myc* protooncogene, multidrug resistance–

associated protein (MRP), CD44, nerve growth factor (NGF), and its associated high-affinity receptor, Trk tyrosine kinase receptor, are several of the crucial molecular markers in neuroblastomas.

Serum markers

Although an elevated serum NSE level is not specific to neuroblastomas, patients who have high levels of NSE (> 100 ng/mL) tend to have advanced-stage neuroblastomas and poor survival rates [14]. Many patients who have neuroblastoma have increased levels of ferritin, the major tissue iron-binding protein. The ferritin levels appear to correlate with the stage of disease. High ferritin level (> 142 ng/mL) is frequently seen in patients who have advanced-stage disease and correlates with worse overall outcome [15]. Serum lactate dehydrogenase level is a nonspecific biochemical marker for neuroblastoma, but increased levels (> 1500 U/mL) are associated with rapid cellular turnover and poor prognosis [16,17].

Molecular markers

Approximately 30% of primary neuroblastomas demonstrate N-*myc* amplification, which is strongly correlated with advanced-stage tumors and poor prognosis, independent of patient age and staging [18]. Typically, less than 5% of neuroblastomas of stages 1, 2, and 4S disease show N-*myc* amplification, whereas nearly half of all advanced-stage tumors demonstrate N-*myc* amplification [19]. Moreover, N-*myc* amplification has been associated with other markers such as high expression of MRP and chromosome 1p deletion, both of which reflect poor outcome for patients who have neuroblastoma [20,21]. The membrane-bound glycoprotein MRP is abundantly expressed in advanced-stage neuroblastomas and contributes to chemoresistance of aggressive tumors [20]. Certainly, the significance of N-*myc* protooncogene and the molecular mechanisms involved in its expression in neuroblastoma remains one of the major areas of research focus. Targeted expression of N-*myc* in transgenic mice results in the development of spontaneous neuroblastoma [22]. In contrast, antisense inhibition of N-*myc* expression in neuroblastoma tissue culture cells has shown to decrease cell proliferation and promote neuron differentiation [23,24]. The potential application of an advanced molecular tool such as small interfering RNA provides hopes of targeting N-*myc* expression in the treatment of advanced-stage neuroblastomas.

CD44 is a cell surface glycoprotein involved in cell-to-cell/matrix interactions and is a marker for aggressive tumor behavior in various cancers [25,26]. It is of interest that higher CD44 expression correlates with less aggressive tumor behavior and improved survival in patients who have neuroblastoma [27]. An inverse relationship exists between the CD44 expression and N-*myc* amplification [28,29]. Recently, a gene expression profiling study using cDNA microarray showed that N-*myc* and CD44 accurately predicted outcome for most of the patients examined, independent of known risk factors [30]. The high expression level of Trk tyrosine kinase receptor for NGF has also shown strong predictability for favorable outcome in patients who have neuroblastoma [31]. A strong correlation was found between early tumor stage, age less than 1 year, normal N-*myc* copy, and Trk expression [31]. Low expression of Trk receptor is associated with N-*myc* amplification and advanced-stage neuroblastomas. Because NGF is a well-known differentiation factor for neuroblastomas [32], the Trk receptors (as cell surface receptors for NGF ligand) may be critical in the regulation of differentiation and potential regression of neuroblastomas.

Clinical presentation

Because most neuroblastomas occur in the retroperitoneum or posterior mediastinum, early symptoms are typically nonspecific (general malaise, weight loss, unexplained fever). Intra-abdominal neuroblastomas often present as an asymptomatic mass that is detected incidentally by parents or a pediatrician during a routine clinic visit. Pelvic tumors may compress the rectosigmoid colon or bladder, producing constipation or urinary retention. In particular, thoracic neuroblastoma typically presents with nonspecific symptoms and is detected as an incidental mass on routine chest radiograph that may be taken for unrelated, mild respiratory symptoms. On occasion, spontaneous hemorrhage occurs in the tumor, resulting in acute onset of abdominal pain with malaise due to anemia. On examination, a firm, relatively fixed mass in the abdomen may be palpated. Hematogenous metastasis is often present at the time of diagnosis. Bone pain with dramatic recent change in activity level may portend bone metastasis. Periorbital ecchymosis or proptosis as a result of skull involvement can be mistakenly attributed to trauma. Painless subcutaneous nodules with distinct bluish discoloration in infants who have stage 4S disease are called blueberry muffin–like spots and indicate a favorable condition with potential for spontaneous tumor regression. Protracted cervical masses in infants and children, routinely considered lymphadenopathy, may represent primary or metastatic neuroblastoma. A paraspinal tumor is at risk for tumor extension through the vertebral foramina and compression of the spinal cord, producing motor deficits and progressive paraplegia.

Syndromes

On rare occasions, patients who have neuroblastoma can present with paraneoplastic syndromes. Opsomyoclonus is characterized by involuntary jerking movements of the limbs and trunk along with rapid, conjugate eye movements. These symptoms are classically described as "dancing eyes, dancing feet" and are thought to be a result of cerebellar responses to antibodies against the neural tissue of the tumor. Although opsomyoclonus is more commonly seen in early-stage tumors with favorable features, symptoms usually persist despite successful treatment of the tumor, resulting in developmental delay [33]. Dehydration and hypokalemia due to intractable secretory diarrhea are hallmark symptoms of neuroblastoma secreting vaso-active intestinal polypeptide [34]. In general, this syndrome occurs more commonly with ganglioneuroblastoma and ganglioneuroma, and symptoms resolve after tumor resection.

Diagnosis

Screening

Elevation of urinary catecholamine metabolites (homovanillic acid and vanillylmandelic acid) is routinely used as a diagnostic screen and for detecting recurrent disease [35,36]. Although the initial enthusiasm for use of homovanillic acid and vanillylmandelic acid for screening infants has subsided due to detection of predominantly favorable tumors that are thought to regress spontaneously, a recent review from Japan showed that 10% of cases had one or more unfavorable biologic markers [37].

Imaging

Plain radiographs and ultrasonography are routinely obtained for patients who have any suspicious mass. Chest radiographs revealing posterior mediastinal mass can narrow the differential diagnoses; calcification is also detected in up to 50% of cases. Ultrasound is helpful to confirm the solid nature of the tumor, which is typically of mixed heterogeneous echo pattern. Contrast-enhanced CT provides details on tumor consistency, extent of local disease, and distant organ involvement. A large perirenal mass with calcification is characteristic of neuroblastoma (Fig. 1). MRI has been particularly useful in discerning the extent of tumor extension into the spinal canal (Fig. 2). Radiolabeled metaiodobenzylguanidine (MIBG) scan is highly specific and sensitive for evaluating bone and bone marrow disease because MIBG is taken up by most neuroblastomas but not by normal bone [38]. The complementary use of technetium 99m

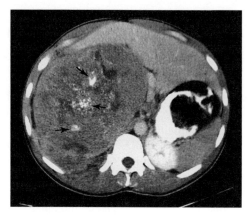

Fig. 1. Neuroblastoma with characteristic calcifications (*arrows*) on CT scan.

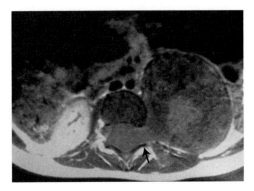

Fig. 2. A dumbbell-shaped left paraspinal neuroblastoma with spinal column extension (*arrow*), visualized with MRI.

methylene diphosphonate bone scan can virtually eliminate any false-negative MIBG results [39]. Ultimately, confirmation of diagnosis for neuroblastoma is made with examination of tissue obtained by bone marrow aspiration or biopsy of primary or secondary disease. Secondary tumor deposits in the skin and lymph nodes are frequently amenable to open biopsy. When dealing with primary tumors, fine needle aspiration can provide reliable diagnosis; however, limitation of tissue sample size usually precludes important immunohistochemical and cytogenetic analyses. Histologic sections are examined using criteria based on the Shimada classification, and tissue samples are assessed for cytogenetic tumor biomarkers.

Staging

The International Neuroblastoma Staging System (Table 1), based on clinical and pathologic criteria, is widely used to stage the disease and to stratify treatment protocols [40].

Treatment

A combined modality of surgery, chemotherapy, and radiotherapy based on disease stage and patient age at presentation is used for neuroblastoma.

Surgical

The goal of surgical intervention is complete resection of tumor. If complete resection is not feasible, then the goal is to perform a biopsy and to stage the tumor. The resectability of primary tumor is assessed using imaging studies, taking into consideration the size of the tumor; adherence or extension into adjacent structures such as vessels and spinal cord; lymph nodal involvement; and the likelihood of surgical cure. For stages 1, 2A, or 2B disease, complete gross excision of tumor is the primary therapeutic goal; however, the surgeon must use sound surgical judgment to avoid preventable complications such as injury to adjacent structures or major blood loss.

Table 1
International Neuroblastoma Staging System

Stage	Definition
1	Localized tumor with complete gross excision, with or without microscopic residual disease; negative ipsilateral lymph nodes
2A	Localized tumor with incomplete gross excision; negative ipsilateral nonadherent lymph nodes
2B	Localized tumor with or without complete gross excision; positive ipsilateral nonadherent lymph nodes; negative contralateral lymph nodes
3	Unresectable unilateral tumor infiltrating across the midline, with or without regional lymph node involvement, or Localized unilateral tumor with contralateral regional lymph node involvement, or Midline tumor with bilateral extension by infiltration (unresectable) or by lymph node involvement
4	Any primary tumor with dissemination to distant lymph nodes, bone, bone marrow, liver, skin, or other organs (except as defined for stage 4S)
4S	Localized primary tumor (as defined for stage 1, 2A, or 2B) with dissemination limited to skin, liver, and bone marrow (limited to infants <1 year old)

For example, the dumbbell tumor with an intraspinal component may be best managed by a staged approach, with adjuvant chemotherapy or initial removal of intraspinal tumor followed by complete surgical resection (see Fig. 2). For advanced stages 3 and 4 disease, initial surgical intervention should be limited to open biopsy for tissue diagnosis along with cytogenetic and tumor biomarker analyses. Delaying surgical resection until adjuvant chemotherapy is given has resulted in decreased morbidity and an increased rate of complete resection. For infants who have stage 4S disease, surgical resection of primary tumor has shown no significant benefit to overall patient survival because these tumors are frequently found to show differentiation and spontaneous regression even without specific treatment.

Chemotherapy

Chemotherapy is the principal treatment for advanced-stage neuroblastomas. When used in combination and based on drug synergy, mechanism of action, and potential drug resistance of tumor, chemotherapy treatment has been effective for patients who have extensive primary, recurrent, or metastatic neuroblastomas. Agents commonly used today are cyclophosphamide, iphosphamide, vincristine, doxorubicin, cisplatin, carboplatin, etoposide, and melphalan. An increase in long-term survival is noted with more intense combination therapy at the expense of toxicities. The quest for intensifying chemotherapy while decreasing side effects has led to bone marrow-ablative therapy, with total body irradiation or melphalan followed by bone marrow transplant for patients who have high-risk disease [41].

Radiotherapy

In general, neuroblastoma is considered radiosensitive. There is little benefit of radiotherapy for stage 1 and 2 tumors despite residual local disease.

Radiotherapy, however, has been shown to decrease the local relapse rate for high-risk neuroblastomas. Local irradiation to the liver is indicated in infants who have stage 4S neuroblastoma and respiratory distress due to hepatomegaly. Irradiation of intraspinal lesions has been less than ideal due to concomitant vertebral body damage resulting in growth arrest and scoliosis. The combination of radiotherapy and chemotherapy has been used recently for advanced-stage disease to enhance resectability. The other use of radiotherapy has been for total body irradiation to achieve bone marrow ablation before autologous bone marrow transplant. Targeted MIBG treatment, used widely in Europe, has shown benefit in the treatment of advanced-stage neuroblastomas as first-line therapy and for refractory neuroblastomas [42–44]; however, a number of complications such as occurrence of secondary malignancy and thyroid dysfunction have been reported [45,46]. High-risk neuroblastomas continue to show poor response to combined treatment modalities and remain a difficult group of tumors in which to achieve local control. Recently, aggressive surgical treatment with local irradiation and myeloablative chemotherapy with stem cell rescue has shown to provide excellent local control in high-risk neuroblastomas [47].

Wilms' tumor

Wilms' tumor is the most common childhood renal tumor, accounting for approximately 6% of all pediatric malignancies. The incidence of Wilms' tumor is 1 in 10,000 children, representing about 650 new cases annually in the United States [1]. This tumor tends to occur between ages 1 and 3 years, with 90% of new cases diagnosed before age 7 years. On rare occasions, Wilms' tumor has been described in teenagers and adults. The significant improvement in survival from 30% several decades ago to a 5- to 7-year survival rate of nearly 90% today is attributed to the success of a multidisciplinary approach and the efforts of cooperative study groups. These groups include the National Wilms' Tumor Study (NWTS) in North America and the International Society of Pediatric Oncology (SIOP) in Europe. Today, Wilms' tumor is one of the most successfully treated pediatric solid malignancies.

Pathology

Histology

Wilms' tumor is an embryonal renal neoplasm that contains blastemal, stromal, and epithelial cells in varying proportions. The diffuse blastemal type is associated with advanced-stage tumors at presentation but considered a good responder to chemotherapy. Analysis of patients in an early NWTS report showed that tumors with anaplastic features, occurring in 5% of patients, represent the most significant marker of adverse prognosis

[48]. Anaplasia occurs primarily in children older than 2 years and is considered a marker of resistance to chemotherapy rather than a predictor factor. Other unfavorable tumor subtypes included in the first two NWTS reports were clear cell sarcoma and rhabdoid tumor of the kidney [49]. Since then, these two sarcomatous lesions have been considered distinct entities separate from Wilms' tumor.

Nephrogenic rests

Nephrogenic rest is defined as the persistence of metanephric tissue in the kidney after the 36th week of gestation. This lesion may be considered a precursor of Wilms' tumor because it is found in 30% to 40% of kidney removed for Wilms' tumor [50,51]. In the NWTS-4 report, nearly half of the unilateral and almost all of the synchronous bilateral Wilms' tumors were associated with the presence of nephrogenic rests [51]. The nephrogenic rests are subclassified into perilobar and intralobar types. The intralobar rests reflect earlier disturbances in nephrogenesis; the perilobar rests are usually multiple and occur far more commonly in the newborn population. The presence of diffuse nephrogenic rests is termed nephroblastomatosis. These nephrogenic rests may involute, undergo hyperplastic overgrowth, or progress to focal neoplastic induction. The structural, epidemiologic, and pathogenetic differences between perilobar rests, intralobar rests, and Wilms' tumor associated with these subtypes imply a substantial degree of pathogenetic heterogeneity for Wilms' tumor.

Cytogenetics

The molecular characterization of Wilms' tumor has significantly contributed to our understanding of cancer cell biology, including the role of tumor suppressor genes. Knudson and Strong [52] originally pioneered the two-hit theory for Wilms' tumor formation, whereby it was thought that a child who had a constitutional lesion (inherited or spontaneous mutation) needed only a single new genetic event for tumorigenesis. Since then, however, research has shown that the formation of Wilms' tumor is a much more complex process, whereby multiple genes and several genetic events are involved. The initial insights into the molecular biology of Wilms' tumor originated from scrutiny of patients who had a complex of anomalies including aniridia, genitourinary malformation, and mental retardation (WAGR syndrome), which was found to be associated with developing Wilms' tumor [53].

Cytogenetic analysis of children who have the WAGR syndrome demonstrated deletions at chromosome 11p13 [54]. This finding provided the first clue to the location of a suppressor gene, *WT1*, involved in the development of Wilms' tumor. In addition, *PAX6*, the gene responsible for aniridia, was found in this region [55]. The *WT1* gene encodes a transcription factor critical to normal kidney and gonadal development [56]. Although several target genes of *WT1* have been identified, its exact role in tumor suppression is still unknown. The Denys-Drash syndrome (pseudohermaphroditism, glomerulopathy, renal failure, and predisposition to Wilms' tumor) is another syndrome associated with *WT1* gene mutation [57]. Only a small number of patients who have sporadic Wilms' tumor have *WT1* mutations, however, suggesting that other genes are involved in the development of Wilms' tumor.

A second Wilms' tumor–suppressor gene, *WT2*, was identified at chromosome 11p15 [58]. Beckwith-Wiedemann syndrome, a collection of congenital abnormalities that includes macroglossia, organomegaly, hemihypertrophy, and hypoglycemia, has been associated with increased susceptibility to development of Wilms' tumor in 5% of patients. This syndrome maps to chromosome 11p15, and a LOH at this locus has been found in Wilms' tumor [59]. In addition to the two genetic loci on chromosome 11, familial Wilms' tumor predisposition at *FWT1* (17q) and *FWT2* (19q) loci has been identified [58]. Moreover, mutation of the p53 tumor suppressor gene also has been found in Wilms' tumor [60]. The NWTS-5 trial reported that LOH at chromosomes 1p and 16q is associated with adverse outcome [61].

Clinical presentation

Various congenital anomalies are known to be associated with Wilms' tumor. Aniridia, hemihypertrophy, genitourinary tract anomalies (eg, cryptorchidism and hypospadias), Beckwith-Wiedemann syndrome, and Denys-Drash syndrome have been reported to confer an increased risk of the development of Wilms' tumor [58]. The frequency of bilaterality and the association with congenital anomalies have led many to believe that Wilms' tumor has a substantial heritable fraction. Most children present with an asymptomatic abdominal mass that is typically first identified by the parent while bathing the child or by the pediatrician during routine physical examination. One third of patients have intermittent abdominal pain that may be exacerbated by abdominal trauma. Gross or microscopic hematuria is found in up to 25% of patients, and hypertension may be present due to an increase in renin secretion by the tumor or from displaced kidney or renal artery by tumor growth. Occasionally, fever, malaise, and anemia occur as a result of tumor necrosis with intraparenchymal bleeding. On examination, a large smooth and firm abdominal mass is encountered. The tumor is usually nontender and immobile and does not cross the midline. Intravascular extension of the tumor may present with cardiac murmur, hepatosplenomegaly, ascites, varicocele, or gonad metastasis.

Diagnosis

Imaging

Few distinguishing radiographic features allow a precise preoperative diagnosis of the renal mass. The chest radiograph is obtained to detect pulmonary metastasis, and linear calcification may be observed on the abdominal radiograph in 3% of Wilms' tumors. Ultrasound examination provides helpful information about the consistency of the mass and potential intravascular involvement. Intravenous pyelogram is rarely used today for the diagnosis of Wilms' tumor. CT scan of the abdomen has been the standard diagnostic modality (Fig. 3). CT discerns information regarding characteristic features of a renal mass, the anatomic extent of the tumor, the presence of a normal-appearing contralateral kidney, and the possibility of bilateral tumor involvement. Intracaval extension of the tumor can be defined on CT scan or ultrasound. The role of chest CT scan for work-up and the subsequent management of pulmonary nodules found only on the chest CT scan have been the subject of much debate and have generated conflicting published reports [62,63]. Traditionally, chest involvements were defined as nodules identified on plain radiographs. In a study by Wilimas and colleagues [63], 78 of 202 chest CT scans were found to be positive by at least one reviewer, resulting in cumulative relapse rate of 13% to 20%. A recent study by the United Kingdom Children's Cancer Study Group, however, showed no difference in prognosis among patients who had positive or negative chest CT scans [62]. A well-designed prospective, randomized study on the role of whole-lung irradiation in patients who have CT-only pulmonary metastasis is still much needed. Recently, MRI has been praised as the imaging modality of choice to determine Wilms' tumor, suggesting it is superior to CT and to ultrasound in defining the extent of intravascular involvement.

Staging

Wilms' tumors are staged on the basis of anatomic involvement of the tumor. Refinement of the inclusion criteria for stages I and II disease was introduced in the NWTS-5 study to include renal sinus vascular invasion. The current NWTS staging system for Wilms' tumor is shown in Table 2.

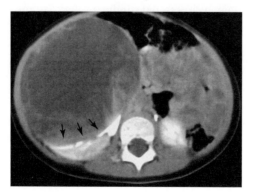

Fig. 3. CT scan of a large Wilms' tumor of the right kidney with characteristic "claw" sign, representing distorted remnant renal parenchyma at the periphery (*arrows*).

Table 2
National Wilms' Tumor Study Group staging system

Stage	Definition
I	Tumor confined to the kidney and completely resected; no penetration of the renal capsule or involvement of renal sinus vessels

II	Tumor extends beyond the kidney but is completely resected (negative margins and lymph nodes; at least one of the following has occurred:
	    Penetration of the renal capsule
	    Invasion of the renal sinus vessels
	    Biopsy of tumor performed before removal
	    Spillage of tumor locally during removal

III	Gross or microscopic residual tumor remains postoperatively, inducing inoperable tumor, positive surgical margins, tumor spillage involving peritoneal surfaces, regional lymph node metastases, or transected tumor thrombus
IV	Hematogenous or lymph node metastases outside the abdomen (eg, lung, liver, bone, and brain)
V	Bilateral renal Wilms' tumors

Treatment

Surgical

Full exploration of the contralateral kidney at the time of surgery has been the NWTS guideline because there is approximately a 7% false-negative rate on CT imaging [64]. A review of the NWTS-4 data showed that the contralateral renal lesions not detected on CT scan were small (<1 cm in six patients; 1–2 cm in three patients) [65]. A chemotherapy regimen of vincristine/dactinomycin or vincristine/dactinomycin/doxorubicin resulted in no tumor recurrences and disease-free status for all patients at 9-year follow-up [64]. This study showed that routine contralateral renal exploration can identify few occult tumors not detected on preoperative imaging. Omission of routine exploration is not likely to affect the outcome or management of newly diagnosed Wilms' tumor, given that adequate preoperative CT or MRI is obtained. These data indicate that the routine contralateral surgical exploration of kidney is no longer necessary.

The transabdominal approach is used to achieve adequate exposure for complete regional staging, which includes thorough inspection of hilar and regional nodes and contralateral kidney if necessary. Gentle handling of the tumor is mandatory to avoid tumor spillage because peritoneal soilage up-stages the tumor and increases the risk of local and abdominal tumor recurrence [66]. Wilms' tumors typically only compress or adhere to the adjacent structure; therefore, en-bloc resection is rarely indicated. Radical nephrectomy is performed with sampling of regional lymph node, but formal lymphadenectomy is not required. Palpation of the renal vein and inferior vena cava should be performed to exclude intravascular tumor extension before vessel ligation. The adrenal gland may be left in situ when the primary tumor involves the lower pole of the kidney. In some patients who have a massive tumor that precludes complete primary resection, performing a biopsy of the tumor, followed by chemotherapy or radiation therapy for subsequent tumor resection, is recommended.

The use of partial nephrectomy for unilateral Wilms' tumor remains controversial. Because the incidence of renal failure from a unilateral nephrectomy is extremely low (0.25%) [67], there must be clear advantages of partial nephrectomy without an increased risk of local recurrence. In an SIOP study, 37 patients who had partial nephrectomy for unilateral tumor demonstrated no difference in relapse-free survival at 5 years compared with the total nephrectomy group (770 patients) [68]. Twenty-two of the 37 patients, however, had received preoperative chemotherapy. Most Wilms' tumors are large or centrally located, making partial nephrectomy difficult at initial presentation. Even after preoperative chemotherapy, only about 10% of unilateral Wilms' tumors are thought to be amenable to partial nephrectomy [69]. Therefore, renal-sparing partial nephrectomy for unilateral Wilms' tumor is considered suitable only for patients who have a solitary kidney, bilateral disease, and renal insufficiency.

Intravascular extension

The inferior vena cava is involved by tumor thrombus in 4% to 10% of Wilms' tumor, but right atrial involvement is rare. Signs and symptoms are variable (hypertension, hematuria, hepatosplenomegaly, ascites, heart failure, and murmur) and depend on the degree of venous obstruction and the extent of vascular involvement. Shamberger and colleagues [70] reported a collaborative study of Wilms' tumor with intravascular extension into the inferior vena cava in 134 patients or into the atrium in 31 patients. These investigators found that preoperative treatment facilitated resection by decreasing the extent of the tumor thrombus, but the overall frequency of complications and the 3-year relapse-free survival were similar between the preoperative group and the primary resection group. When dealing with intracardiac tumor extension, a combined thoracoabdominal approach including the use of cardiopulmonary bypass is the safest and most effective method. A recent SIOP study reported uncomplicated resection of nine intracardiac Wilms' tumors with cardiopulmonary bypass and hypothermia [71]. Overall survival of children who have cavoatrial tumor extension is not different from survival with intrarenal lesion of similar stage and histology.

Bilateral Wilms' tumor

Synchronous bilateral disease occurs in about 5% to 8% of children who have Wilms' tumor. Girls are affected more frequently, and the patients are 20 months younger at diagnosis than those who have unilateral tumors. Bilateral Wilms' tumor is also more frequently associated with hemihypertrophy and genitourinary anomalies. The current management guidelines dictate that patients undergo bilateral renal biopsies, with staging of each kidney. Biopsy specimens should be obtained from all discrete bilateral lesions because discordant pathology can occur and adequate lymph node sampling is essential for accurate staging. After 6 to 8 weeks of chemotherapy, follow-up imaging studies are obtained to determine the feasibility of renal-sparing procedures. Patient survival has not been found to be compromised by attempting to conserve native renal function with renal-sparing operations [72]. The primary resection of bilateral tumors is not recommended. In the NWTS-4 study, 98 children who had bilateral Wilms' tumor underwent partial nephrectomy, with complete gross disease resection in 88%, renal preservation in 72%, a local relapse rate of 8%, and a 4-year survival rate of 81.7% [73].

Chemotherapy

The first-line chemotherapeutic agents for Wilms' tumor are dactinomycin, vincristine, and doxorubicin. For those who relapse or are resistant to the initial regimen, a combination of cyclophosphamide, ifosfamide, carboplatin, and etoposide is considered. The NWTS-3 protocol allowed an 11-week regimen of vincristine and dactinomycin for stage I tumors, resulting in an 89% 4-year relapse-free survival rate [74]. This study also found a beneficial addition of doxorubicin for stage III tumors but not for stage II. The addition of cyclophosphamide did not benefit treatment of children who have stage IV tumors [74]. NWTS-4 addressed the issue of dose intensification. Dactinomycin and doxorubicin, administered in single, moderately high doses, produced comparable outcomes [75]. The study also showed that a short interval therapy of 18 to 26 weeks was effective [76]. For stage III disease, doxorubicin resulted in more than a 50% decrease in tumor relapse, but the long-term risk of cardiomyopathy from doxorubicin remains unclear. The use of doxorubicin was found to be associated with cumulative rate of 4.4% of congestive heart failure [77]. To reduce complications and toxicity from chemotherapy, vincristine/dactinomycin or vincristine alone therapy was tried for stage I tumors, producing encouraging results [78].

Radiation therapy

NWTS-2 and -3 showed that radiation therapy offers no additional advantages to relapse-free or overall survival when treatment is combined with vincristine and dactinomycin [79,80]. NWTS-3 also demonstrated that for children who had stage III favorable-histology tumors, 10-Gy radiotherapy with vincristine/dactinomycin/doxorucibin was comparable to 20-Gy radiotherapy with vincristine/dactinomycin [79]. The current guideline suggests local abdominal irradiation (10 Gy) for stage III favorable-histology tumors and for stage II, III with diffuse anaplastic Wilms' tumors. Whole lung irradiation is administered to children who have pulmonary metastasis. NWTS-3 demonstrated 4-year relapse-free and overall survival rates of 72% and 78%, respectively, in children who had favorable-histology

Wilms' tumor and pulmonary metastasis [74]. The role for whole-lung irradiation in children who have CT-only pulmonary metastasis remains unclear. In such patients treated in the NWTS-3 and -4, there was no statistical difference in the 4-year relapse-free survival rates of 89% with irradiation and 80% with chemotherapy alone [81].

Preoperative therapy

In general, preoperative therapy is considered for Wilms' tumors that are not completely resectable at initial operation, such as tumors with bilaterality, cavoatrial extension, or metastatic lesions. A significant number of patients are down-staged after chemotherapy. In their review of 30 patients, Greenberg and colleagues [82] reported that preoperative chemotherapy resulted in down-staging of disease in 41% of patients, therefore allowing easier removal of tumors and less radiation exposure. A potential problem of preoperative therapy is the inability to accurately classify and stage tumors. Zuppan and colleagues [83], however, reported that preoperative chemotherapy did not alter the recognizable anaplastic element. Preoperative therapy has also been used to allow partial nephrectomy with unilateral Wilms' tumor, with some debate. Percutaneous biopsy followed by 4 to 6 weeks of chemotherapy was reported to successfully treat 9 children who had Wilms' tumor (4 who had unilateral tumor) [84]. In a retrospective study from the St. Jude Children's Research Hospital, however, only 2 of 43 children who had unilateral tumor had lesions amenable to partial nephrectomy [85]. Although the current NWTS guidelines recommend primary surgical treatment of Wilms' tumor, they also point out that preoperative therapy may be of benefit in children who have bilateral involvement, extensive intravascular involvement, and inoperable massive tumors.

References

[1] Gurney JG, Severson RK, Davis S, et al. Incidence of cancer in children in the United States. Sex-, race-, and 1-year age-specific rates by histologic type. Cancer 1995;75: 2186–95.

[2] Hicks MJ, Mackay B. Comparison of ultrastructural features among neuroblastic tumors: maturation from neuroblastoma to ganglioneuroma. Ultrastruct Pathol 1995;19:311–22.

[3] Peuchmaur M, d'Amore ES, Joshi VV, et al. Revision of the International Neuroblastoma Pathology Classification: confirmation of favorable and unfavorable prognostic subsets in ganglioneuroblastoma, nodular. Cancer 2003;98:2274–81.

[4] Chatten J, Shimada H, Sather HN, et al. Prognostic value of histopathology in advanced neuroblastoma: a report from the Childrens Cancer Study Group. Hum Pathol 1988;19: 1187–98.

[5] Shimada H. Tumors of the neuroblastoma group. Pathology (Phila) 1993;2:43–59.

[6] Shimada H, Ambros IM, Dehner LP, et al. The International Neuroblastoma Pathology Classification (the Shimada system). Cancer 1999;86:364–72.

[7] Brodeur GM, Green AA, Hayes FA, et al. Cytogenetic features of human neuroblastomas and cell lines. Cancer Res 1981;41:4678–86.

[8] Gilbert F, Balaban G, Moorhead P, et al. Abnormalities of chromosome 1p in human neuroblastoma tumors and cell lines. Cancer Genet Cytogenet 1982;7:33–42.

[9] Brodeur GM, Fong CT, Morita M, et al. Molecular analysis and clinical significance of N-myc amplification and chromosome 1p monosomy in human neuroblastomas. Prog Clin Biol Res 1988;271:3–15.

[10] Srivatsan ES, Ying KL, Seeger RC. Deletion of chromosome 11 and of 14q sequences in neuroblastoma. Genes Chromosomes Cancer 1993;7:32–7.

[11] Attiyeh EF, London WB, Mosse YP, et al. Chromosome 1p and 11q deletions and outcome in neuroblastoma. N Engl J Med 2005;353:2243–53.

[12] Gilbert F, Feder M, Balaban G, et al. Human neuroblastomas and abnormalities of chromosomes 1 and 17. Cancer Res 1984;44:5444–9.

[13] Look AT, Hayes FA, Nitschke R, et al. Cellular DNA content as a predictor of response to chemotherapy in infants with unresectable neuroblastoma. N Engl J Med 1984;311: 231–5.

[14] Berthold F, Engelhardt-Fahrner U, Schneider A, et al. Age dependence and prognostic impact of neuron specific enolase (NSE) in children with neuroblastoma. In Vivo 1991; 5:245–7.

[15] Silber JH, Evans AE, Fridman M. Models to predict outcome from childhood neuroblastoma: the role of serum ferritin and tumor histology. Cancer Res 1991;51:1426–33.

[16] Joshi VV, Cantor AB, Brodeur GM, et al. Correlation between morphologic and other prognostic markers of neuroblastoma. A study of histologic grade, DNA index, N-myc gene copy number, and lactic dehydrogenase in patients in the Pediatric Oncology Group. Cancer 1993; 71:3173–81.

[17] Woods WG. The use and significance of biologic markers in the evaluation and staging of a child with cancer. Cancer 1986;58:442–8.

[18] Brodeur GM, Seeger RC, Schwab M, et al. Amplification of N-myc in untreated human neuroblastomas correlates with advanced disease stage. Science 1984;224:1121–4.

[19] Look AT, Hayes FA, Shuster JJ, et al. Clinical relevance of tumor cell ploidy and N-myc gene amplification in childhood neuroblastoma: a Pediatric Oncology Group study. J Clin Oncol 1991;9:581–91.

[20] Bordow SB, Haber M, Madafiglio J, et al. Expression of the multidrug resistance-associated protein (MRP) gene correlates with amplification and overexpression of the N-myc oncogene in childhood neuroblastoma. Cancer Res 1994;54:5036–40.

[21] Norris MD, Bordow SB, Marshall GM, et al. Expression of the gene for multidrug-resistance-associated protein and outcome in patients with neuroblastoma. N Engl J Med 1996;334:231–8.

[22] Weiss WA, Aldape K, Mohapatra G, et al. Targeted expression of MYCN causes neuroblastoma in transgenic mice. EMBO J 1997;16:2985–95.

[23] Negroni A, Scarpa S, Romeo A, et al. Decrease of proliferation rate and induction of differentiation by a MYCN antisense DNA oligomer in a human neuroblastoma cell line. Cell Growth Differ 1991;2:511–8.

[24] Whitesell L, Rosolen A, Neckers LM. Episome-generated N-myc antisense RNA restricts the differentiation potential of primitive neuroectodermal cell lines. Mol Cell Biol 1991;11: 1360–71.

[25] Esteban F, Bravo JJ, Gonzalez-Moles MA, et al. Adhesion molecule CD44 as a prognostic factor in laryngeal cancer. Anticancer Res 2005;25:1115–21.

[26] Kashyap MK, Kumar A, Emelianenko N, et al. Biochemical and molecular markers in renal cell carcinoma: an update and future prospects. Biomarkers 2005;10:258–94.

[27] Comito MA, Savell VH, Cohen MB. CD44 expression in neuroblastoma and related tumors. J Pediatr Hematol Oncol 1997;19:292–6.

[28] Combaret V, Gross N, Lasset C, et al. Clinical relevance of CD44 cell surface expression and MYCN gene amplification in neuroblastoma. Eur J Cancer 1997;33:2101–5.

[29] Kramer K, Cheung NK, Gerald WL, et al. Correlation of MYCN amplification, Trk-A and CD44 expression with clinical stage in 250 patients with neuroblastoma. Eur J Cancer 1997; 33:2098–100.

[30] Wei JS, Greer BT, Westermann F, et al. Prediction of clinical outcome using gene expression profiling and artificial neural networks for patients with neuroblastoma. Cancer Res 2004; 64:6883–91.

[31] Nakagawara A, Arima-Nakagawara M, Scavarda NJ, et al. Association between high levels of expression of the TRK gene and favorable outcome in human neuroblastoma. N Engl J Med 1993;328:847–54.

[32] Matsushima H, Bogenmann E. Expression of trkA cDNA in neuroblastomas mediates differentiation in vitro and in vivo. Mol Cell Biol 1993;13:7447–56.

[33] Hiyama E, Yokoyama T, Ichikawa T, et al. Poor outcome in patients with advanced stage neuroblastoma and coincident opsomyoclonus syndrome. Cancer 1994;74:1821–6.

[34] El Shafie M, Samuel D, Klippel CH, et al. Intractable diarrhea in children with VIP-secreting ganglioneuroblastomas. J Pediatr Surg 1983;18:34–6.

[35] LaBrosse EH, Com-Nougue C, Zucker JM, et al. Urinary excretion of 3-methoxy-4-hydroxymandelic acid and 3-methoxy-4-hydroxyphenylacetic acid by 288 patients with neuroblastoma and related neural crest tumors. Cancer Res 1980;40(6):1995–2001.

[36] Laug WE, Siegel SE, Shaw KN, et al. Initial urinary catecholamine metabolite concentrations and prognosis in neuroblastoma. Pediatrics 1978;62:77–83.

[37] Tajiri T, Suita S, Sera Y, et al. Clinical and biologic characteristics for recurring neuroblastoma at mass screening cases in Japan. Cancer 2001;92:349–53.

[38] Andrich MP, Shalaby-Rana E, Movassaghi N, et al. The role of 131 iodine-metaiodobenzylguanidine scanning in the correlative imaging of patients with neuroblastoma. Pediatrics 1996;97:246–50.

[39] Gordon I, Peters AM, Gutman A, et al. Skeletal assessment in neuroblastoma–the pitfalls of iodine-123-MIBG scans. J Nucl Med 1990;31:129–34.

[40] Brodeur GM, Pritchard J, Berthold F, et al. Revisions of the international criteria for neuroblastoma diagnosis, staging, and response to treatment. J Clin Oncol 1993;11:1466–77.

[41] Matthay KK, O'Leary MC, Ramsay NK, et al. Role of myeloablative therapy in improved outcome for high risk neuroblastoma: review of recent Children's Cancer Group results. Eur J Cancer 1995;31A:572–5.

[42] De Kraker J, Hoefnagel CA, Caron H, et al. First line targeted radiotherapy, a new concept in the treatment of advanced stage neuroblastoma. Eur J Cancer 1995;31A:600–2.

[43] Kang TI, Brophy P, Hickeson M, et al. Targeted radiotherapy with submyeloablative doses of 131I-MIBG is effective for disease palliation in highly refractory neuroblastoma. J Pediatr Hematol Oncol 2003;25:769–73.

[44] Mairs RJ, Fullerton NE, Cosimo E, et al. Gene manipulation to enhance MIBG-targeted radionuclide therapy. Nucl Med Biol 2005;32:749–53.

[45] Garaventa A, Gambini C, Villavecchia G, et al. Second malignancies in children with neuroblastoma after combined treatment with 131I-metaiodobenzylguanidine. Cancer 2003; 97:1332–8.

[46] van Santen HM, de Kraker J, van Eck BL, et al. High incidence of thyroid dysfunction despite prophylaxis with potassium iodide during (131)I-meta-iodobenzylguanidine treatment in children with neuroblastoma. Cancer 2002;94:2081–9.

[47] von Allmen D, Grupp S, Diller L, et al. Aggressive surgical therapy and radiotherapy for patients with high-risk neuroblastoma treated with rapid sequence tandem transplant. J Pediatr Surg 2005;40:936–41.

[48] Bonadio JF, Storer B, Norkool P, et al. Anaplastic Wilms' tumor: clinical and pathologic studies. J Clin Oncol 1985;3:513–20.

[49] Beckwith JB. Wilms' tumor and other renal tumors of childhood: a selective review from the National Wilms' Tumor Study Pathology Center. Hum Pathol 1983;14:481–92.

[50] Beckwith JB. Precursor lesions of Wilms tumor: clinical and biological implications. Med Pediatr Oncol 1993;21:158–68.

[51] Beckwith JB, Kiviat NB, Bonadio JF. Nephrogenic rests, nephroblastomatosis, and the pathogenesis of Wilms' tumor. Pediatr Pathol 1990;10:1–36.

[52] Knudson AG Jr, Strong LC. Mutation and cancer: a model for Wilms' tumor of the kidney. J Natl Cancer Inst 1972;48:313–24.

[53] Miller RW, Fraumeni JF Jr, Manning MD. Association of Wilms's tumor with aniridia, hemihypertrophy and other congenital malformations. N Engl J Med 1964;270: 922–7.

[54] Riccardi VM, Sujansky E, Smith AC, et al. Chromosomal imbalance in the aniridia-Wilms' tumor association: 11p interstitial deletion. Pediatrics 1978;61:604–10.

[55] Miles C, Elgar G, Coles E, et al. Complete sequencing of the Fugu WAGR region from WT1 to PAX6: dramatic compaction and conservation of synteny with human chromosome 11p13. Proc Natl Acad Sci U S A 1998;95:13068–72.

[56] Roberts SG. Transcriptional regulation by WT1 in development. Curr Opin Genet Dev 2005;15:542–7.

[57] Dharnidharka VR, Ruteshouser EC, Rosen S, et al. Pulmonary dysplasia, Denys-Drash syndrome and Wilms tumor 1 gene mutation in twins. Pediatr Nephrol 2001;16:227–31.

[58] Coppes MJ, Egeler RM. Genetics of Wilms' tumor. Semin Urol Oncol 1999;17:2–10.

[59] Steenman M, Westerveld A, Mannens M. Genetics of Beckwith-Wiedemann syndrome-associated tumors: common genetic pathways. Genes Chromosomes Cancer 2000;28: 1–13.

[60] Malkin D, Sexsmith E, Yeger H, et al. Mutations of the p53 tumor suppressor gene occur infrequently in Wilms' tumor. Cancer Res 1994;54:2077–9.

[61] Grundy PE, Telzerow PE, Breslow N, et al. Loss of heterozygosity for chromosomes 16q and 1p in Wilms' tumors predicts an adverse outcome. Cancer Res 1994;54:2331–3.

[62] Owens CM, Veys PA, Pritchard J, et al. Role of chest computed tomography at diagnosis in the management of Wilms' tumor: a study by the United Kingdom Children's Cancer Study Group. J Clin Oncol 2002;20:2768–73.

[63] Wilimas JA, Kaste SC, Kauffman WM, et al. Use of chest computed tomography in the staging of pediatric Wilms' tumor: interobserver variability and prognostic significance. J Clin Oncol 1997;15:2631–5.

[64] Ritchey ML, Green DM, Breslow NB, et al. Accuracy of current imaging modalities in the diagnosis of synchronous bilateral Wilms' tumor. A report from the National Wilms Tumor Study Group. Cancer 1995;75:600–4.

[65] Ritchey ML, Shamberger RC, Hamilton T, et al. Fate of bilateral renal lesions missed on preoperative imaging: a report from the National Wilms Tumor Study Group. J Urol 2005; 174(4):1519–21.

[66] Shamberger RC, Guthrie KA, Ritchey ML, et al. Surgery-related factors and local recurrence of Wilms tumor in National Wilms Tumor Study 4. Ann Surg 1999;229:292–7.

[67] Ritchey ML, Green DM, Thomas PR, et al. Renal failure in Wilms' tumor patients: a report from the National Wilms' Tumor Study Group. Med Pediatr Oncol 1996;26:75–80.

[68] Haecker FM, von Schweinitz D, Harms D, et al. Partial nephrectomy for unilateral Wilms tumor: results of study SIOP 93–01/GPOH. J Urol 2003;170:939–42.

[69] Moorman-Voestermans CG, Aronson DC, Staalman CR, et al. Is partial nephrectomy appropriate treatment for unilateral Wilms' tumor? J Pediatr Surg 1998;33:165–70.

[70] Shamberger RC, Ritchey ML, Haase GM, et al. Intravascular extension of Wilms tumor. Ann Surg 2001;234:116–21.

[71] Szavay P, Luithle T, Semler O, et al. Surgery of cavoatrial tumor thrombus in nephroblastoma: a report of the SIOP/GPOH study. Pediatr Blood Cancer 2004;43:40–5.

[72] Montgomery BT, Kelalis PP, Blute ML, et al. Extended followup of bilateral Wilms tumor: results of the National Wilms Tumor Study. J Urol 1991;146:514–8.

[73] Horwitz JR, Ritchey ML, Moksness J, et al. Renal salvage procedures in patients with synchronous bilateral Wilms' tumors: a report from the National Wilms' Tumor Study Group. J Pediatr Surg 1996;31:1020–5.

[74] D'Angio GJ, Breslow N, Beckwith JB, et al. Treatment of Wilms' tumor. Results of the Third National Wilms' Tumor Study. Cancer 1989;64:349–60.

[75] Green DM, Breslow NE, Beckwith JB, et al. Comparison between single-dose and divided-dose administration of dactinomycin and doxorubicin for patients with Wilms' tumor: a report from the National Wilms' Tumor Study Group. J Clin Oncol 1998;16:237–45.

[76] Green DM, Breslow NE, Beckwith JB, et al. Effect of duration of treatment on treatment outcome and cost of treatment for Wilms' tumor: a report from the National Wilms' Tumor Study Group. J Clin Oncol 1998;16:3744–51.

[77] Green DM, Grigoriev YA, Nan B, et al. Congestive heart failure after treatment for Wilms' tumor: a report from the National Wilms' Tumor Study group. J Clin Oncol 2001;19: 1926–34.

[78] Pritchard-Jones K, Kelsey A, Vujanic G, et al. Older age is an adverse prognostic factor in stage I, favorable histology Wilms' tumor treated with vincristine monochemotherapy: a study by the United Kingdom Children's Cancer Study Group, Wilm's Tumor Working Group. J Clin Oncol 2003;21:3269–75.

[79] Thomas PR, Tefft M, Compaan PJ, et al. Results of two radiation therapy randomizations in the third National Wilms' Tumor Study. Cancer 1991;68:1703–7.

[80] Thomas PR, Tefft M, Farewell VT, et al. Abdominal relapses in irradiated second National Wilms' Tumor Study patients. J Clin Oncol 1984;2:1098–101.

[81] Meisel JA, Guthrie KA, Breslow NE, et al. Significance and management of computed tomography detected pulmonary nodules: a report from the National Wilms Tumor Study Group. Int J Radiat Oncol Biol Phys 1999;44:579–85.

[82] Greenberg M, Burnweit C, Filler R, et al. Preoperative chemotherapy for children with Wilms' tumor. J Pediatr Surg 1991;26:949–53.

[83] Zuppan CW, Beckwith JB, Weeks DA, et al. The effect of preoperative therapy on the histologic features of Wilms' tumor. An analysis of cases from the Third National Wilms' Tumor Study. Cancer 1991;68:385–94.

[84] McLorie GA, McKenna PH, Greenberg M, et al. Reduction in tumor burden allowing partial nephrectomy following preoperative chemotherapy in biopsy proved Wilms tumor. J Urol 1991;146:509–13.

[85] Wilimas JA, Magill L, Parham DM, et al. Is renal salvage feasible in unilateral Wilms' tumor? Proposed computed tomographic criteria and their relation to surgicopathologic findings. Am J Pediatr Hematol Oncol 1990;12:164–7.

SURGICAL
CLINICS OF
NORTH AMERICA

Surg Clin N Am 86 (2006) 489–503

Germ Cell Tumors

Deborah F. Billmire, MD

Section of Pediatric Surgery, JW Riley Hospital for Children, Suite 2500,
Barnhill Drive, Indianapolis, IN 46202, USA

The category of germ cell tumors includes a broad array of histologic subtypes ranging from the benign, mature teratoma to the primitive, aggressive embryonal carcinoma (Box 1). These tumors share their origin in a primordial germ cell with multipotent capacity for differentiation along a variety of pathways. Several theories have been proposed to explain the origin and location of these tumors. Some investigators support the theory of aberrant migration of primitive germ cells originating in the embryonic yolk sac [1,2]. An alternative theory is that these tumors arise from totipotent cells originating in the primitive knot and primitive streak that invaginate between the layers of the bilaminar disc to form the mesoderm [3]. Germ cell tumors tend to occur in the midline or para-axial locations of the body. Sacrococcygeal tumors are the most common, followed by gonadal, mediastinal, retroperitoneal, and multiple other rare sites. Germ cell tumors may also occur in the brain but are not included in this review. Germ cell tumors are seen at all ages in childhood, with different age peaks for the various anatomic sites. In any given tumor, there may be a mixture of the various benign and malignant subtypes of germ cell histologies. Two of the malignant cell types secrete proteins that may be detected in the systemic circulation. Endodermal sinus tumors secrete alpha fetoprotein (AFP) and choriocarcinomas secrete beta human chorionic gonadotropin (β-HCG). The development of sensitive assays for these tumor markers has improved diagnostic accuracy and monitoring of therapy for these subtypes of malignant germ cell tumors. In the prechemotherapy era, survival of patients who had malignant germ cell tumors treated with surgery alone was rare. The advent of multiagent regimens such as vincristine/dactinomycin/cyclophosphamide (VAC) resulted in some progress, but the development of platinum-based regimens in the 1980s and 1990s dramatically improved survival. Children who have malignant germ cell tumors currently have

E-mail address: dbillmir@iupui.edu

Box 1. Spectrum of histologic types included in the category of germ cell tumors

1. Teratoma (mature, immature; has elements of all three germ layers: endoderm, mesoderm, ectoderm)
2. Germinoma (formerly called dysgerminoma in girls and women; seminoma in boys and men)
3. Endodermal sinus tumor (also called yolk sac tumor)
4. Choriocarcinoma
5. Embryonal carcinoma

---

survival rates of 70% to 90% depending on age, site, and histology [4–7]. Future studies will focus on maintaining high survival rates and on reducing toxicity of chemotherapy and surgical morbidity. The characteristic features of each site are discussed separately.

Sacrococcygeal tumors

The sacrococcygeal region is the most common site for germ cell tumors in childhood. Girls predominate, with a female-to-male ratio of 4:1 [8]. Three fourths of tumors present in the neonatal period, with most becoming evident by age 4 years [9]. A commonly used anatomic classification system was developed by Altman and colleagues [10] in a survey of the Surgical Section of the American Academy of Pediatrics and reported in 1974. Type I tumors are almost entirely external, type II tumors are primarily external with a small presacral component, type III tumors are primarily presacral with a small external component, and type IV tumors are entirely presacral. The overall risk of malignancy is 13% to 27%, but a strong correlation of malignancy with age at presentation is apparent. Benign tumors are seen in greater than 90% of children younger than age 2 months but present in less than half of children older than 2 months at presentation [10].

Over the past 15 years, increasing attention has focused on the frequency and impact of prenatal diagnosis for sacrococcygeal teratomas [11–16]. As prenatal diagnosis has become more common, there has been an increased request for the pediatric surgeon to undertake prenatal counseling for families with fetal diagnosis. A series of sacrococcygeal teratomas with fetal diagnosis was recently reported by Hedrick and colleagues in 2004 [16]. In their cohort of 30 fetuses seen in Philadelphia over a 7-year period, there was an overall mortality of 53%. There were five episodes of fetal demise, most from overt cardiac failure and hydrops. Four pregnancies were terminated. Of the 21 live births, 7 died as neonates. Most fatalities were related to tumor rupture during preterm labor at 25 to 27 weeks' gestation or to premature delivery at 30 to 32 weeks, with intraoperative rupture and bleeding during resection. Fourteen fetuses had fetal intervention, including 4 that had fetal tumor resection. Three of 4 fetuses who had tumor debulking before delivery survived; all delivered at 27 to 29 weeks' gestation and had complicated neonatal courses. A series of 17 consecutive fetuses evaluated in San Francisco also had mortality of nearly 50%, with most deaths due to hydrops [14]. The series reported by Holterman and colleagues in 1998 focused exclusively on cases that had prenatal diagnosis as an incidental finding without maternal symptoms and still found a significant overall mortality of 33% [12]. These investigators found that the presence of a purely solid tumor was the most important predictor of mortality and that the sudden development of hydramnios was a negative prognostic factor. These series clearly reflect the high mortality and challenging management of this group of patients. Close fetal monitoring is required for diagnosis of sacrococcygeal tumor in utero. Patients who have solid lesions with evolving evidence of polyhydramnios, hydrops, and high-output cardiac failure are at extremely high risk of mortality.

The principles of resection for sacrococcygeal teratoma are largely unchanged since the early description by Gross and coworkers in 1951 [17]. Complete tumor resection, removal of the coccyx, and preservation of muscle and neural structures remain the central features. Several investigators have described techniques for securing early vascular control in solid, highly vascular lesions, including aortic occlusion [18], ligation of the internal iliac and middle sacral arteries in a premature infant [19], and aortic control with ligation of blood supply to the tumor [20,21]. In addition to devascularization, Kamata and colleagues [21] proposed maintaining the supine position during resection of the tumor to provide improved control of hemorrhage and respiratory management.

The extreme distortion and thinning of the muscle layers by large tumors contribute to difficulty in preservation and reapproximation of sphincter and gluteal structures. Use of the muscle stimulator commonly applied in reconstructive procedures for imperforate anus can be helpful in this regard. In addition to sphincter reconstruction, proper placement of the anal opening on the perineum is an important goal. It is common for the anus to be within the sphincter but secured in a posteriorly displaced position toward the sacrum, posing difficulty in defecation [22]. The classic skin closure is a chevron configuration. Fishman and colleagues [22] recently described a variant with right-angled flaps that restores a more normal buttock contour and avoids scars below the gluteal crease. This reconstruction also provides more tissue between the anus and coccyx while respecting the limits of the sphincter complex.

Malignant sacrococcygeal germ cell tumors occur most often in infants and toddlers. They are almost exclusively of yolk sac histology, with variable frequency of associated mature or immature teratoma components. These malignant tumors may arise de novo but are also seen in infants who have previously undergone resection of a benign sacrococcygeal teratoma. The incidence of recurrent tumor in neonates and infants who have previously undergone resection of a benign teratoma is 4% to 21%. Approximately 50% to 70% of these recurrences are malignant endodermal sinus tumors [23]. This finding underscores the importance of continued careful follow-up with periodic digital rectal examination and AFP level in all patients who have had previous resection of a benign sacrococcygeal teratoma. Frequency of monitoring has been recommended at 1- to 3-month intervals for the first year and at 3- to 6-month intervals for at least 3 years [23,24]. Patients who have de novo tumors often have a type IV configuration and present with progressive bowel or bladder complaints. Advanced-stage disease is seen in 59% to 80% of malignant sacrococcygeal germ cell tumors at diagnosis [25,26]. Current survival is excellent with platinum-based chemotherapy, and most patients are optimally treated with a neoadjuvant approach. Complete tumor resection is an important component of therapy and is accomplished with a higher success rate and less morbidity after shrinkage of the tumor by chemotherapy [25]. Survival rates with current regimens range from 81% to 90% [4,6,26].

The success of current chemotherapy regimens for malignant sacrococcygeal tumors and the favorable survival rates of liveborn neonatal patients who have sacrococcygeal tumors have produced a population of long-term survivors. Quality of life and functional outcome are aspects of care that have received limited attention [8,24,27–31]. Symptomatic impairment of urinary function has been noted in 16% to 50% of children. Neurogenic bladder with incontinence, multiple urinary tract infections, and vesicoureteral reflux are most often seen. In Lahdenne and colleagues' [29] series of 45 patients, urodynamic abnormalities were seen in 78% of patients, with subjective complaints by history in only 18%. Bowel dysfunction ranging from constipation to fecal soiling and patulous anus has been reported in 5% to 27% of patients [8,24,30]. Multiple factors contribute to this problem. In some series, larger tumors with pelvic extension have had increased association with long-term sequelae [27,31]. Other series have not confirmed this association [28,30]. Additional congenital anomalies that are seen in some patients may also contribute to dysfunction. Boemers and colleagues' [31] series of 11 children included 2 who had tethered spinal cord and 1 who had unilateral renal agenesis and obstructed contralateral megaureter. Long-standing compression or stretching of the pelvic nerves during gestation may play a role in fetal-onset cases. Dilation of the urinary tract has been described in up to 43% of fetuses with prenatal imaging [16]. Operative trauma may also contribute. The importance of meticulous dissection with aid of the muscle stimulator may be helpful in identifying and preserving the attenuated muscle structures. In the past, initial therapy for large invasive tumors consisted of an aggressive attempt at surgical resection prior to chemotherapy. This practice frequently resulted in the need for second look procedures for positive margins or residual mass. The success of current chemotherapy in producing marked shrinkage of the tumor and a shift to encouraging postchemotherapy resection may also provide improved results in future cases. A review of the German MAKEI experience with malignant sacrococcygeal germ cell tumors by Göbel and coworkers [25] demonstrated an improved outcome for those patients treated with up-front chemotherapy and delayed resection. Event-free survival and overall survival were improved in patients treated with complete tumor resection. Surgical resection was more successful in obtaining clear margins when undertaken after chemotherapy was given. Continued follow-up, with attention to bowel and bladder function and monitoring for recurrent tumor, is an important aspect of care for these children.

Testis tumors

Testis is the primary site for germ cell tumors in only 4% of children [9]. Malignant tumors of the testis account for approximately 1% of childhood cancer [32]. The most common presentation is a painless scrotal mass, and almost all series include several children who had an incorrect preoperative diagnosis of hydrocele or testicular torsion [33–35]. Transillumination is positive in 15% to 25% of cases from coexisting hydrocele or a cystic component of the tumor [36]. Although rare, the possibility of tumor should be kept in mind when evaluating children who have scrotal swelling. Ultrasound should be obtained whenever a normal testis is not palpable on physical examination.

Approximately 85% of testicular tumors in children are of germ cell histology (Table 1). The frequency of malignancy ranges from 22% to 63%. There are two age peaks: one in infancy and one in adolescence. Malignant germ cell tumors in infants are almost uniformly due to pure endodermal sinus (yolk sac) histology. The adolescent malignant tumors are most often mixed germ cell tumors or germinoma (seminoma).

A concept that has become increasingly applied to certain pediatric testis tumors over the past decade is testicular-preserving surgery [32,34,37–39]. This approach may be appropriate for benign teratomas in prepubertal boys and for epidermoid cysts. When considering this technique, it is important to adhere to careful preoperative work-up and oncologic principles.

The initial evaluation of a boy who has suspected testis tumor includes scrotal ultrasound and serum AFP and β-HCG. If serum markers are

Table 1
Distribution of testis neoplasms in the pediatric age group in selected series

Author	Teratoma	Malignant germ cell tumor	Other testis neoplasm	Epidermoid cyst
Ross et al [39]	92	244	41	13
Ciftci et al [33]	9	26	3	3
Metcalfe et al [34]	43	16	4	10
Total	144	286	48	26

elevated or inguinal adenopathy is present, then an abdominal and pelvic CT scan should be obtained preoperatively. Interpretation of retroperitoneal adenopathy may be more difficult after orchiectomy due to reactive enlargement of regional lymph nodes from the procedure. Prepubertal boys who have normal serum markers and ultrasound findings consistent with teratomas or epidermoid cysts may be considered for testis-sparing surgery. Inguinal approach with early vascular control is recommended before mobilization of the testis into the field. Most investigators do not comment specifically on the technique of warm or cold ischemia. In their series of 32 testis-preserving resections in adults, Steiner and colleagues [40] advocate 5 minutes of immersion of the testis in crushed ice before occlusion of the spermatic cord. If there is a clear demarcation between normal testicular parenchyma and neoplasm, then enucleation of the tumor or excision of the tumor with a rim of normal parenchyma may be undertaken. It is important not to violate the tumor capsule in situ. If no clear definition is seen between normal parenchyma and neoplasm, then orchiectomy should be undertaken. For those lesions confirmed to be benign by frozen-section analysis, the remnant testis may be returned to the scrotum. For malignant lesions, high ligation of the cord and orchiectomy should be completed. In one series, 13 boys, including 7 who had teratomas, were treated with testis-preserving surgery [34]. Follow-up ranged from 11 months to 14 years with no evidence of recurrence. Eight boys had follow-up ultrasound, with mean testicular volume of 85% on the operated side compared with the undisturbed side. The concept of testis-sparing resection has not been recommended in postpubertal boys who have suspected germ cell tumors due to the increased incidence of mixed tumors with malignant elements, the high incidence of carcinoma in situ (CIS), and the risk of recurrence as malignancy after resection of previous teratoma [34,39]. CIS of the testis is also called testicular intraepithelial neoplasia. It is the acknowledged precursor of testicular germ cell tumors in men but is rare in infantile testis tumor patients. CIS is found in testicular tissue adjacent to testis tumors in up to 90% of adults [41]. If left untreated, 50% will progress to invasive malignancy within 5 years. It is not sensitive to systemic chemotherapy but can be obliterated by radiotherapy. Endocrine function is preserved in about 75% of men who have testicular radiation for CIS but infertility should be expected [41]. The concept of testis-sparing surgery in postpubertal males who have germ cell tumors has been selectively considered in some centers for patients who have a solitary testis to preserve endocrine function and occasionally fertility. Steiner and colleagues [40] in Austria reported 32 testis-sparing procedures in adults, and Heidenreich and coworkers [42] in Germany reported similar procedures in 73 men who had single testis or bilateral testicular tumors. Monorchism may be congenital or a consequence of torsion, trauma, or previous testicular neoplasm. The incidence of synchronous or metachronous bilaterality for testis tumors is 3.5% [43]. Steiner and colleagues' [40] series of 30 men followed strict criteria for size and location of tumor, preoperative endocrine function, and management of coexisting CIS. The high prevalence of CIS in men who have germ cell tumor of the testis mandates radiation in most patients. Because CIS is a manifestation of early malignancy with very high prevalence, orchiectomy is still recommended for patients who have a healthy contralateral testis. In Heidenreich's series, the testis-sparing approach was only considered in patients who had isolated testis, favorable characteristics for preserved endocrine function, and anticipated compliance with need for long-term follow-up.

For prepubertal boys who have suspected malignancy and all postpubertal boys who have any germ cell tumors, radical orchiectomy is recommended with early high ligation of the cord. A scrotal approach is not advised and has been associated with a significant incidence of scrotal recurrence in most reported series [33,35].

Stage I tumors are those localized to the testis with intact capsule, negative margins, and appropriate fall in tumor markers after removal. For boys who have stage I tumors, radical orchiectomy and close follow-up without chemotherapy are recommended. The recently completed Pediatric Oncology Group (POG)/Children's Cancer Study Group (CCG) intergroup protocol using this approach included 63 boys who had stage I disease [35]. All had endodermal sinus (yolk sac) tumor and only 2 had associated immature teratoma components. The mean age in this series was 16 months, with age ranging from 1 month to 5.6 years. The overall survival rate at 6-year follow-up was 100%. Fifty boys (78.8%) had event-free survival and were spared exposure to chemotherapy. The remaining 13 boys had relapse with tumor and were successfully salvaged with platinum-based chemotherapy. For boys who have stage III to IV malignant germ cell tumors of the testis, radical orchiectomy followed by platinum-based chemotherapy is recommended. Routine retroperitoneal lymph node dissection is not required [7,39,44]. Previous studies have documented low yield, no survival benefit, and significant complication rates from routine retroperitoneal lymph node dissection in prepubertal patients [45]. The POG/CCG intergroup study for high-risk malignant germ cell tumors in children and adolescents included 60 boys who had stage II to IV testicular germ cell tumors [7]. All were treated with radical orchiectomy and chemotherapy including cisplatin, etoposide, and bleomycin (PEB). Routine retroperitoneal lymph node dissection was not recommended. Patients who had persistent evidence of disease after chemotherapy underwent surgical exploration with excisional biopsy or dissection. Age ranged from 0.6 to 19.3 years. Histology varied by age, with pure yolk sac tumor in 82% of boys younger than 15 years and mixed malignant germ cell tumors in 80% of boys 15 years or older. The overall survival rate was 93.3%, with no significant difference by platinum dose. It is important to note that five of six failures from tumor progression were seen in boys over age 15 years who had mixed malignant germ cell tumors.

A persisting area of controversy in testicular germ cell tumors is determination of the threshold for management using adult standards. Urologic reviews often refer to puberty as the determining factor, with histologic confirmation of pubertal changes in the resected specimen in transitional age groups [34,39]. The stage I and II pediatric intergroup trials sponsored by POG and CCG offered eligibility to patients younger than 10 years; all enrolled subjects were younger than 6 years. The stage III and IV POG/CCG protocols were open to patients up to age 21 years and included subjects ranging from less than 1 to 19 years. It will be important in future studies to design study arms for adolescents and to track not only age but pubertal staging and biologic data as demographic information.

Ovarian germ cell tumors

Germ cell tumors are the most common neoplasms of the ovary in childhood and adolescence, representing 67% to 87% of pediatric ovarian tumors [46–48]. If the neonatal age group is excluded, the risk of germ cell malignancy in pediatric and adolescent ovarian neoplasms is 20% [49]. This relatively high incidence of malignancy means that all pediatric ovarian neoplasms should be approached with the possibility of malignancy in mind. The preoperative finding of elevated AFP or β-HCG confirms malignancy, but tumors with pure germinoma or embryonal carcinoma have normal markers. Approximately 11% [49,50] of girls present with an acute abdomen secondary to torsion or rupture of an ovarian tumor; however, serum markers are not available at time of operation to aid in decision making. Most of the remaining pediatric ovarian tumors are benign teratomas. These tumors occur throughout childhood but are most frequent in school-aged girls and adolescents.

Assessment of information regarding ovarian tumors in the pediatric age group is difficult because of the low incidence of these tumors, the heterogeneity of inclusion parameters in reported series (neonatal patients, nonneoplastic cysts), and series deliberately focused on only one histologic subtype. The entity of immature teratoma without overt malignant elements is also problematic due to their unpredictable behavior. Several European series include high-grade immature teratoma in their series of malignant ovarian tumors [5,6,51]. Adult ovarian cancer principles are often applied to children even though adult ovarian cancer is generally epithelial based with different patterns of spread and sensitivity to chemotherapy.

An example of this confusion is seen in the frequently quoted malignancy risk of 2% for cystic ovarian lesions. This statistic is often mentioned in pediatric reviews of ovarian tumors [52–54] without confirmation in the data presented. The data supporting this statement were derived from a single series of mainly women thought to have benign cystic teratomas. At histologic examination, 2% were found to have secondary malignant degeneration of epithelial elements [55]. The true risk of malignancy in pediatric ovarian neoplasms with a cystic component is unknown. In the recently reported

POG/CCG series of 131 girls younger than 20 years who had malignant germ cell tumors, at least 75 had a grossly cystic component to their tumor. This subgroup included patients who had pure malignant histology and many who had mixed tumors including benign teratoma elements. Overall, 60 of 131 girls had malignant tumors that contained some areas of benign teratoma [49]. In the absence of direct invasion of neighboring structures, there were no gross features that helped to distinguish these tumors from purely benign lesions.

The POG/CCG study also examined yield of the various staging maneuvers at laparotomy for ovarian tumors in children. The previous guidelines had been based on adult principles and were seldom followed completely. Ascitic cytology was obtained in 100 girls and was positive for malignant cells in 25%. Random biopsy samples of normal-appearing omentum, lymph nodes, peritoneum, and contralateral ovary were consistently negative. Biopsy of abnormal structures had variable confirmation of malignancy. Based on these findings, the surgical guidelines for future Children's Oncology Group studies of ovarian germ cell tumors in pediatric patients have been modified (Box 2).

Before the advent of chemotherapy, the prognosis for malignant germ cell tumors of the ovary in children was dismal, even for patients suspected to have limited disease. Some of the fatalities in girls believed to have limited disease may have been due to failure to recognize overtly malignant elements in large immature teratomas. The availability of the tumor markers AFP and β-HCG has allowed more accurate inclusion of endodermal sinus and choriocarcinoma-containing tumors in the malignant category and provides a mechanism to monitor for persistent or recurrent occult disease. The continuing evolution of platinum-based chemotherapy has been extremely effective in treating these tumors. The TGM 85 and 90 protocols in France for nonseminomatous ovarian germ cell tumors [50] used a six-drug regimen

---

Box 2. Children's Oncology Group surgical guidelines for ovarian germ cell tumors in pediatric patients

1. Ascites for cytology or peritoneal washings if no ascites present
2. Inspect omentum; resect only if abnormal
3. Inspect and palpate iliac and para-aortocaval nodes; perform biopsy only if abnormal
4. Inspect and palpate contralateral ovary; perform biopsy only if abnormal
5. No violation of tumor capsule in situ for resectable tumors
6. Primary resection for localized tumors; perform biopsy only if resection would require sacrifice of other organs and plan for postchemotherapy resection

including VAC and carboplatin/etoposide/bleomycin (JEB) or PEB. Conservative surgery was strongly encouraged. The 5-year overall survival rate for secreting tumors was 84%. The United Kingdom experience with JEB therapy revealed a 5-year survival rate of 93.2% for ovarian tumors [6]. The POG/CCG intergroup study using PEB therapy with randomization of platinum dose in stage III and IV patients had overall survival rates of 95.1% for stage I, 93.8% for stage II, 98.3% for stage III, and 93.3% for stage IV ovarian tumors [49].

The European studies have pioneered the concept of surgery and careful follow-up without chemotherapy for stage I malignant germ cell tumors at sites other than the infant testis [4–6,51,56]. Dark and colleagues [56] reported 9 girls who had germinoma and six who had endodermal sinus tumor treated initially with surgery only. Recurrence was seen in 2 of 6 with endodermal sinus and 3 of 9 with germinoma. One died of pulmonary embolus while on chemotherapy, but all others survived. The TGM studies in France [50] included 12 girls who had secreting tumors treated with surgery only; 6 relapsed. Five of 6 were salvaged with chemotherapy. The current Children's Oncology Group protocol for malignant germ cell tumors is also evaluating the role of surgery and surveillance for well-documented stage I malignant germ cell tumors of the ovary. Eligibility for the observation arm requires that all staging guidelines be followed completely.

The concept of fertility preservation and organ-sparing surgery for ovarian tumors should be considered in girls in a similar manner to the concept of testis preservation in boys for selected tumors. The risk of synchronous or metachronous benign teratomas of the ovary in childhood is around 5% [9]. The POG/CCG series of 131 girls who had malignant ovarian germ cell tumors included 4 patients who had a contralateral teratoma and 7 who had a contralateral malignancy. With relatively small tumors, it is often possible to dissect a plane between the tumor capsule and normal ovarian parenchyma. In Templeman and colleagues' series of 52 girls who had mature cystic teratoma, 48% were able to undergo removal of the tumor with ovary preservation [57]. In girls who have small tumors suggestive of teratoma and normal preoperative serum markers, enucleation of the tumor with preservation of the ovary may be considered. There is an increased risk of tumor rupture with enucleation, especially in laparoscopic cases. In Templeman and colleagues' [57] series of teratomas, rupture occurred in 92.8% of laparoscopic cases and in 36.8% of open cases. If the tumor is large, if markers are elevated or unknown, or if no clear demarcation exists between tumor and normal parenchyma, then oophorectomy should be done.

Other extragonadal germ cell tumors

Germ cell tumors may occur in many other anatomic locations and are most often para-axial. Although the sacrococcygeal site is most common, most of the remaining extragonadal tumors occur in the mediastinum, retroperitoneum, and genital regions. Other rare sites include neck, oral cavity, and stomach [58–60].

Germ cell tumors arising in the mediastinum and retroperitoneum tend to be undetected until they have reached a very large size. Most of these will be benign teratomas [61], which provides a therapeutic surgical challenge because tumor shrinkage by chemotherapy may not be an option. As in all other cases of suspected germ cell tumor, AFP and β-HCG should be obtained preoperatively. Initial biopsy samples should be obtained for tumors that are large and for which resection is considered to be hazardous. Needle biopsy has been successful in some reported cases [62]. Chemotherapy has been extremely successful in reducing tumor bulk and in facilitating complete resection of tumors that have malignant components identified by markers or histology. In the POG/CCG intergroup study of malignant mediastinal germ cell tumors, 22 patients had initial biopsy only. Three early deaths occurred. One had complete resolution of the mass with chemotherapy and survived without definitive surgery. The remaining 18 patients had sufficient reduction in tumor size to allow complete resection after chemotherapy [62]. In a similar fashion, the POG/CCG intergroup study of retroperitoneal malignant germ cell tumors included 25 children, with 20 initially treated with partial debulking or biopsy only. Chemotherapy was again successful in most of these children, with complete resolution of the mass in 5 and successful resection in 12. There were two early deaths and one in a child in whom a large mass persisted (biopsy samples showed areas of benign teratoma, and further resection was not attempted, with eventual death) [63].

The general philosophy for surgical approach to germ cell tumors of the mediastinum and retroperitoneum should be conservative at diagnosis, with biopsy only for large tumors. For those with elevated tumor markers or histologic confirmation of malignancy, neoadjuvant chemotherapy should be undertaken before attempt at resection (with high expectation of tumor shrinkage). For benign tumors and for persisting masses after chemotherapy, an aggressive surgical approach should be undertaken. Mixed tumors with components of malignant and mature teratoma are more common in mediastinal (61%) than in retroperitoneal (16%) sites.

Germ cell tumors of the genital region are most often endodermal sinus tumors in girls younger than 3 years. These tumors present with vaginal bleeding or symptoms of bowel and bladder dysfunction. Previous experience with malignant germ cell tumors at this site consisted of radical resection at diagnosis, and poor outcome was expected. As in all other sites of malignant germ cell tumors in children, current platinum therapy has dramatically changed survival and functional outcome. Of 13 children who had genital primary in the POG/CCG intergroup study, 11 had extensive tumors at diagnosis and had initial biopsy with neoadjuvant chemotherapy. Two had complete resolution of mass and 9 underwent conservative surgical procedures with organ preservation and successful outcome [64].

Summary

Germ cell tumors in childhood are heterogeneous in histology, age at presentation, and anatomic site. Although most are benign, the possibility of malignancy should be considered at all sites. The overall prognosis for malignant germ cell tumors has improved dramatically with the advent of platinum-based therapy. Current surgical approach to malignant tumors at all sites should be conservative at diagnosis, with resection of only those tumors that can be removed without excessive risk of hemorrhage or damage to surrounding structures. Surgical approach for malignant tumors that persist after chemotherapy should be aggressive, with many having only residual benign teratoma components. For benign gonadal tumors, the possibility of enucleation with gonad preservation should be considered in select cases. The prognosis for sacrococcygeal teratoma is lower when diagnosed in utero than when it is diagnosed postnatally. Solid tumors and evidence of hydrops are poor prognostic factors.

References

[1] Teilum G. Classification of endodermal sinus tumor (mesoblastoma vitellinum) and so called "embryonal carcinoma" of the ovary. Acta Pathol Microbiol Scand 1965;64:407–29.

[2] Sobis H, Vandeputte M. Sequential morphological study of teratomas derived from displayed yolk sac. Dev Biol 1975;45:276–90.

[3] Brown NJ. Teratomas and yolk sac tumors. J Clin Pathol 1976;29:1021–5.

[4] Baranzelli MC, Flamant F, De Lumley L, et al. Treatment of non-metastatic, non-seminomatous malignant germ-cell tumour in childhood: experience of the "Société Francaise d'Oncologie Pédiatrique" MGCT 1985–1989 Study. Med Pediatr Oncol 1993;21:395–401.

[5] Göbel U, Schneider DT, Calaminus G, et al. Germ-cell tumors in childhood and adolescence. Ann Oncol 2000;11(3):263–71.

[6] Mann JR, Raafat F, Robinson K, et al. The United Kingdom Children's Cancer Study Group's second germ cell tumor study: carboplatin, etoposide, and bleomycin are effective treatment for children with malignant extracranial germ cell tumors, with acceptable toxicity. J Clin Oncol 2000;18(22):3809–18.

[7] Cushing B, Giller R, Cullen J, et al. Randomized comparison of combination chemotherapy with etoposide, bleomycin, and either high-dose or standard-dose cisplatin in children and adolescents with high-risk malignant germ cell tumors: a Pediatric Intergroup Study (POG 9049 and CCG 8882). J Clin Oncol 2004;22(13):2691–700.

[8] Schmidt B, Haberlik A, Uray E, et al. Sacrococcygeal teratoma: clinical course and prognosis with a special view to long-term functional results. Pediatr Surg Int 1999;15:573–6.

[9] Grosfeld JL, Billmire DF. Teratomas in infancy and childhood. Cur Prob Cancer 1985;1(9): 1–53.

[10] Altman RP, Randolph JG, Lilly JR. Sacrococcygeal teratoma: American Academy of Pediatrics Surgical Section Survey—1973. J Pediatr Surg 1974;9:389–98.

[11] Flake AW. Fetal sacrococcygeal teratoma. Sem Pediatr Surg 1993;2(2):113–20.

[12] Holterman AX, Filliatrault D, Lallier M, et al. The natural history of sacrococcygeal teratomas diagnosed through routine obstetric sonogram: a single institution experience. J Pediatr Surg 1998;33(6):899–903.

[13] Chisholm CA, Heider AL, Kuller JA, et al. Prenatal diagnosis and perinatal management of fetal sacrococcygeal teratoma. Am J Perinatol 1999;16(1):47–50.

[14] Westerburg B, Feldstein VA, Sandberg PL, et al. Sonographic prognostic factors in fetuses with sacrococcygeal teratoma. J Pediatr Surg 2000;35(2):322–6.

[15] Olutoye OO, Johnson MP, Coleman BG, et al. Abnormal umbilical cord dopplers may predict impending demise in fetuses with sacrococcygeal teratoma: a report of 2 cases. Fetal Diagn Ther 2003;18:428–31.

[16] Hedrick HL, Flake AW, Crombleholme TM, et al. Sacrococcygeal teratoma: prenatal assessment, fetal intervention, and outcome. J Pediatr Surg 2004;39(3):430–8.

[17] Gross RE, Clatworthy HW, Mecker IA. Sacrococcygeal teratomas in infants and children: a report of 40 cases. Surg Gynecol Obstet 1951;92:341–54.

[18] Lindahl H. Giant sacrococcygeal teratoma: a method of simple intraoperative control of hemorrhage. J Pediatr Surg 1988;23(11):1068–9.

[19] Robertson FM, Crombleholme TM, Frantz ID III, et al. Devascularization and staged resection of giant sacrococcygeal teratoma in the premature infant. J Pediatr Surg 1995; 30(2):309–11.

[20] Angel CA, Murillo C, Mayhew J. Experience with vascular control before excision of giant, highly vascular sacrococcygeal teratomas in neonates. J Pediatr Surg 1998;33(12): 1840–2.

[21] Kamata S, Imura K, Kubota A, et al. Operative management for sacrococcygeal teratoma diagnosis in utero. J Pediatr Surg 2001;36(4):545–8.

[22] Fishman SJ, Jennings RW, Johnson SM, et al. Contouring buttock reconstruction after sacrococcygeal teratoma resection. J Pediatr Surg 2004;39(3):439–41.

[23] Rescorla FJ, Sawin RS, Coran AG, et al. Long-term outcome for infants and children with sacrococcygeal teratoma: a report from the Children's Cancer Group. J Ped Surg 1998;33(2): 171–6.

[24] Huddart SN, Mann JR, Robinson K, et al. Sacrococcygeal teratomas: the UK Children's Cancer Study Group's experience. I. Neonatal. Pediatr Surg Int 2003;19:47–51.

[25] Göbel U, Schneider DT, Calaminus G, et al. Multimedia treatment of malignant sacrococcygeal germ cell tumors: a prospective analysis of 66 patients of the German Cooperative Protocols MAKEI 83/86 and 89. J Clin Oncol 2001;19(7):1943–50.

[26] Rescorla F, Billmire DF, Stolar C, et al. The effect of cisplatin dose and surgical resection in children with malignant germ cell tumors at the sacrococcygeal region: a pediatric intergroup trial (POG/CCG 8882). J Pediatr Surg 2001;36:12–7.

[27] Malone PS, Spitz L, Kiely EM, et al. The functional sequelae of sacrococcygeal teratoma. J Pediatr Surg 1990;25(6):679–80.

[28] Havránek P, Hedlund H, Rubenson A, et al. Sacrococcygeal teratoma in Sweden between 1978 and 1989: long-term functional results. J Pediatr Surg 1992;27(7):916–8.

[29] Lahdenne P, Wikström S, Heikinheimo M, et al. Late urologic sequelae after surgery for congenital sacrococcygeal teratoma. Pediatr Surg Int 1992;7:195–8.

[30] Rintala R, Lahdenne P, Lindahl H, et al. Anorectal function in adults operated for a benign sacrococcygeal teratoma. J Pediatr Surg 1993;28(9):1165–7.

[31] Boemers TML, van Gool JD, de Jong TPVM, et al. Lower urinary tract dysfunction in children with benign sacrococcygeal teratoma. J Urol 1994;151:174–6.

[32] Walsh C, Rushton HG. Diagnosis and management of teratomas and epidermoid cysts. Ped Urol Oncol 2000;27(3):509–18.

[33] Ciftci AO, Bingöl-Koloğu M, Senocak ME, et al. Testicular tumors in children. J Pediatr Surg 2001;36(12):1796–801.

[34] Metcalfe PD, Farivar-Mohseni H, Farhat W, et al. Pediatric testicular tumors: contemporary incidence and efficacy of testicular preserving surgery. J Urol 2003;170:2412–6.

[35] Schlatter M, Rescorla F, Giller R, et al. Excellent outcome in patients with stage I germ cell tumors of the testes: a case study of the Children's Cancer Group/Pediatric Oncology Group. J Pediatr Surg 2003;35:319–24.

[36] Ravitch MM. Embryonal carcinoma of testicle in childhood: review of literature and presentation of 2 cases. J Urol 1966;96:501–7.

[37] Rushton HG, Belman AB, Sesterhenn I, et al. Testicular sparing surgery for prepubertal teratoma of the testis: a clinical and pathological study. J Urol 1990;144:726–36.

[38] Pearse I, Glick RD, Abramson SJ, et al. Testicular-sparing surgery for benign testicular tumors. J Pediatr Surg 1999;34(6):1000–3.

[39] Ross JH, Rybicki L, Kay R. Clinical behavior and a contemporary management algorithm for prepubertal testis tumors: a summary of the prepubertal testis tumor registry. J Urol 2002;168:1675–9.

[40] Steiner H, Holtl L, Maneschg C, et al. Frozen section analysis-guided organ-sparing approach in testicular tumors: technique, feasibility, and long-term results. Urology 2003; 62(3):508–13.

[41] Dieckmann KP, Skakkebaek NE. Carcinoma in situ of the testis: review of biological and clinical features. Int J Cancer 1999;l83:815–22.

[42] Heidenreich A, Weißbach L, Höltl W, et al. Organ sparing surgery for malignant germ cell tumors of the testis. J Urol 2001;166:2161–5.

[43] Bokemeyer C, Schmoll HJ, Schöffski P, et al. Bilateral testicular tumours: prevalence and clinical implications. Eur J Cancer 1993;29A(6):874–6.

[44] Grady RW. Current management of prepubertal yolk sac tumors of the testis. Pediatr Urol Oncol 2000;27(3):503–8.

[45] Grady RW, Ross JH, Kay R. Patterns of metastatic spread in prepubertal yolk sac tumor of the testis. J Urol 1995;153:1259–61.

[46] von Allmen D. Malignant lesions of the ovary in childhood. Sem Pediatr Surg 2005;14: 100–5.

[47] Cass DL, Hawkins E, Brandt ML, et al. Surgery for ovarian masses in infants, children, and adolescents: 102 consecutive patients treated in a 15-year period. J Pediatr Surg 2001;36: 693–9.

[48] Morowitz M, Huff D, von Allmen D. Epithelial ovarian tumors in children: a retrospective analysis. J Pediatr Surg 2003;38(3):331–5.

[49] Billmire D, Vinocur C, Rescorla F, et al. Outcome and staging evaluation in malignant germ cell tumors of the ovary in children and adolescents: an intergroup study. J Pediatr Surg 2004;39(3):424–9.

[50] Baranzelli MC, Bouffet E, Quintana E, et al. Non-seminomatous ovarian germ cell tumours in children. Eur J Cancer 2000;36:376–83.

[51] Baranzelli MC, Kramar A, Bouffet E, et al. Prognostic factors in children with localized malignant nonseminomatous germ cell tumors. J Clin Oncol 1999;17(4):1212–8.

[52] Silva PD, Ripple J. Outpatient minilaparotomy ovarian cystectomy for benign teratomas in teenagers. J Pediatr Surg 1996;31:1383–6.

[53] Cohen Z, Shinhar D, Kopernik G, et al. The laparoscopic approach to uterine adnexal torsion in childhood. J Pediatr Surg 1996;31(11):1557–9.

[54] Nezhat C, Winer WK, Nezhat F. Instruments and methods—laparoscopic removal of dermoid cysts. Obstet Gynecol 1989;73:278–80.

[55] Peterson WF, Prevost EC, Edmunds FT, et al. Benign cystic teratomas of the ovary; a clinico-statistical study of 100 cases with a review of literature. Am J Obstet Gynecol 1955;70(2):368–82.

[56] Dark GG, Bower M, Newlands ES, et al. Surveillance policy for stage I ovarian germ cell tumors. J Clin Oncol 1997;15(2):620–4.

[57] Templemann CL, Hertweck SP, Scheetz JP, et al. The management of mature cystic teratomas in children and adolescents: a retrospective analysis. Hum Reprod 2000;15(12): 2669–72.

[58] Elmasalme F, Giacomantonio M, Clarke KD, et al. Congenital cervical teratomas in neonates: case report and review. Eur J Pediatr Surg 2000;10(4):252–7.

[59] Corapcioglu F, Ekingen G, Sarper N, et al. Immature gastric teratomas of childhood: a case report and review of the literature. J Pediatr Gastroenterol Nutr 2004;39(3): 292–4.

[60] Maeda K, Yamamoto T, Yoshimara H, et al. Epignathus: a report of two neonatal cases. J Pediatr Surg 1989;24(4):395–7.

[61] Lack EE, Travis WD, Welch KJ. Retroperitoneal germ cell tumors in childhood: a clinical and pathologic study of 11 cases. Cancer 1985;56:602–8.

[62] Billmire D, Vinocur C, Rescorla F, et al. Malignant mediastinal germ cell tumors: an intergroup study. J Pediatr Surg 2001;36(1):18–24.

[63] Bilmire D, Vinocur C, Rescorla F, et al. Malignant retroperitoneal and abdominal germ cell tumors: an intergroup study. J Pediatr Surg 2003;38(3):315–8.

[64] Rescorla F, Billmire D, Vinocur C, et al. The effect of neoadjuvant chemotherapy and surgery in children with malignant germ cell tumors of the genital region: a pediatric intergroup trial. J Pediatr Surg 2003;38(6):910–2.

SURGICAL
CLINICS OF
NORTH AMERICA

ELSEVIER
SAUNDERS

Surg Clin N Am 86 (2006) 505–514

Bowel Management for Patients with Myelodysplasia

Edward Doolin, MD

Children's Hospital of Pennsylvania, 34th & Civic Center Blvd., University of Pennsylvania,
Philadelphia, PA 19104, USA

Children born with menigomyelocele have a compendium of neurologic disorders including a disrupted defecation process. Many of the multiple factors that contribute to an effective bowel movement are altered in meningomyelocele [1,2]; however, aggressive and proactive management using mechanical and pharmacologic therapies can result in functional and continent patients.

The normal bowel movement requires a balance of many factors. Anal tone is the most obvious component, whereby the internal anal sphincter function is controlled by a balance of the sympathetic and parasympathetic nervous system. This creates a tonic anal tone, which can relax to allow defecation. The extent and nature of this dysfunction is variable and difficult to measure [3]. Stool consistency depends on colon function and transit. Slow colon transit, variable absorption, and stasis can result in stool retention, which in turn can lead to stool dehydration, bacterial overgrowth, and impaction.

The Valsalva maneuver is a mechanical effort that can facilitate the passage of feces. Although the colon and rectum have an intrinsic motility, it is weak and often less effective when large amounts of stool dilate the organ. A Valsalva maneuver is an adjunct that creates a large transanal pressure gradient. The diaphragm, abdominal musculature, and pelvic floor all contribute to this pressure; however, the skeletal muscles of the abdomen are weak in patients who have meningomyelocele, which makes the Valsalva maneuver less effective.

Intrinsic motility, mobility, and stool consistency—all are tools to optimize bowel function and can be assessed and modified to create a management program [4–6].

E-mail address: doolin@email.chop.edu

0039-6109/06/$ - see front matter © 2006 Elsevier Inc. All rights reserved.
doi:10.1016/j.suc.2005.12.009   *surgical.theclinics.com*

Mechanical purgatives

Mechanical purgatives take advantage of the use of high volumes of a solution to induce colon evacuation. This approach may seem like the most aggressive and invasive of the cleansing regimens; however, because the main mechanisms by which it works are volume and hydrostatic pressure as opposed to bowel stimulation, it is one of the gentler approaches to bowel cleansing. In addition, this technique does not depend on bowel motility and a strong abdominal compartment to be effective [7,8].

The fundamentals of this technique are simple and straightforward. A high volume of an isotonic solution is placed within the rectum or the proximal colon. The voluminous solution has the effect of dissolving and softening the stool. It also has the effect of increasing the hydrostatic pressure proximal to the stool, which causes the stool to be evacuated.

There are three basic approaches to deliver this program. The first is the use of an enema (Fig. 1). A child who has myelodysplasia often has a good functioning internal anal sphincter but poorly functioning pelvic skeletal muscles. The skeletal muscles are important for the ability to voluntarily contract the anus and retain an enema. Children who have myelodysplasia find this voluntary contraction difficult, if not impossible. A method that may be useful is to temporarily obstruct the anus with a large balloon (Fig. 2) [9]. This method allows the infusion of the high-volume solution with minimal leakage around the anus, and the solution can be delivered well up into the transverse colon. The balloon can be maintained after the solution has been delivered to allow for dissolving the stool. When the balloon is released, the solution is evacuated. Evacuation can be assisted with voluntary Valsalva maneuver and manual abdominal compressions.

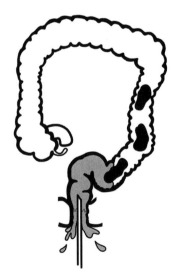

Fig. 1. Retrograde enema using a routine nonobstructing catheter.

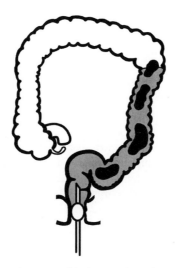

Fig. 2. Retrograde enema with the use of an obstructing balloon.

The second technique is to deliver the solutions transrectally by using an elongated enema tube to deliver the solution to the transverse colon (Fig. 3) [10]. The tortuosity of the sigmoid colon sometimes makes this delivery difficult; however, when it is possible, it is easier and safer to deliver a large-volume enema proximal to the stool to be evacuated. After the solution is delivered, voluntary Valsalva maneuver or evacuation with manual abdominal compressions can be performed.

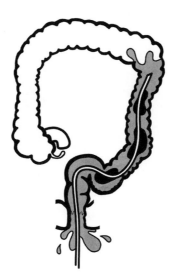

Fig. 3. The delivery of an enema solution using an elongated tube to directly place the solution in the transverse colon.

The ability to deliver the enemas using the previous techniques can be compromised if the patient has to do it on his or her own. Mobility often inhibited in the patient who has lumbosacral myelodysplasia, and the difficulty in transferring from a wheelchair and in reaching the perineal area without assistance often makes these enemas challenging to administer. Because of physical disabilities or body habitus, many of these patients have difficulty reaching the anus or attempting to manipulate a catheter into the anus. An option, when the independence of the patient and the setting in which the enema is given are restrictive, is to offer an antegrade continent enema (ACE) [11–13]. An antegrade enema is a method that allows the delivery of a large-volume enema to the ascending and transverse colon (Fig. 4). The advantage of this method is easy access so that a patient who has myelodysplasia can perform it alone.

The techniques for the ACE are multiple. A popular technique is to create an appendicostomy with a reversed appendix [14,15]. Tube cecostomy and appliances can also be used with equal success [16]. Each has their advantages and disadvantages. The advantages of an appendicostomy are that it minimizes leakage and avoids the need for an appliance. The disadvantages are that it often narrows, is sometimes difficult to catheterize, and occasionally requires revision. The appliances are easy to use but have to be changed from time to time and, in the long run, often leak.

The prerequisites for a successful ACE procedure include an anatomically correct cecum and appendix or appliance, the ability to deliver the enema, a uniformly dynamic colon that will propel the affluent, and finally and most important, previous success on a retrograde transrectal bowel regimen. It is critical to realize that the ACE procedure only offers a convenient way to deliver an enema to the right and transverse colon. It does not improve the effectiveness of the enema. The patient who fails the use of retrograde

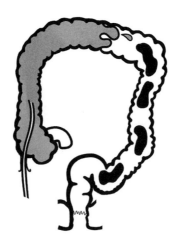

Fig. 4. An antegrade enema that delivers an enema to the ascending and transverse colon using a catheter or stoma placed in the proximal colon.

enemas for nontechnical reasons will likely not have a better outcome with the ACE procedure.

Diet and fiber

The use of dietary supplements is important in the optimal management of children who have myelodysplasia. As mentioned earlier, these patients have an inherent dysmotility and an inherent sensation abnormality. A certain amount of "organ training" is required to allow the bowel to function optimally, which necessitates minimal variability in the volume, consistency, and nature of the stool. In addition, the propensity for bacterial overgrowth must be minimized by maintaining the proper transit and water content of the stool. The easiest way to accomplish this is through dietary supplementation of soluble fiber. The addition of soluble fiber is effective in the control of the water content of the stool and in optimizing the volume and consistency of the stool [17].

Fiber is the part of food that is an indigestible complex sugar. Most children do not eat enough fiber on a daily basis to influence bowel habits. As a result, a child who has myelodysplasia may require supplements. There are two types of fiber: soluble and insoluble. Soluble fiber retains water in the intestines, which optimizes the transit time of stool. This time allows the stool to bulk up and evacuate from the colon. Insoluble fiber draws water into the intestine and increases the transit time of stool. As a result, the amount and frequency of stools may increase. When insoluble fiber is taken in excess, it can lead to cramping.

Although it is important to include both types of fiber in one's diet, successful management in children who have constipation requires adequate intake of soluble fiber. In children who have constipation, it is important that they receive 10 g of soluble fiber per day. This amount may be difficult to obtain from diet alone, and a dietary supplement is often necessary. Table 1 lists fiber supplements that are effective and easy to use.

Table 1
Fiber supplements

Brand name	Soluble fiber	Source
Benefiber	3/packet	Powder (tasteless)
Citrucil	2 g/dose	Powder
CVS brand fiber powder	2 g/Tbsp	Powder
Fiber Choice	4 g/tablet	Chewable tablets
Juice and Fiber	10 g	Juice
Juice and Fiber Cookie	3 g	Cookie (choc. chip, vanilla, oatmeal)
Metamucil (orange flavor)	2.4 g/Tbsp	Powder
Metamucil Wafer (apple or cinnamon)	3 g/2 wafers	Wafer
Metamucil (regular flavor)	2.4 g/tsp	Powder
Rite Aid brand fiber	2 g/Tbsp	Powder

Abbreviations: choc., chocolate; Tbsp, tablespoon; tsp, teaspoon.

Using natural sources of fiber is another option; however, it is difficult for many reasons. First, the ability to completely delineate and understand the type and amount of fiber in various natural foods can be challenging. How recipes are prepared, including the type and extent of cooking, also complicates the calculation of fiber. Second, there is a difficult lifestyle issue in trying to constantly control a diet when the circumstances are constantly changing, such as being at work, at school, and so forth. Finally, trying to develop such an optimal diet can be expensive. The regular use of these foods, however, aids colon health and stool consistency. Foods containing soluble and insoluble fiber are listed in Table 2.

The use of diet is a prerequisite, not a treatment, for the dysmotility of the bowel in myelodysplasia. The diet itself is not effective; purgatives and laxatives are always needed. Trying to "compromise" good function leads to deterioration of the colon.

Table 2
Fiber component of foods

Source	Amount
Soluble fiber	
Oat bran	2 g/oz
Whole wheat bread	0.3 g/slice
White bread	0.3 g/slice
Spaghetti	1.3 g/2 oz
Beans, kidney	2.9 g/0.5 cup
Carrots	1.1 g/0.5 cup
Broccoli	1.4 g/0.5 cup
Bananas	0.7 g/medium size
Grapefruit	2.3 g/medium size
Grapes	0.6 g/cup
Apricots	2 g/cup
Strawberries	3.4 g/cup
Apples	1 g/medium size
Pear (with peel)	2.2 g/medium
Blackberries	1.4 g/cup
Insoluble fiber	
Bran cereal	8.9 g/oz
Corn flakes	1 g/oz
Whole wheat bread	1.6 g/slice
White bread	0.3 g/slice
Broccoli	1.4 g/0.5 cup
Carrots	1.5 g/0.5 cup
Peas	3.1 g/0.5 cup
Potatoes, brown (with skin)	0.9 g/0.5 cup
Green beans	0.8 g/0.5 cup
Apple (with skin)	2.8 g/medium size
Blueberries	3.5 g/cup
Banana	2.1 g/medium size
Pears (with skin)	1.8 g/medium size

Laxatives

In children who have mild disease, laxatives can be effective and allow for easier management. It must be understood, however, that the colon is the end organ of the laxative, and the defective end organ attenuates the effectiveness of the laxatives. There are several different types of laxatives (Table 3), each with pros and cons.

Bulking agents simply add fiber to the stool to improve transit and make the water content of the stool more consistent, which are important factors in helping these patients who have compromised colon function. The colons of these patients do not have the reserve to deal with stress such as a hard stool or diarrhea. Bulking agents should be part of every patient's management. They are prepared in combination with gentle stimulants. Although this preparation is convenient, it can be difficult to titrate the two components separately when there are changes in the patient's condition.

Emollients such as mineral oil can ease the passage of stool, which may be more important in inflammatory anal disease such as fissure or hemorrhoids. If the anus is normal, other than the meningomyelocoele, then this treatment is not usually needed. Stimulants cause contraction of the colon; they do not add to the relaxation of the sphincter as in a normal child. For low defects with good colon function or in children who have mild symptoms, stimulants can be a good resource. The colons of children who have high lesions and severe constipation, however, do not usually respond to this treatment. High-volume enemas and hyperosmolar stimulants are often the mainstay of treatment in such children. Paradoxically, they are gentler and remain more successful than the stimulants [18].

Adjunctive therapy

Botulinum toxin type A

Botulinum toxin type A has been used successfully in treating detrusor spasm [19–21]. In addition, it has been used successfully to treat Hirschsprung's disease, anal fissure, and constipation. These patients, however, had abnormal anal function as the primary problem. In meningomyelocele,

Table 3
Laxatives

Bulking Agents	Emollients	Softeners in Combination	Stimulants	Hyperosmolar
Benefiber	Mineral Oil	Colace	Ducolax	Saline
Citrucel		Ducolax	ExLax	Fleet Phosphosoda
Fibercon		Kaopectate	Senokot-S	Soap water
Metamucil		Senokot		Glycerine and water
		Pericolace		Milk and Molasses

the sphincter is normal and there is no good published experience with this therapy.

Biofeedback

It has long been speculated that the use of outside stimulation can restore the function of denervated organs. The bladder has been studied extensively and is discussed elsewhere [22,23].

Defecation has a more complex set of stimuli and responses. The nature of stool, activity, voluntary input, and extrinsic and intrinsic stimuli all affect the patient but have never been modified with external stimuli such as electromagnetic field energy or biofeedback [24].

Surgical adjuncts

Children who have memingomyelocoele have a lifelong struggle because of an imbalance between the sluggish colon and the tone of the anus. This imbalance results in chronic constipation. The medical support described previously aids greatly in keeping the person comfortable and regular, affording a normal lifestyle. Over time, however, significant deterioration of the colon is observed. It becomes no longer possible to medically support the patient because of the total lack of responsiveness of the organs. This condition is seen in other settings such as anal fissure, functional constipation, Hirschsprung's disease, and anal atresia. Procedures such as colon reduction, sphincterotomy, and myomectomy have been used in these settings. Although it is occasionally useful to apply these techniques to children who have spina bifida, caution should be applied because of significant but subtle differences among these patients. Acquired megacolon in children who have anal atresia is a problem that causes them to be resistant to medical therapy. Colon reduction is a successful therapy [25]; however, these children have normally functioning proximal colons, and the megacolon is usually only in the sigmoid colon. Children who have myelodysplasia often acquire a diffuse megacolon, which is not as responsive to surgery [26]. Sphincterotomies and myomectomies likewise do not addresss the complex imbalance between the anal muscle and the dystonic colon. The results are usually poor at best and cause complications of incontinence at worst [27].

Summary

Children who have meningomyelocele have a complex and variable problem with neurogenic bowel. Deficits that cause the dysfunction are difficult to quantitate because they have an unpredictable effect on each other and on function. Using diet, medication, activity, and volume purgatives, a good clinical lifestyle can be achieved, but this requires individual tailoring and a great deal of trial and error. Aggressive and careful management by a knowledgeable caretaker can help the myelodysplastic patient who has neurogenic bowel stay clean and maintain a relatively normal social lifestyle.

References

[1] Forsythe WI, Kinley JG. Bowel control of children with spina bifida. Dev Med Child Neurol 1970;12(1):27–31.

[2] Nash DF. Bowel management in spina bifida patients. Proc R Soc Med 1972;65(1):70–1.

[3] Liebman WM. Disorders of defecation in children: evaluation and management. Postgrad Med 1979;66(2):105–10.

[4] Leibold S. A systematic approach to bowel continence for children with spina bifida. Eur J Pediatr Surg 1991;1(Suppl 1):23–4.

[5] Leibold S, Ekmark E, Adams RC. Decision-making for a successful bowel continence program. Eur J Pediatr Surg 2000;10(Suppl 1):26–30.

[6] Doraisamy P. Bowel management in patients with spinal cord lesions. Singapore Med J 1984; 25(2):70–2.

[7] Scholler-Gyure M, Nesselaar C, van Wieringen H, et al. Treatment of defecation disorders by colonic enemas in children with spina bifida. Eur J Pediatr Surg 1996;6(Suppl 1):32–4.

[8] Eire PF, Cives RV, Gago MC. Faecal incontinence in children with spina bifida: the best conservative treatment. Spinal Cord 1998;36(11):774–6.

[9] Shandling B, Gilmour RF. The enema continence catheter in spina bifida: successful bowel management. J Pediatr Surg 1987;22(3):271–3.

[10] Pena A. Advanced in the management of fecal incontinence secondary to anorectal malformations. Surg Annu 1990;22:143–67.

[11] Castellan MA, Gosalbez R, Labbie A, et al. Outcomes of continent catheterizable stomas for urinary and fecal incontinence: comparison among different tissue options. BJU Int 2005; 95(7):1053–7.

[12] Calado AA, Macedo A Jr, Barroso U Jr, et al. The Macedo-Malone antegrade continence enema procedure: early experience. J Urol 2005;173(4):1340–4.

[13] Perez M, Lemelle JL, Barthelme H, et al. Bowel management with antegrade colonic enema using a Malone or a Monti conduit—clinical results. Eur J Pediatr Surg 2001;11(5):315–8.

[14] Tackett LD, Minevich E, Benedict JF, et al. Appendiceal versus ileal segment for antegrade continence enema. J Urol 2002;167(2 pt 1):683–6.

[15] Levitt MA, Soffer SZ, Pena A. Continent appendiscostomy in the bowel management of fecally incontinent children. J Pediatr Surg 1997;32(11):1630–3.

[16] Duel BP, Gonzalez R. The button cecostomy for management of fecal incontinence. Pediatr Surg Int 1999;15(8):559–61.

[17] Forrest D. Management of bladder and bowel in spina bifida. Clin Dev Med 1976;57:122–54.

[18] Wicks K, Shultleff D. Stool management in myelodysplasias and extrophies. In: Shultleff DB, editor. Grune & Stratton; 1986. p. 221–42.

[19] Marte A, Vessella A, Cautiero P, et al. Efficacy of toxin-A botulinum for treating intractable bladder hyperactivity in children affected by neuropathic bladder secondary to myelomeningocele: an alternative to enterocystoplasty. Minerva Pediatr 2005;57(1):35–40.

[20] Riccabona M, Koen M, Schindler M, et al. Botulinum-A toxin injection into the detrusor: a safe alternative in the treatment of children with myelomeningocele with detrusor hyperreflexia. J Urol 2004;171(2 Pt 1):845–8.

[21] Schulte-Baukloh H, Michial T, Schobert J, et al. Efficacy of botulinum-A toxin in children with detrusor hyperreflexia due to myelomeningocele: preliminary results. Urology 2002; 59(3):325–7.

[22] Katona F, Eckstein HB. Treatment of the neuropathic bowel by electrical stimulation of the rectum. Dev Med Child Neurol 1974;16(3):336–9.

[23] Han SW, Kim MJ, Kim JH, et al. Intravesical electrical stimulation improves neurogenic bowel dysfunction in children with spina bifida. J Urol 2004;171(6 pt 2):2648–50.

[24] Marshall DF, Boston VE. Altered bladder and bowel function following cutaneous electrical field stimulation in children with spina bifida—interim results of a randomized double-blind placebo-controlled trial. Eur J Pediatr Surg 1997;7(Suppl 1):41–3.

[25] Pena A, elBehery M. Advances in the management of fecal incontinence secondary to anorectal malformations. Surg Annu 1990;22:143–67.

[26] Mingin GC, Baskin LS. Surgical management of the neurogenic bladder and bowel. Int Braz J Urol 2003;29(1):53–61.

[27] Hardcastle JD, Parks AG. A study of anal incontinence and some principles of surgical treatment. Proc R Soc Med 1970;63(Suppl):116–8.

SURGICAL
CLINICS OF
NORTH AMERICA

ELSEVIER
SAUNDERS

Surg Clin N Am 86 (2006) 515–523

Bladder Management for Patients with Myelodysplasia

Michael C. Carr, MD, PhD[a,b,*]

[a]The Children's Hospital of Philadelphia, Division of Urology, 3rd Floor Wood Center,
34th Street and Civic Center Boulevard, Philadelphia, PA 19104-4399, USA
[b]University of Pennsylvania School of Medicine, 295 John Morgan Building,
3620 Hamilton Walk, Philadelphia, PA 19104-6055, USA

Bladder function can simply be defined by two simple processes: storage and emptying. For children born with myelodysplasia, the developmental anomaly can affect both these processes, leading in some situations to upper tract deterioration unless myelodysplasia is recognized in a timely fashion. Pioneering work by Lapides and colleagues demonstrated that clean intermittent catheterization can be employed to empty the bladder, thus improving the situation for children with poor bladder emptying [1]. Pharmacologic measures have been used to improve bladder storage and the combination of pharmacotherapy and clean intermittent catheterization has become the mainstay technique in the management of children with myelodysplasia.

The distribution of the myelomeningocele level is depicted in Fig. 1 [2]. Most bony abnormalities occur in the lumbosacral region. The actual level of the meningocele may not correspond to the distribution of the injured nerve roots. In general, nerves opposite the level of the bony defect or those more caudally positioned are affected. Occasionally, the injury may affect more cranially positioned nerve roots and there may be differences on opposite sides of the spinal cord even at the same level [3]. Often, a lipoma of the filum terminala, or dura, is associated with the meningocele compressing or stretching the nerve roots. These patients, too, have an Arnold-Chiari malformation, which affects both the brain and brain stem, so that the majority of children require placement of a ventriculoperitoneal shunt. All of this leads to a considerable variation in the type and extent of neurologic injury. There remains ongoing debate concerning the appropriate evaluation,

* The Children's Hospital of Philadelphia, 34th Street and Civic Center Boulevard, Third Floor, Wood Building, Philadelphia, PA 19104-4399.
E-mail address: Carr@email.chop.edu

0039-6109/06/$ - see front matter © 2006 Elsevier Inc. All rights reserved.
doi:10.1016/j.suc.2006.01.003   *surgical.theclinics.com*

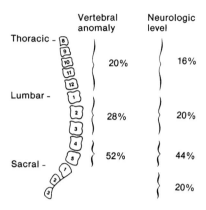

Fig. 1. Distribution of level of lesion in children with myelodysplasia. Most lesions involve the lumbosacral area. (*From* Bauer SB. Neurologic anomalies: myelodysplasia. In: Krane RJ, Siroky MB, editors. Clinical neuro-urology. Philadelphia: Lippincott Williams & Wilkins; 1991. p. 376, with permission.)

management, and treatment of patients with myelomeningocele [4–6]. Urodynamic investigation, which is the best way of assessing the function of the bladder, was commonly performed in children after they reached school age. It was deemed important to achieve social continence. Increasingly, the evaluation of the newborn has been favored once the back has been closed and the child's neurosurgical condition stabilized [7]. The initial assessment provides a baseline so that subsequent studies can look for evidence of progressive deterioration.

The prenatal diagnosis of myelomeningocele is now more common, with a triple screen being performed to look for the presence of a neural tube defect [8]. Confirmation of the myelomeningocele occurs with ultrasonography so that appropriate prenatal counseling can take place and a thorough explanation of the various sequelae of spina bifida provided to expectant parents. Currently the National Institutes of Health is sponsoring a randomized prospective trial, the Management of Myelomeningocele Study trial, which will provide a critical assessment of the outcome of infants born with myelomeningocele and repaired in utero during mid-gestation, as compared to those infants who have postnatal closure in the first 24 hours of life [9].

Bladder evaluation

The evaluation of the lower urinary tract can be accomplished by evaluating the kidneys and bladder ultrasonographically. As long as the bladder stores urine at low pressure with coordination between the detrusor and the external sphincter, then effective emptying should occur and the kidneys should remain normal. When this process is somehow circumvented, the compliance of the bladder may be altered, bladder emptying worsens, and the child is at greater risk for urinary tract infections and, potentially, upper tract changes. Compliance is simply defined as the overall pressure in the bladder at a given volume [10]. Bladders have the unique property of maintaining a low pressure that is generally less than 10 cm of water pressure over a variable volume. Once the bladder becomes full, the signal is transferred via the afferent nerves to the pontine micturition center. These signals are then processed allowing for appropriate relaxation of the pelvic floor musculature and external sphincter, which are innervated by the pudendal nerve so that there is coordinated relaxation of these muscles before the detrusor muscle begins to contract. The urodynamic evaluation becomes critical in defining the activity of the external sphincter looking for evidence of synergy, dyssynergy, or the absence of activity. Bauer and colleagues performed an evaluation of newborn infants and found that 55% of babies had detrusor sphincter dyssynergia, 18% had synergy, and 27% had absent activity [7]. The urodynamic evaluation is further able to assess the bladder capacity, overall compliance, and bladder emptying. The external sphincter is designed to provide a resting tone that maintains urinary continence. Alteration of this function can contribute to persistent incontinence (ie, low leak-point pressure, external sphincter denervation) or detrusor sphincter dyssynergia that leads to detrusor hypertrophy of the bladder due to a functional obstruction (Fig. 2). These changes alter the storage capability of the bladder, with progressive loss of bladder capacity and compliance. The use of urodynamics allows the early detection of potentially injurious conditions so that the appropriate intervention occurs.

Further work in this cohort of newborns determined that 79% of children with detrusor sphincter dyssynergy developed deterioration of the urinary tract within the first 3 years of life. Children with synergic sphincter activity rarely show deterioration. In fact, only those who converted to a dyssynergic pattern on subsequent studies did so and usually within a year of the alteration from synergic to dyssynergic [11]. Similarly, children with complete denervation of the sphincter were unlikely to show signs of urinary tract deterioration. Those children who did were presumed to develop increased outlet resistance due to progressive fibrosis of the denervated skeletal muscle component of the external sphincter [12].

Bauer and colleagues proposed a set of guidelines for the surveillance of infants and children who were born with myelomeningocele [2]. These guidelines were based on the premise that those infants and children with dyssynergia are at greatest risk for upper tract deterioration and require the greatest amount of surveillance. Renal ultrasonography has supplanted the use of intravenous pyelograms since it provides an assessment of the upper tracts, ureteral dilation, bladder wall changes, and bladder emptying. The dyssynergic group is monitored with a post-void residual urine volume and urine culture every 3 months, renal ultrasonography every 6 months, and urodynamic studies annually to look for evidence of deterioration. Urodynamics following closure of the myelomeningocele need to be interpreted carefully because some infants manifest spinal shock and show evidence of

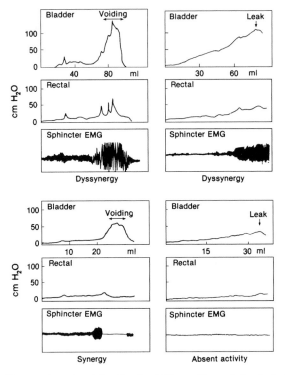

Fig. 2. Types of lower urinary tract function in children with myelodysplasia. The activity of the external urethral sphincter is classified as dyssynergic, synergic, or absent, according to its response during a detrusor contraction or a sustained increase in intravesical pressure. Absent activity implies complete denervation of the sphincter. (*From* Bauer SB, Neurologic anomalies: myelodysplasia. In: Krane RJ, Siroky MB, editors. Clinical neuro-urology. Philadelphia: Lippincott Williams & Wilkins; 1991. p. 378, with permission.)

a flaccid bladder that does not empty well. Generally, the spinal shock resolves within several weeks so that it may be best to defer the initial urodynamic study until this resolves. In the interim, infants are placed on intermittent catheterization. If the external sphincter is synergic, then annual renal ultrasound and urodynamic studies should be performed. Those patients who have complete denervation of the detrusor and external sphincter require annual renal ultrasounds to monitor the urinary tract.

Therapeutic options

Intervention is necessary when there are signs of outflow obstruction or elevated detrusor pressure on filling or both. High bladder-filling and voiding pressures, particularly in the face of uncoordinated external sphincter activity, are worrisome signs, suggesting that either bladder decompensation or upper urinary tract deterioration will occur. Thus, newborn infants who demonstrate these worrisome features are begun on intermittent catheterization [13]. Additionally, they are placed on anticholinergic therapy to potentially decrease intravesical pressures and also to minimize the occurrence of uninhibited bladder contractions [14].

Once the bladder function can be characterized as synergic, dyssynergic, or a relative absence of external electromyographic activity, then the subsequent evaluation can be tailored according to the patient. At least until the children are of school age, annual ultrasounds can be alternated with urodynamic evaluations. In situations in which children develop recurrent urinary tract infections or have changes in their continence patterns, then urodynamic studies can be employed to look for changes in overall bladder compliance and external sphincter activity.

Newer methods of dealing with this situation include the use of urethral dilation of the external sphincter [15] or the injection of botulinum toxin type A directly into the external sphincter. Bloom and colleagues have shown that urethral dilation can be effective in altering the guarding reflex so that infants or children with evidence of detrusor sphincter dyssynergy will empty their bladders more effectively and lessen the chance of upper tract deterioration [16]. Credé voiding, which involves applying pressure to the suprapubic region to facilitate bladder emptying, is contraindicated in those infants or children with an intact sacral reflex function. Such children have a reflexic increase in external urethral sphincter electromyographic activity during a Credé maneuver. Failure of such conservative approaches may lead to a cutaneous vesicostomy as an alternative option.

Video urodynamic studies that combine the use of fluoroscopic imaging and monitoring of intravesical, intraabdominal, and electromyographic activity of the external sphincter have become the best tools for assessing infants and children with a neurogenic bladder (Fig. 3). Such studies are particularly helpful in the evaluation of a child with persistent urinary incontinence with a neurogenic bladder. Such a child with persistent incontinence may have uninhibited detrusor contractions, elevated intravesical pressures, a low urethral resistance, or excessive urine volume. The institution of anticholinergic therapy (eg, oxybutynin, tolterodine) may lower detrusor tone and contractility. Newer agents that are long-acting improve overall patient compliance for the medication and increase the likelihood of success. Patients who have a diminished leak-point pressure may benefit from alpha-sympathomimetic agents, such as ephedrine and phenoxybenzamine (Fig. 4).

The child with denervation of the external sphincter may not empty well because of a fixed urethral resistance due to fibrosis. Such a patient would benefit from intermittent catheterization to facilitate bladder emptying. That same patient may only be plagued with stress incontinence due to the fixed nature of the external sphincter.

The use of botulinum toxin type A has become more popular because it treats both the external urethral sphincter and the detrusor muscle. Promising results in adult patients have led to the use of botulinum toxin type A in

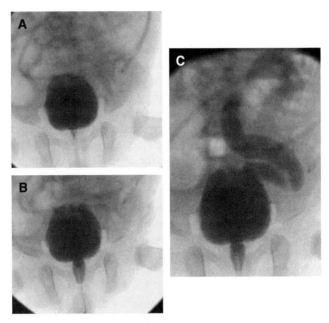

Fig. 3. Videourodynamic evaluation of a 2-month-old with postnatal repair of mylomeningo-cele. (*A*) Funneling of bladder neck. (*B*) Evidence of contrast in prostatic urethral associated with bladder contraction. (*C*) Evidence of left vesicoureteral reflux during a bladder contraction in which dyssynergy is present.

pediatric patients, again with encouraging outcomes [17]. Detrusor sphincter dyssynergy due to a lack of coordination of the external sphincter muscle and detrusor muscle may be overcome by injecting the external sphincter with botulinum toxin type A. Typically, injections performed at the 12-, 3-, 6- and 9-o'clock positions use 20 international units per injection site. Botulinum toxin type A has also been injected directly into the detrusor [18]. This technique has been used when anticholinergic therapy is ineffective and the bladder still manifests evidence of uninhibited bladder contractions. Success has been achieved for as long as 6 to 9 months following the initial injection, but longer success following a single injection into the detrusor remains unknown.

The final option in the management of patients who have either persistent urinary incontinence despite maximal pharmacotherapy or an intermittent catheterization regimen involves reconstructive surgery. Such surgery ultimately represents a failure of medical management and the hope is that early and aggressive management of such patients in the future will limit the need for reconstructive surgery. These patients require an increase in bladder capacity and improvement in overall bladder compliance, which can be accomplished by augmenting the bladder with a segment of intestine [19]. For those patients with persistent incontinence, this alone will not render

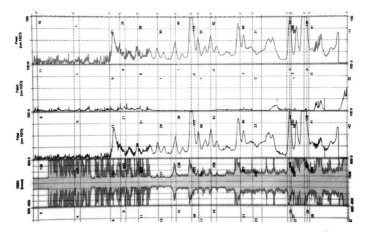

Fig. 4. Urodynamic tracing demonstrates intravesical pressure in the first panel, intraabdominal pressure in the second panel, true intravesical pressure in the third panel, and electromyographic activity in the fourth panel. This specific tracing shows patient-generated pressures of well over 80 cm of water with dyssynergy and failure of relaxation of the external sphincter.

the patient dry because many have a diminished leak-point pressure. Several surgical procedures have been devised to increase the outlet resistance. However, none seems to have universal applicability and overall success.

Female patients can be managed by injecting a bulking agent at the bladder neck, trying to coapt the tissues more effectively as urethral resistance is increased [20]. If reconstructive surgery is needed to increase bladder capacity, then a combination of a urethral sling and a catheterizable channel would be necessary to maximize the success of the surgery [21].

Male patients with decreased urethral resistance pose an even greater surgical challenge, since there is no surgical procedure that has been proven to be uniformly successful. Attempts at bladder neck reconstruction include such procedures as the Kropp procedure [22], the Pippi Salle procedure [23], bladder neck suspensions, and slings and artificial urinary sphincters [24]. Each procedure has advantages and disadvantages that need to be carefully explored with the patient and family.

In the past, an indwelling Foley catheter has been used to address the problem. This technique has been modified. Typically the catheter is left in place only at night, so that the patient resumes clean intermittent catheterization during the day. The use of a catheter for anywhere from 8 to 12 hours can decrease the postobstructive diuresis that occurs in some patients who have not been catheterized overnight. Their urine output is not as great during the day, increasing the likelihood that they will remain dry with their clean intermittent catheterization regimen during the day [25].

Patients born with myelomeningocele need a coordinated team approach to maximize their management. Success requires that treatment be tailored and closely monitored for each period of childhood. That is, for the newborn, toddler, school-aged child and adolescent. Successes in the pediatric population contribute to emerging challenges as these children mature, bringing with them management issues into adulthood.

References

[1] Lapides J, Diokno AC, Silber SJ, et al. Clean intermittent self-catheterization in the treatment of urinary tract disease. J Urol 1971;107:458.

[2] Bauer SB. Pediatric neurology. In: Krane RJ, Siroky MB, editors. Clinical neuro-urology. Boston: Little, Brown and Company; 1979. p. 279.

[3] Barson AJ. The vertebral level of termination of the spinal cord during normal and abnormal development. J Anat 1970;106:489.

[4] Johnston JH, Farkas A. Congenital neuropathic bladder: practicalities and possibilities of conservative management. Urology 1975;5:729.

[5] McGuire EJ, Woodside JR, Bordon TA, et al. Prognostic value of urodynamic testing in myelodysplasia patients. J Urol 1981;126:205.

[6] Webster GD, et al. The urological evaluation and management of patients with myelodysplasia. Br J Urol 1986;58:261.

[7] Bauer SB, Hallett M, Khoshbin S, et al. Predictive value of urodynamic evaluation in newborns with myelodysplasia. JAMA 1984;252:650.

[8] Adzick NS, Walsh DS. Myelomeningocele: prenatal diagnosis, pathophysiology and management. Semin Pediatr Surg 2003;12(3):168.

[9] Rintoul NE, Sutton LN, Hubbard AM, et al. A new look at myelomeningoceles: functional level, vertebral level, shunting and the implications for fetal intervention. Pediatrics 2002; 109(3):409.

[10] Ghoniem GM, Bloom DA, McGuire EJ, et al. Bladder compliance in myelomeningocele children. J Urol 1989;141:1404.

[11] van Gool JD, et al. Detrusor sphincter dyssynergia in children with myelomeningocele: a prospective study. Z Kinderchir 1982;37:148.

[12] Bauer SB, Spindel MR. The changing neurological lesion in myelodysplasia. JAMA 1987; 258:1630.

[13] Hopps CV, Kropp KA. Preservation of renal function in children with myelomeningocele managed with basic newborn evaluation and close follow-up. J Urol 2003;169(1):305.

[14] Goessl C, Knispel HH, Fiedler U, et al. Urodynamic effects of oral Oxybutynin chloride in children with myelomeningocele and detrusor hyperreflexia. Urol 1998;51:94.

[15] Bloom DA, Knechtel JM, McGuire EJ. Urethral dilation improves bladder compliance in children with myelomeningocele and high leak point pressures. J Urol 1990;144:430.

[16] Park JM, McGuire EJ, Koo HP, et al. External urethral sphincter dilation for the management of high risk myelomeningocele: 15-year experience. J Urol 2001;165:2383.

[17] Schulte-Baukloh H, Michael T, Schobert J, et al. Efficacy of botulinum-a toxin in children with detrusor hyperreflexia due to myelomeningocele: preliminary results. Urol 2002;59:325.

[18] Riccabona M, Koen M, Schindler M, et al. Botulinum-a toxin injection into the detrusor: a safe alternative in the treatment of children with myelomeningocele with detrusor hyperreflexia. J Urol 2004;171:845.

[19] Kass EJ, Koff SA. Bladder augmentation in the pediatric neuropathic bladder. J Urol 1983; 129:552.

[20] Misseri R, Casale AJ, Cain MP, et al. Alternative uses of dextranomer/hyaluronic acid copolymer: the efficacy of bladder neck injection for urinary incontinence. J Urol 2005; 174(4 Pt 2):1691.

[21] Dik P, Klijn AJ, van Gool JD, et al. Transvaginal sling suspension of bladder neck in female patients with neurogenic sphincter incontinence. J Urol 2003;170(2 Pt 1):580 [discussion: p. 581].

[22] Kropp KA. Bladder neck reconstruction in children. Urol Clin North Am 1999;26(3):661.

[23] Pippi Salle JL. Surgical management of urinary incontinence in children with neurogenic sphincteric incompetence. J Urol 2000;164(5):1668.

[24] Gonzalez R, Merino FG, Vaughn M. Long-term results of the artificial urinary sphincter in male patients with neurogenic bladder. J Urol 1995;154(2 Pt 2):769.

[25] Koff SA, Gigax MR, Jayanthi VR. Nocturnal bladder emptying: a simple technique for reversing urinary tract deterioration in children with neurogenic bladder. J Urol 2005; 174(4 Pt 2):1629.

ELSEVIER
SAUNDERS

Surg Clin N Am 86 (2006) 525–535

SURGICAL
CLINICS OF
NORTH AMERICA

Index

Note: Page numbers of article titles are in **boldface** type.

0039-6109/06/$ - see front matter © 2006 Elsevier Inc. All rights reserved.
doi:10.1016/S0039-6109(06)00035-1

Changing Your Address?

Make sure your subscription changes too! When you notify us of your new
address, you can help make our job easier by including an exact copy of your
Clinics label number with your old address (see illustration below.) This
number identifies you to our computer system and will speed the processing of
your address change. Please be sure this label number accompanies your old
address and your corrected address—you can send an old Clinics label with
your number on it or just copy it exactly and send it to the address listed below.

We appreciate your help in our attempt to give you continuous coverage.
Thank you.

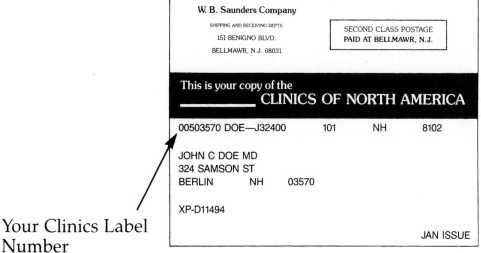

Your Clinics Label Number

Copy it exactly or send your label
along with your address to:
Elsevier Periodicals Customer Service
6277 Sea Harbor Drive
Orlando, FL 32887-4800
Call Toll Free 1-800-654-2452

Please allow four to six weeks for delivery of new subscriptions and for
processing address changes.